Osteoporosis Research

Gustavo Duque • Ken Watanabe
(Editors)

Osteoporosis Research

Animal Models

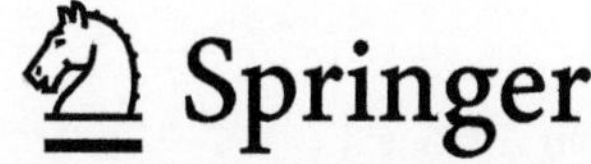

Editors
Gustavo Duque, M.D., Ph.D., FRACP
Department of Geriatric Medicine
Ageing Bone Research Centre
Sydney Medical School – Nepean Campus
The University of Sydney
Penrith, NSW
Australia

Ken Watanabe, Ph.D
Department of Bone and Joint Disease
National Center for Geriatrics
and Gerontology
Obu, Aichi
Japan

ISBN 978-0-85729-292-6 e-ISBN 978-0-85729-293-3
DOI 10.1007/978-0-85729-293-3
Springer London Dordrecht Heidelberg New York

British Library Cataloguing in Publication Data
A catalogue record for this book is available from the British Library

Library of Congress Control Number: 2011922531

Cover design: eStudioCalamar, Figueres/Berlin

Printed on acid-free paper

Springer is part of Springer Science+Business Media (www.springer.com)

To Erasto, for all his support.
Gustavo Duque

Foreword

Research into the causes and treatments for osteoporosis has expanded exponentially over the last decade. The development of novel drugs and new therapeutic targets for the skeleton have forced an evolution in our understanding of skeletal physiology. But, nowhere have the advances been so rapid as in animal models, a forerunner for all human studies and a requirement for ultimate new drug approval by regulatory agencies. The spectrum of animal model research in skeletal biology has grown at the same trajectory as cellular and molecular techniques such that numerous species are now used in research settings. In particular, the genetically engineered mouse has been one of the greatest advances in translational science, and this holds for skeletal biology as well as other disciplines. This book, *Osteoporosis Research: Animal Models*, is the first of its kind book as a "stand alone" manual for students, residents, fellows and laboratory associates. This multi-authored textbook provides an accurate roadmap of the landscape in experimental skeletal biology and the application of model systems to different experimental approaches. Drs. Duque and Watanabe should be congratulated. They have selected authors for individual chapters that are recognized as leaders in their respective field. In sum, this book promises to be a regular staple in bone biology laboratories around the world. In an era when printed text is fading, a textbook such as this will still find a home, and will be widely used in the foreseeable future.

Clifford J. Rosen, M.D.
Past-President, American Society for Bone
and Mineral Research,
Senior Scientist,
Maine Medical Center Research Institute

Preface

It usually starts with a wonderful hypothesis but could be suddenly stopped by the wrong choice of the animal model to test it. Biomedical research is a dynamic process that initiates with a hypothesis, continues with the selection of an appropriate experimental model and ends with the publication of data confirming or rejecting that initial hypothesis. Thanks to biomedical research the human race has found the cure for multiple diseases, has alleviated pain and suffering and has prolonged its life span to levels unimaginable hundred years ago.

An important step in biomedical research is the selection of the appropriate animal model that fulfils the required characteristics to test a specific hypothesis. For years, experimental animals have been used in biomedical research since it is widely accepted that a living organism provides an interactive, dynamic system that can be observed and manipulated experimentally in order to investigate mechanisms of normal function and of disease. As a result, a greater understanding of living systems can be attained and this knowledge can be generalized to other species including humans, facilitating the development of effective therapies. Several aspects of using experimental animals, such as life conditions and ethical issues, have become pivotal in biomedical research always looking for the best and more humane care for these animals.

Osteoporosis research has not been the exception. Numerous animal models have been used to understand the mechanisms of osteoporosis and age-related bone loss as well as to test new therapies to prevent osteoporosis and fractures. Animal models of osteoporosis, going from murine to non-human primates, are now established. In addition, diagnostic techniques have significantly advanced due to the fact that they have been tested in these animals prior to their validation in humans.

In this very diverse field of experimental animal models for osteoporosis, the bone researcher has to decide the most suitable model to assess a hypothesis and to provide valid and reliable data. Selecting the appropriate animal model could be confusing and time consuming. This book attempts to solve this challenge by providing the bone researcher with a handy and practical guide on how to select the appropriate animal model and what type of experimental approach would be more suitable for that specific model.

The book starts with a chapter on how to select your animal model. This chapter describes the particular characteristics of most animal models in terms of bone structure, changes in bone cellularity and the role of hormones and growth factors in their bone metabolism. After reviewing this chapter, the reader would find that using models other than the usual murine ones could be a good choice for their particular experimental approach.

From Chaps. 2–6, we have focused on the most common techniques in bone research and their particular characteristics and requirements for each animal model. These chapters describe in detail how to manipulate the samples and how to obtain the best results from every particular model. We expect that the readers will find these chapters extremely useful when selecting their experimental techniques and when interpreting their results.

Chapter 7 is dedicated to the impact of cancer on bone. Metastatic cancer directly affects bone structure and cellularity and therefore preventing bone metastasis is a subject of intense research. Considering that animal models for cancer research have very specific features and requirements, a chapter has been fully dedicated to this subject. The authors explain in detail how to select an appropriate model of metastatic bone disease as well as the particular features of the most common animal models used for this purpose.

Moving from the diagnostic methods to the use of animal models to assess potential therapeutic targets of osteoporosis in Chap. 8, the authors provide with a very useful guide on how to test treatments for osteoporosis in experimental animals. Using the wrong experimental model to assess new compounds would prevent potential major advances in osteoporosis research. Therefore, in this chapter the authors guide the reader on the selection of the right experimental model and the most appropriate techniques to administrate osteoporosis medications without affecting the quality of life of the experimental animals.

The later chapters of this book highlight the two most common models of osteoporosis: the oophorectomized (OVX) and the aged mice and rats. Chapter 9 describes the advantages and disadvantages of the OVX model and provides some useful tips to obtain the best results from this model.

A particular unique component of this book is the inclusion of animal models of normal and accelerated aging (Chaps. 10 and 11). In an "estrogen centered" field, which is slowly moving into accepting the very relevant role of aging in the pathogenesis of osteoporosis, the description of the unique characteristics, advantages and disadvantages of the aging animal model constitutes one of the major strengths of this book giving it a major relevance for osteoporosis research in the near future.

In Chaps. 12 and 13, we wanted to include other large animal models and non-human primate models of osteoporosis. Although less commonly used due to costs and logistic issues, these animal models provide a closer approach to the features of osteoporosis in humans and therefore could be the optimal models when assessing new therapeutic targets.

Finally, in addition to the use of animal models to test therapeutic targets of osteoporosis, animal models are also useful to assess the characteristics of fracture healing and fracture fixation. Chapter 14 elegantly describes the animal models and techniques used to assess different approaches to fracture healing and fixation. With multiple figures, the authors illustrate to the reader with the most advanced techniques and their practicalities in a very descriptive and didactic manner.

In summary, this book is expected to constitute the most practical guide for the selection of animal models as well as the identification of the most appropriate techniques for bone research. Due to the importance of using animal models in a very ethical manner, throughout its pages the reader would find the Editors' particular emphasis on human treatment to experimental animals. In fact, we would like to highlight that experimental animals should be used only when *in vitro* techniques are limited, and that ethical care of experimental animals should be pivotal in every aspect of biomedical research. The best way of thanking our animals for the evidence and medical advances they are providing us is to treat them as humanly as possible. At the end we are the same creatures in the eyes of a Great Architect.

Gustavo Duque, M.D., Ph.D., FRACP
Ken Watanabe, Ph.D.

Acknowledgments

The Editors would like to thank Mrs. Leigh Bambury for her assistance in the preparation of this work. We remain grateful to Melissa Morton from Springer for her outstanding support to this project. To Nadine Firth for her gentle guidance in the development of this project. Finally, we would like to thank all the authors of these book chapters who, like us, share the same interest in the development of a cure for osteoporosis. Without their collaboration this project would have never been successful.

Gustavo Duque, M.D., Ph.D., FRACP
Ken Watanabe, Ph.D.

Contents

Contributors

Jameela Banu, Ph.D. Department of Medicine, Physiology and Medical Research Division, Edinburg Regional Academic Center, University of Texas Health Science Center at San Antonio, Edinburgh, TX, USA

Stephen Becker, MD. Department of Trauma, Hand and Reconstructive Surgery, University of Saarland, Saarland, Germany

Mary L. Bouxsein, Ph.D. Center for Advanced Orthopedic Studies, Beth Israel Deaconess Medical Center, Boston, MA, USA

David B. Burr, Ph.D. Department of Anatomy and Cell Biology, Indiana University School of Medicine, Indianapolis, IN, USA

Blaine A. Christiansen, Ph.D. University of California-Davis Medical Center, Department of Orthopaedics, Sacramento, CA

Natalie Dion, Ph.D. CRCHUM – Hôpital Saint-Luc, East René-Lévesque Blvd, Montréal (Québec), Canada

Gustavo Duque, M.D., Ph.D., FRACP Discipline of Geriatric Medicine, Ageing Bone Research Centre, Sydney Medical School – Nepean Campus, The University of Sydney, Penrith NSW, Australia

Audray Fortin, B.Sc. Laboratory of Metabolic Bone Diseases, CRCHUM – Hôpital Saint-Luc, Montréal, Québec, Canada

Chan Gao, M.B.B.S. Department of Experimental Medicine, McGill University Health Centre, McGill University, Montréal, Québec, Canada

Patric Garcia, M.D. Department of Trauma, Hand and Reconstructive Surgery, University of Saarland, Saarland, Germany

Edward J. Harvey, M.D., M.Sc., FRCSC Department of Surgery, McGill University Health Centre, McGill University, Montréal, Quebec, Canada

Janet E. Henderson, Ph.D. Department of Medicine and Surgery, Orthopaedic Research and JTN Wong Labs for Bone Engineering, McGill University and Research Institute – McGill University Health Centre, Montreal General Hospital, Montréal, Québec, Canada

Markus Herrmann, M.D. Ageing Bone Research Centre, Sydney Medical School – Nepean Campus, The University of Sydney, Penrith, NSW, Australia

Tina Histing, M.D. Department of Trauma, Hand and Reconstructive Surgery, University of Saarland, Saarland, Germany

Joerg H. Holstein, M.D. Department of Trauma, Hand and Reconstructive Surgery, University of Saarland, Saarland, Germany

Jacquelin Jolette, DVM, Dipl. ACVP Department of Bone Pathology, Charles River Preclinical Services, Montréal, Québec, Canada

Moritz Klein, M.D. Department of Trauma, Hand and Reconstructive Surgery, University of Saarland, Saarland, Germany

Lee Wei Li, M.Sc., M.B.A. Department of Medicine, Ageing Bone Research Centre, Sydney Medical School – Nepean Campus, The University of Sydney, Penrith, NSW, Australia

Michael D. Menger, M.D. Institute for Clinical and Experimental Surgery, University of Saarland, Saarland, Germany

Tim Pohlemann, M.D. Department of Trauma, Hand and Reconstructive Surgery, University of Saarland, Saarland, Germany

Susan Reinwald, Ph.D. Department of Anatomy and Cell Biology, Indiana University School of Medicine, Indianapolis, IN, USA

Markus J. Seibel, M.D., Ph.D. Bone Research Program, ANZAC Research Institute, The University of Sydney, Concord, NSW, Australia

Antonio C. Shimano, M.D., Ph.D. Department of Biomechanics, Medicine and Rehabilitation of the Locomotor System, University of São Paulo, Ribeirão Preto School of Medicine, Ribeirão Preto, São Paulo, Brazil

Susan Y. Smith, M.Sc. Department of Bone Research and General Toxicology, Charles River Preclinical Services, Montréal, Québec, Canada

Louis-Georges Ste-Marie, M.D. Department of Medicine, CRCHUM – Hôpital Saint Luc, Montréal, Québec, Canada

A. Simon Turner, BVSc, MS, Dipl. AVCS Department of Clinical Sciences, Colorado State University, Fort Collins, CO, USA

Robert J. van 't Hof, B.Sc., M.Sc., Ph.D. Department of Rheumatology, Molecular Medicine Centre, Institute of Genetics and Molecular Medicine, University of Edinburgh, Western General Hospital, Edinburgh, Midlothian, UK

Aurore Varela, DVM, DABT Department of Bone Research, Charles River Preclinical Services, Montréal Québec, Canada

José B. Volpon, M.D., Ph.D. Department of Biomechanics, Medicine and Rehabilitation of the Locomotor System, University of São Paulo, Ribeirão Preto School of Medicine, Ribeirão Preto, São Paulo, Brazil

Ken Watanabe, Ph.D. Department of Bone and Joint Disease, National Center for Geriatrics and Gerontology, Obu, Aichi, Japan

Yu Zheng, M.D., Ph.D. Bone Research Program, ANZAC Research Institute, The University of Sydney, Concord, NSW, Australia

Hong Zhou, M.D., Ph.D. Bone Research Program, ANZAC Research Institute, The University of Sydney, Concord, NSW, Australia

How to Select Your Animal Model for Osteoporosis Research

1

A. Simon Turner

1.1 Introduction

The rising burden of osteoporotic fractures increases morbidity and mortality in the aging population, imposing a significant cost on society.[1,2] This means there is a never-ending search for new therapies for osteoporosis as well as increasing interest in the biology and behavior of orthopedic implants in osteoporotic bone.[3] Therefore, there will always be a need for both small and large animal models for osteoporosis research. While there is no perfect animal model that mimics all the physiologic characteristics of osteoporosis in humans, some valuable and essential information on new therapies can be derived from the selection of the appropriate animal model, along with careful experimental design. An animal model can provide uniform experimental material for testing and minimize the limitations associated with studying the disease in humans, where there is considerable behavioral variability among test subjects. Furthermore, evaluation of new therapies requires both the clinical dose and five times the clinical dose to give an indication of the margin of safety. The high cost and long time frame for clinical testing are additional reasons why various animal models play a crucial role in osteoporosis research.

The aim of this chapter is to introduce the reader to the fundamental and practical differences that exist between animal models most commonly used for osteoporosis research. The chapter (an overview) presents the reader with many important questions that must be answered before selecting a model. After reading the overview provided in this chapter, the investigator should seek further specific details from earlier studies in the appropriate animal model, including the less-characterized models (mice, lactating rats, rabbits, marmosets, ferrets, guinea pigs, hibernating bears, etc.) from other chapters of this book and from additional citations.

A.S. Turner
Department of Clinical Sciences, Colorado State University, 300 West Drake Rd., Fort Collins, CO 80523, USA
e-mail: sturner@colostate.edu

1.2 Food and Drug Administration (FDA) Requirements

The guidelines proposed by the United States Food and Drug Administration (FDA) suggest two species needed for testing new therapies for osteoporosis.[4] The first is the well-characterized ovariectomized (OVX) rodent model.[5] This model shares many of the characteristics of postmenopausal bone loss in women as well as response to drugs such as bisphosphonates, estrogen, parathyroid hormone, and calcitonin.[5,6] Although this widely studied model mimics postmenopausal bone loss over a short period of time (with bone resorption exceeding bone formation), the lack of a Haversian system in cortical bone and absence of the basic multicellular unit–based remodeling in young animals are limitations.[7] Following proof of concept in a rodent model, investigators must consider a large animal model, higher up the phylogenetic scale (e.g., dog, pig, sheep, goat, primate) with intracortical bone remodeling resembling that of humans.

G. Duque and K. Watanabe (eds.), *Osteoporosis Research*,
DOI: 10.1007/978-0-85729-293-3_1,

1.3 Collaboration with Veterinarians, Veterinary Schools, and Private Laboratories

Collaboration with the veterinary profession and well-trained staff is strongly advised for many reasons. Apart from having a more thorough understanding of the species-specific anatomy, physiology, and overall health issues, veterinarians and veterinary technicians can assist investigators with potential inconveniences such as handling, housing, dietary needs, ethical implications, and availability, to name a few. Keeping up to date with advances in animal anesthesia and analgesia (discussed later) is also a reason to collaborate with these individuals. They will be able to present information to the investigator and sponsor of the study about the habits and behaviors of the animals being used. During the study period, veterinarians and their technicians may provide important end points for therapies being evaluated for treatment of osteoporosis. These end points may be requested by regulatory agencies. Veterinarians experienced with various animals are likely to have access to existing databases of biological information about the different species.

Another advantage of veterinary assistance is help in preparation of the Institutional Animal Care and Use Committee (IACUC) protocol, which is now mandatory for use of research animals in most biomedical research institutions in the United States and in many other countries. Some animal research is unregulated but likely will not be funded by governmental agencies. It is in the best interest of the investigator (and the animals intended for use in a study) to work with facilities that have a well-organized IACUC in place. Readers interested in the organization and management of IACUCs are referred to some current texts.[8,9] Many funding agencies and scientific journals require documentation of IACUC review and approval, without which a grant will not be considered or data published.

1.4 Laws on Use of Animals for Research

It is not the purpose of this chapter to present the laws pertaining to the procurement and care of animals for research, as they do vary among different countries. There is increasing public awareness about the humane use of animals for research and it is the responsibility of the investigator(s) and staff to be well versed in the regulations and ethics of animal use.[10] In the United States the federal Animal Welfare Act (AWA), which has been amended numerous times since it was first signed into law in 1966, must be studied and understood by investigators and their support staff. There are numerous texts and websites dealing with this subject.[11] In the United States, investigators must be well aware of the Public Health Service Policy on Humane Care and Use of Laboratory Animals (PHS policy) and the United States Department of Agriculture (USDA) Animal Welfare Act Regulations.

One factor in deciding what animal to use is availability of support staff. For primate studies, working with veterinarians and other trained personnel experienced in this area is essential.[12,13] Appropriate husbandry of primates requires additional skill sets regarding handling and feeding, making animal care a very important link in the success of the experiments. An initial overview of practical aspects of the different animal models is shown in Table 1.1.

Table 1.1 Overview of initial practical aspects of animals commonly used for osteoporosis research

Animal	Cost	Availability	Manageability – handling	Life span (years)	Social and ethical issues	References
Rats	Low	Readily	Easy	2.5–3	Minimal	Lelovas et al.,[5] Harkness and Wagner[17]
Dogs	Moderate	Readily	With care	10–12	Sensitive	
Domestic and minipigs	Moderate	Readily	Loud and noisy Can be aggressive	10–15	Less critical	
Sheep/goats	Moderate	Readily	Easy	10–15	Less critical	
Primates	High	Difficult (especially in wild state)	DifficultVeterinary involvement essential	30–40	Sensitive	Watts[26]

Some initial questions regarding choice of an animal model, fundamental to osteoporosis as well as other areas of orthopedic research, include:

- Is it an appropriate analog?
- Has the model been used before?
- How well characterized is it?
- Can the results be translated to the human condition?
- Can modification of an existing model yield more answers?
- What is the availability of skeletally mature individuals?
- How easy is it to adapt the animal to experimentation?
- What is the cost of the animals and cost of housing?
- What are the societal and ethical considerations?

Some animals are well-accepted animal models in certain fields. For example, pigs are very desirable for studies involving wound healing, cardiothoracic procedures, and xenotransplantation. However, this does not mean they are perfectly suited to osteoporosis research (because of handling, housing, temperament, and size of adult farm breeds), although smaller breeds have been very useful in some studies on occasions[14,15] (see Chap. 13 of this book).

Of all the large animals, the OVX monkey remains the best characterized of the large animal models of osteopenia and has been an important model in the evaluation of many new drugs for osteoporosis.[13] Much of the physiology (skeletal, reproductive, immunologic, etc.) is similar to that of humans, making it the model of choice. However, the cost, availability, and ethical concerns, to name a few issues, will always limit the use of primates in research.

1.5 What Can You Derive from Animal Models Used for Osteoporosis Studies?

A fundamental question for an osteoporosis researcher is: Does the bone resemble the bone of the target population? Unlike rodents, which are a modeling species and lack intracortical remodeling, skeletally mature and aged large animals have osteonal remodeling which is relevant to bone of humans.

The larger bones of rapidly growing terrestrial animals (e.g., sheep, goats, pigs) contain a plexiform bone whose brick-like pattern surprises some histologists unfamiliar with animal tissues. Having plexiform bone is an efficient way for a growing animal to obtain mechanical strength, thereby avoiding pathological fracture while fleeing from potential predators. However, as large animals age, Haversian remodeling begins to appear in different areas of the long bones, although the Haversian systems of humans are usually larger than those of mammals.[16] Some physiological characteristics of the different animal models commonly used are shown in Table 1.2.

1.6 Husbandry

It is beyond the scope of this chapter to describe all the necessary requirements for housing (housing dimensions, climate, lighting, etc.) the animals commonly used for osteoporosis research. However, this cannot

Table 1.2 Physiological characteristics of animals commonly used for osteoporosis research

Animal	Reproductive cycle	Skeletal maturity (years; approx.)	Digestive tract	Number of offspring (average)	References
Rats (*Rattus norvegicus*)	Polyestrus (4–5 days)	>10 Months	Monogastric – omnivore	6–12	Lelovas et al.,[5] Harkness and Wagner[17]
Dogs (*Canis familiaris*)	Monoestrus (nonseasonal) 1–2 cycles/year	1.3 Years	Monogastric – carnivore	6–7	Reinwald and Burr[16]
Domestic and minipigs (*Sus scrofa*)	Nonseasonal, polyestrus (19–21 days)	>2.5 Years	Monogastric – omnivore	5	Reinwald and Burr[16]
Sheep/goats (*Ovis aries, Capra hircus*)	Seasonal polyestrus (17 days)	>3.5 Years	Ruminant – herbivore	1–3	Reinwald and Burr[16]
Primates (*Macaca fasicularis*)	Polyestrus (28 days)	>5 Years (female) >6 Years (male)	Monogastric – omnivore	1	Smith et al.[13]

be ignored when embarking on an animal study because of the various animal protection acts, regulatory agencies, etc. that now exist in most countries. Of the animals discussed in this chapter, rats are the easiest to house in large numbers, contributing to their popularity for all forms of biomedical research. They are housed in either metal cages with mesh floors or plastic cages with solid floors,[17] and the ambient temperature and the 12:12 light/dark cycle can be conveniently controlled. Complete, commercially available pelleted diets are easily obtained.

When an investigator considers the use of a larger animal for osteoporosis research, a number of very important issues will arise, the first being husbandry. Ease of housing, availability of commercially available dog chow diets, and familiarity of handling and training make many investigators consider dogs first after they have done rodent studies. Most IACUCs require daily "enrichment time" when dogs are used in studies although some type of "enrichment" is encouraged or required for all species. Sheep and goats (flock animals) must be housed with at least one or more of the same species visible or in the same pen. They are among the easiest of the large animals to house and handle and their popularity as research animals has been increasing steadily. Sheep can adapt to a very wide range of climates and environments. Although genetically quite similar to sheep, goats have more sociable and interactive personalities than sheep. They are not as nervous as sheep, are very inquisitive, and do not tolerate close confinement for long periods as well.[18]

Osteoporosis research is almost exclusively performed on adult animals, making use of skeletally mature farm pig breeds impractical because of their enormous size. Young pigs may be easier to work with, but are not a good model for osteoporosis research because of the immature bone and continued growth of the animal as the study continues. Those eager to use farm pigs should first enquire about the body weight of the skeletally mature animal. They should then enquire about the availability of special equipment and technicians trained to work with these larger breeds. Difficulties in handling large pigs have led to the popularity of the miniature and micropig breeds (Göttingen, Yucatan, Sinclair, etc.) for osteoporosis research. Despite the greater expense of these smaller pig breeds, the advantages of greater ease in housing and handling, their omnivorous diet, and the anatomy of the gastrointestinal tract have made research using small pigs more popular.

If primates are to be used for a study, the housing and handling requirements as dictated by regulatory agencies become even more critical than those for the species discussed above. These are the main reasons why the use of primates (despite the similarities to humans) is limited and restricted to well-designed facilities, tailored specifically for these animals.

Other animal models for osteoporosis research such as hibernating bears[19,20] present practical and logistical husbandry issues that are beyond reach for most investigators. This does not mean they are unavailable or should be ignored, because some laboratories do have experienced personnel and animal-handling skills. This makes networking, close collaboration, and an advanced understanding about publication and authorship between groups essential.

1.7 Availability of Older Animals and Male Animals

Before beginning a study, an investigator will need access to skeletally mature animals. Much research in the past has been flawed because immature animals were used. It is well known that bone biology in growing animals is very different from that of skeletally mature animals. Skeletal maturity can be verified with radiographs to evaluate growth plate closure or from veterinary texts.[21]

Sexually mature female animals are used most frequently in bone studies in general. However, of the approximately ten million people affected by osteoporosis each year, 20% of these are men.[22] Mature male animals, specifically rams (sheep), bucks (goats), and boars (pigs) can be difficult to obtain because these are generally kept by livestock operations only to be used as breeding stock to enhance certain genetic characteristics of the flock or herd. However, investigators could potentially locate a source of a limited number of skeletally mature intact boars, rams, or bucks if essential to the study. Handling of intact, potentially aggressive male farm animals requires experienced veterinary and technical personnel and well-designed facilities.

The most practical animal model to begin searching for new therapies for male hormone deficiency is unquestionably the orchidectomized (ORX) adult rat.[23] If a treatment effect is observed in rats, a realistic dose of the drug can then be determined with the appropriate end points (bone mineral density (BMD), biochemical markers, histomorphometry, etc.) for use in a larger animal.

Rats are easily trained to a treadmill for evaluation of exercise on bone metabolism before studies in larger animals are contemplated. For example, aged male rats have been used as a model of osteoporosis in men, to study the effect of physical exercise and nutrition on bone structure and metabolism.[24]

1.8 Knockout Animals

When it comes to genetic engineering, the laboratory mouse has no competitors, although models of transgenic mice and congenitally osteoporotic mice are limited. Examples include the senescence-accelerated mouse (SAM) and the SAM-resistant (SAMR) inbred strains. The SAMP6 strain is characterized by accelerated aging and senile osteoporosis and may be useful for some studies.[25] For further details of accelerated aging animals, refer to Chap. 11 of this book.

1.9 Hormonal Differences in Animals

For relevance to human osteoporosis, an animal model should demonstrate bone loss associated with estrogen deficiency. Most animals do not experience natural menopause as do women, so in order to accelerate bone loss, ovariectomy or castration is performed to approximate the bone loss associated with human menopause. An exception would be elderly Old World primates[26] but the impracticality and expense of keeping primates until natural menopause occurs sometime after 30 years of age is obvious.[13]

The estrus cycles (length, frequency, initiating stimulus, etc.) of animal models used for osteoporosis studies vary widely, presenting a challenge to the researcher investigating what model to use. An overview of the different cycles is presented in Table 1.2. The details of the estrus cycles and sex hormone levels of the commonly used models are presented in the appropriate chapters.

Many other questions associated with surgical castration and the animal model of choice need to be asked. One issue to consider is how long it takes for castration to produce significant bone loss. Bone loss is most readily detected in cancellous bone because of the greater surface area it presents for remodeling. Large animals have an inherent resilience and castration alone does not result in a continuous unchecked bone loss that results in the severe bone loss seen in elderly women. There are instances where additional intervention (Ca restriction, metabolic acidotic diet, corticosteroid therapy) will be needed to produce a greater or more rapid bone loss, so that a therapeutic effect of a particular drug will be significant.[15,27-30] When such perturbation of the model is necessary, inclusion of a group of intact animals may be needed in a study to distinguish the skeletal effects of estrogen insufficiency alone.[16]

A question that is sometimes overlooked is whether ovariectomy alone is effective at all? Despite numerous advantages (bone structure and composition) in orthopedic research and the similarity between dog cortical bone microstructure and human bone[31] the most controversial model is the castrated (OVX or ORX) dog. It has been the most popular model for arthroplasty, cruciate ligament, meniscus, and fracture healing studies.[16,25] Readers of this chapter know that there are millions of neutered female dogs in the world that have been deficient of sex hormones and fairly sedentary throughout most of their lives, yet pathological fractures associated with decreased bone volume are unheard of in the veterinary profession. Some may even question the validity of using the OVX dog model at all.[25]

Large farm animals (pigs, goats, sheep) do lose bone following OVX but their day-to-day activities rarely incur spontaneous fracture of vertebral bodies or femoral neck. Strictly speaking, they truly are models of *osteopenia* rather than models of *osteoporosis*.[3,32,33]

Another potential complicating issue that investigators may need to consider is whether there is a seasonal variation in BMD, as encountered in humans. This may not be a problem with a rat study where exposure to light can be carefully regulated. However, season needs to be taken into account in long-term studies with sheep or goats that are housed outdoors and that experience changes in day length that influence their reproductive cycles.[34,35] One advantage of the rat model is the convenience of being able to standardize the exposure to light (a 12:12 hour light–dark cycle), ambient temperature, and humidity. Such standardization can be difficult but nevertheless achievable for farm animals such as sheep, goats, and pigs.

1.10 Animal Models for Osteoporosis Drug Therapy Evaluation

When selecting an animal model for testing drugs, some initial questions should be addressed:

- Can the therapy for the osteoporosis be administered in a practical manner?
- Can it be given orally or is an injection necessary?
- Is additional technical support needed to administer the drug(s)?
- What is the dose and would this be the equivalent dose in humans?
- Will it be absorbed and metabolized in the animal as it would in humans?

Some drugs may require a pharmacokinetic study to determine if therapeutic levels are obtained before embarking on an expensive trial involving castrated animals. Some drugs can be given orally in monogastric animals (rats, dogs, and pigs) but are not effective when given orally to ruminants (sheep and goats) because of metabolism and inactivation by the rumen microflora.

Another question to be asked is: What is the duration of therapy in the animal model? This is based upon the rate of bone turnover, which varies between animal species, and treatment should be the equivalent of 4 years of human exposure. Details of remodeling rates and therapy duration can be obtained in chapters on the specific animal models.

A final question is: When should the anti-osteoporotic drug being tested be administered? Is it a prevention study or a response to therapy (interventional) study? Should the treatment be continuous (e.g., selective estrogen receptor modulators (SERMS)) or intermittent (e.g., bisphosphonates)? As mentioned above, FDA guidelines recommend two doses: one that is clinically effective and the other five times greater, thereby providing a margin of safety and enhancing the likelihood of detecting toxicities.

1.11 Study End Points

Important issues to consider when selecting animal models for osteoporosis research are the end points to be measured, which are discussed in detail in Chaps. 2–6 of this book. Some of these end points may be dictated by regulatory agencies. Static and dynamic bone histomorphometry, aided by fluorochrome labeling of mineralizing surfaces, is one of the most common end points and has been used for many years in animal studies. There are ample publications concerning rats,[5,36] sheep,[37] and primates[12] as well as textbooks available for investigators to determine fluorochrome doses and their schedules. The most commonly used labels in animals are the veterinary drug tetracycline (TC), calcein, alizarin complex one, xylenol orange, and calcein blue. More details about histomorphometry can be found in Chap. 4 of this book. An overview of basic bone biology of animals commonly used for osteoporosis research is shown in Table 1.3.

Table 1.3 Overview of basic bone biology of animals commonly used for osteoporosis research

Animal	Bone structure	Osteonal remodeling	Sustained post-OVX bone loss (time)	Bone depletion period following OVX	Likeness of bone composition	References
Rats	Lamellar	No (modeling)	Yes	14 Days (proximal tibial metaphysis), 60 days (lumbar vertebrae)	Differs most	Lelovas et al.[5]
Dogs	Lamellar	Yes	Variable and controversial	Decreased (e.g., 1–4 months) or unchanged	Most similar	Reinwald and Burr,[16] Egermann et al.[25]
Domestic and minipigs	Plexiform when young	Yes when mature	Yes	>6 Months	Quite similar	Reinwald and Burr[16]
Sheep/goats	Plexiform when young	Yes, more when mature	No (>12 months)	>6 Months	Somewhat	Wu et al.[53]
Primates	Lamellar	Yes	Yes	9 Months	Most similar	Smith et al.[13]

Cost may be an issue when using some fluorochromes, especially in the larger animals, because dosage is determined by body weight. Other issues are toxicity (rapid chelation of serum calcium), and to obviate this some labels (e.g., calcein) must be given as a slow intravenous drip unless given subcutaneously. The mucous membrane color may change from pink to purple with some fluorochromes (e.g., Alizarin complexone), alarming some handlers. TC is a common antibacterial, which is sometimes used both therapeutically (mainly in sheep, goats, and swine) and prophylactically (mainly in swine). Such prior administration can cause fluorescing bands on the mineralizing surfaces that could interfere with other labels used in dynamic histomorphometry, thereby affecting study results. Investigators should avoid procuring farm animals that have been treated with TC.

To document longitudinal changes throughout a study, biopsies of the left and right iliac crests are useful, but this usually requires general anesthesia and additional cost.

Dogs, sheep, goats, and swine have sizable iliac crests that are amenable to several biopsies throughout a study. Following appropriate fluorochrome labeling, data from these samples can be compared to that from humans. Iliac crest biopsy is a simple procedure, well tolerated, the morbidity is low, and the histomorphometric data can be supportive to the hypotheses of the study. However, the iliac crest is not a weight-bearing bone and may not reflect what is happening in other parts of the animal's skeleton.[16]

Sometimes, the biopsy can be performed while the animal is anesthetized for other noninvasive imaging procedures such as peripheral quantitative computed tomography (pQCT) or dual energy X-ray absorptiometry (DEXA). Other bones may not be available for histomorphometry until necropsy.

The most widely used method of noninvasive measurement of BMD is DEXA followed by pQCT. These are discussed in greater detail in Chap. 5 of this book. Investigators must be aware that, aside from the anatomical difference between human and quadruped vertebral bodies and long bones, none of the absolute BMD values in healthy animals are similar to those in humans.[25] An important question investigators must first address, regardless of the imaging technique being used, is at what site (lumbar vertebrae, proximal femur, etc.) the BMD should be measured. For repeated measuring using DEXA and pQCT, movement-free positioning of the animal (usually under general anesthesia) is essential. General anesthesia can add to the expense of a study, although the newer pQCT scanners allow faster data acquisition in spiral scan mode, which means anesthetic times and doses (and therefore costs) for the animals are considerably reduced. Some bones of the human skeleton such as the proximal femur and lumbar vertebrae can be imaged with the patient in one position on the table. This does not apply to the same region in the quadruped. For example, positioning sheep and goats for BMD or pQCT images of the proximal femur in a longitudinal study can be a challenge because of the difficulty in abducting the pelvic limbs. Positioning for the same images of the lumbar vertebrae is more reliable.

pQCT is an excellent imaging technique compared to DEXA because of its three-dimensional (3D) image and ability to analyze cortical and cancellous regions of the femur, lumbar vertebrae, etc., separately. It is a useful complement to histomorphometry. Microcomputerized tomography (μCT) of explanted bones (e.g., vertebral bodies) to determine in 3D the bone volume, trabecular number, and trabecular thickness, combined with dynamic histomorphometry, are now useful end points for animal studies.[12] Further details are available in Chap. 5 of this book.

Many bone loss studies in animals have used a cross-sectional study design with end points being classic histomorphometry or conventional μCT studies.[38] The drawbacks of cross-sectional study design can be overcome by novel in vivo μCT in rat and mouse models using image registration methods, visualizing architectural changes at the level of individual trabeculae.[38] The obvious advantage of longitudinal study designs is that the same animal can be monitored over different time points enabling researchers to obtain comparable levels of information from fewer animals.[6]

For successful longitudinal studies, an identical region of interest (ROI) of trabecular bone (where active remodeling is seen) must be available at each time point. The lumbar spine is probably one of the most reliable sites for repeated measurements of the same bone and same ROI, without issues over precise positioning of the anesthetized animal. Bone densities in some large animals (pigs especially) are significantly higher than those observed in humans, but this should not discount the use of large animals as experimental subjects.

What tissues must be harvested at necropsy to verify safety? The reproductive tract should be of prime importance, especially in studies of synthetic estrogens because of the potential for tumorigenicity.

Measuring at least one biochemical marker of bone turnover has been recommended. Urinary pyridinium cross-links (a marker of bone resorption), bone-specific alkaline phosphatase (BSAP; a bone-specific isoenzyme), or osteocalcin (a marker of bone formation) have all been used in animal studies. All of these have advantages, but other considerations arise such as the practicality of collection of urine from large animals such as sheep or pigs. Most readers will be unfamiliar with the methods used by veterinarians or technicians to collect urine from large animals.

Bending torsional and compressive testing of explanted bone to document changes in fragility should be part of the study. Collaboration with a facility experienced with biomechanical testing of animal bones is essential. Before testing the actual bones from experimental animals it is wise to practice with similar bones from other sources, to allow bioengineers time to perfect their testing apparatus. Initial pilot studies are helpful in determining what sort of variance can be expected and to determine sample size to detect group differences in treatments. Further details of biomechanics can be found in Chap. 3 of this book.

1.12 Osteoporosis Models Associated with Glucocorticoid Administration

Glucocorticoid (GC)-induced bone loss severely affects human patients' health and quality of life.[15] It is seen in patients on long-term therapy for conditions such as asthma, rheumatoid arthritis, autoimmune disorders, Crohn's disease, or organ transplantation. To understand the pathophysiology of the bone loss as well as response to therapy, animal models such as dogs,[39] sheep,[29,30] and adult and growing minipigs[14,15] have been used to study GC osteoporosis. Corticosteroid administration (methylprednisolone is often used) can be combined with OVX to accelerate bone loss. Investigators must select a dose that will exhibit a bone loss effect of the GC but not cause profound immunosuppression, which may result in loss of animals due to exacerbations of subclinical disease. For example, some sheep flocks have a high incidence of mesenteric abscessation that might have remained clinically silent for the entire life of the animal but can cause a serious illness with prolonged immunosuppression associated with GC therapy.[40] The bacterium *Corynebacterium pseudotuberculosis* is a frequent pathogen. Careful withdrawal of steroid administration is recommended but some animals can develop withdrawal symptoms and some may have to be excluded from the study. Joint pain and partial lameness has been associated with steroid withdrawal in sheep, and anti-inflammatory therapy was used for a brief period for humane reasons.[29]

While on steroid therapy, sheep and goats need close veterinary attention to skin conditions (alopecia), potential abscess formation, weight loss, anorexia, and infection of other body systems (e.g., lungs). To avoid local skin infections different muscles of the shoulder, neck, and gluteal regions should be utilized for multiple injections.[30] Reports of studies using GC-treated animals often fail to disclose the losses or health problems of subjects in their studies. Investigators should allow for some potential loss when determining group sizes and statistical power.

1.13 Osteoporosis Models Associated with Dietary Manipulation

One advantage of using an animal such as the minipig is that the diet can be prepared such that it resembles the average human diet. Most investigators interested in animal models will first think of chronic calcium deficiency and its effect on the skeleton over time. This seems obvious, but is difficult to implement in some animal models. For example, commercial dog chows routinely have excessive calcium, and restriction of calcium intake, as well as surgical castration, may be essential when using dogs.

What is being fed to sheep or goats during studies of osteopenia must be carefully scrutinized. Naturally occurring phytoestrogens in certain clovers fed to sheep can act like selective estrogen receptor modulators, introducing an unwanted variable.

Calcium deficiency is very difficult to produce in sheep and goats because the rumen is an efficient absorber of calcium and therefore calcium deficiency with dietary change alone is difficult. An osteopenic goat model (OVX plus low-calcium diet) has been shown to induce osteopenia at the iliac crest, L2, L7, calcaneus, and humeral head with deterioration of trabecular microarchitecture and mechanical properties of cancellous bone.[41] Carefully designed studies feeding Ca-deficient diets to estrogen-deficient animals ideally should have a group that remains intact, to determine the contribution of the hormone deficiency versus the dietary contribution.

The cause of osteoporosis in humans is multifactorial and, apart from genetic, lifestyle, and life-stage factors, nutrition is a well-recognized cause. Several studies in people have implicated a dietary-induced metabolic acidosis (DIMA) as a contributing factor to osteoporosis.[42,43] This finding prompted some studies using OVX sheep consuming a diet that induces metabolic acidosis.[27,28] Sheep are sensitive to DIMA and this model would be useful to study mechanisms involving bone loss related to acidifying diets. More practical aspects of animals commonly used for osteoporosis research are shown in Table 1.2.

1.14 Evaluation of Implants in an Osteoporotic Environment

The search for an ideal implant for use in bones is being conducted for years, with emphasis on biocompatibility, resistance to wear and corrosion, and neoplastic tissue response.[18] There is also an increasing interest in implant–bone interaction and design of orthopedic devices (screws, pins, prostheses, etc.) for osteoporotic bone. The goal is to optimize biomaterial surfaces and avoid complications when used in clinical cases, both in the axial and appendicular skeleton as well as the maxillofacial region.[44-46] In osteoporotic bone, the decreased BMD may not provide the firm primary mechanical stabilization required for long-term success.[46] Because of the inherent size of the animal, testing of implants destined for the human skeleton is often impossible in rats, mice, or even rabbits. However, smaller animals might be perfect for an initial screening and test of concept for certain implant coatings (e.g., hydroxyapatite) and biomaterials designed to promote osteointegration and fracture fixation in mechanically weakened bone.[47] Much initial in vitro pilot work can be done in osteoporotic cadaveric human bone, if it is available. Ultimately an animal of appropriate size relative to the implant will be needed to simulate the biomechanical and biological environment of the large bones of human patients. The osteopenic environment must be documented as the study progresses, following OVX $\pm$ dietary manipulation either with sequential BMD measurements of the axial or appendicular skeleton and/or iliac crest biopsy histomorphometry. Larger animals allow investigators to look at numerous different implants in trabecular bone (e.g., distal femur) or cortical bone (e.g., radius, femur, tibia), all within the same animal. However, animal behavior can be unpredictable, especially that of goats, sheep, and pigs. Such behavior can lead to either pathological fracture of a long bone or implant loosening, necessitating euthanasia and loss of data points.

Investigators should avoid the temptation of trying to get too much data from one animal by inserting many implants in one bone (especially the tibia), only to lose the animal because of pathological fracture through one of the implant sites, necessitating early euthanasia.

1.15 Use of Animal Models for Evaluation of Spine Fusion

Because of the altered state of bone formation in osteoporosis, there is need for animal models to study the relationship between fracture healing and osteoporosis.[48] There is also interest in evaluating therapies to enhance fracture healing and spine fusion, and the OVX rat is ideal for use as a screening model before more expensive large animals are used. For evaluating growth factors (e.g., BMP-2, BMP-7) to enhance dorsolateral ("posterolateral" in humans) lumbar spinal fusion, rat, rabbit, dog, and sheep models are now well characterized. However, only skeletally mature, larger-sized animals (sheep, goats, pigs, certain breeds of dogs, and, if required, nonhuman primates) will be useful if commercially available spine instrumentation (pedicle screws, rods, etc.) is being evaluated in an osteopenic environment, largely because of vertebral body dimensions.

1.16 Other Practical Issues of Animal Models of Osteoporosis

1.16.1 Pilot Studies

Pilot studies using abattoir or cadaver specimens are often invaluable. It is also desirable to network with colleagues at other facilities who may have unwanted bones from animals that would otherwise be disposed of. This shows a certain respect for animals that have been sacrificed for research. Care must be taken to ensure that the animals are disease-free, and the parts packaged and shipped carefully and stored appropriately.

Preliminary screening of screw holding can be performed using young animal bones before such implants are used in skeletally mature animals where ovariectomy and or dietary manipulation will be performed. Demineralized calf vertebrae, mimicking osteomalacia rather than osteoporosis, have some biomechanical properties that are useful for screw pullout screening tests.[49]

Access to osteoporotic human cadaveric specimens can be difficult and impractical but deserves consideration in some cases.

1.17 Anesthesia and Analgesia in Animal Models

1.17.1 General Anesthesia

General anesthesia in veterinary medicine has made considerable strides over the past 10–20 years as far as safety and efficacy are concerned, with better and more effective drugs. It is beyond the scope of this chapter to provide details of animal anesthesia. There are many veterinary texts available that cover anesthesia of virtually all domestic animals used in research, including nonhuman primates.[50]

Most readers of this textbook will have very little, if any, experience with safely anesthetizing animals other than perhaps mice and rats. When anesthesia of larger animals discussed in this chapter is needed, then conducting the study takes on a new dimension and challenge. Some of the drugs for larger animals are different, and more expensive; intraoperative monitoring is strongly recommended; and special equipment (such as laryngoscopes and appropriate endotracheal tubes) may be necessary. This will mean enlisting either veterinarians or veterinary technicians experienced in animal anesthesia. What is perplexing is that anesthesia and analgesia of the animals are often underserved even in many well-funded studies. Too frequently, publications about animal research in reputable journals will attempt to excuse anesthesia deaths. Such explanations range from vague, meaningless statements such as "anesthesia death due to an allergic reaction to the anesthetic" or "anesthetic complications." Most of these losses can be attributable to overdosing and too great depth of anesthesia, and/or insufficient monitoring of vital signs. Ruminant (sheep/goats) anesthesia can be especially challenging because of regurgitation and potential aspiration pneumonia. Ruminants must be held off feed (not water) for at least 24 h before anesthesia, and oro-tracheal intubation during general anesthesia is mandatory. Occasionally an animal may have a subclinical respiratory infection with compromise to the lungs that is exacerbated by the stress of anesthesia and surgery, and these losses are understandable. Animals in poor health should be screened and not be used if they appear to be under anesthetic risk.

With the veterinary anesthetic drugs, delivery systems, and monitoring equipment currently available, loss of an animals while under general anesthesia is generally due to inexperience and is largely inexcusable. Unfortunately, loss of a data point in the middle of a long-term study is very expensive, both in money and time lost, if some of the study has to be repeated.

1.17.2 Postoperative Pain Control

Another field that has advanced is the understanding and treatment of animal pain.[51,52] Many investigators who have little or no training in analgesia in research animals need to collaborate more closely with veterinarians and veterinary technicians. It is especially important that animals be evaluated frequently by someone familiar with their species-specific behavior and habits. Research publications are still appearing with statements that say "postoperative analgesia was provided as needed." It is far better to provide analgesics regardless. Determining whether an animal is in pain and whether the therapy is effective has been a challenge to the veterinary profession for many years; however, advances have been made as we are now understanding what behavioral signs animals show when they are in pain. What type and duration of analgesic therapy should be used will depend upon the degree of injury or insult experienced by the animals and how much their comfort and behavior has been affected (drinking, eating, activity).

Some journals publishing studies that have used animal models are now demanding details (drug names, doses used, etc.) about postoperative pain management.

1.18 Summary

This chapter has presented some of the initial issues that investigators must address when considering using an animal model for osteoporosis research. When these are overlooked, money and animals will be wasted. Collaboration and communication with laboratories and other investigators experienced with these animals (especially the larger farm animals and primates) are not only essential for the initiation and success of a study, but a requirement by many IACUCs around the world. Other chapters in this book will discuss the different models, and their strengths and weaknesses in more detail.

Acknowledgments I am grateful to Drs. Sue VandeWoude and Ann Wagner, Colorado State University, for helpful suggestions for this chapter.

References

1. Karlsson MK, Gerdhem P, Ahlborg HG. The prevention of osteoporotic fractures. *J Bone Joint Surg Br*. 2005;87-B:1320-1327.
2. Burge R, Dawson-Hughes B, Solomon DH, et al. Incidence and economic burden of osteoporosis-related fractures in the United States, 2005–2025. *J Bone Miner Res*. 2007;22: 465-475.
3. Turner AS. Animal models of osteoporosis – necessity and limitations. *Eur Cells Mater*. 2001;1:66-81.
4. Thompson DD, Simmons HA, Pirie CM, Ke HZ. FDA guidelines and animal models for osteoporosis. *Bone*. 1995; 17:125S-133S.
5. Lelovas PP, Xanthos TT, Thoma SE, et al. The laboratory rat as an animal model for osteoporosis research. *Comp Med*. 2008;58(5):424-430.
6. Leitner MM, Tami AE, Montavon PM, et al. Longitudinal as well as age-matched assessments of bone changes in the mature ovariectomized rat model. *Lab Anim*. 2009;43(3): 266-271.
7. Sigrist IM, Gerhardt C, Alini M, et al. The long-term effects of ovariectomy on bone metabolism in sheep. *J Bone Miner Res*. 2007;25:28-35.
8. Podolsky LM, Lukas VS. *The Care and Feeding of an IACUC*. Boca Raton: CRC; 1999.
9. Silverman J, Suckow MA, Murthy S. *The IACUC Handbook*. Boca Raton: CRC; 2000.
10. Hart LA, ed. *Responsible Conduct with Research Animals*. New York: Oxford University Press; 1998.
11. International regulations and resources. http://www.aaalac.org/resources/internationalregs.cfm
12. Fox J, Newman MK, Turner CH, et al. Effects of treatment with parathyroid hormone 1-84 on quantity and biomechanical properties of thoracic vertebral trabecular bone in ovariectomized rhesus monkeys. *Calcif Tissue Int*. 2008; 82(3):212-220.
13. Smith SY, Jolette J, Turner CH. Skeletal health: primate model of postmenopausal osteoporosis. *Am J Primatol*. 2009;71(9):752-765.
14. Akahoshi S, Sakai A, Arita S, et al. Modulation of bone turnover by alfacalcidol and/or alendronate does not prevent glucocorticoid-induced osteoporosis in growing minipigs. *J Bone Miner Metab*. 2005;23:341-350.
15. Glüer CC, Scholz-Ahrens KE, Helfenstein A, et al. Ibandronate treatment reverses glucocorticoid-induced loss of bone mineral density and strength in minipigs. *Bone*. 2007; 40:645-655.
16. Reinwald S, Burr D. Perspective: review of nonprimate large animal models for osteoporosis research. *J Bone Miner Res*. 2008;23:1353-1368.
17. Harkness JE, Wagner JE. *The Biology and Medicine of Rabbits and Rodents*. 4th ed. Baltimore: Williams & Wilkins; 1995.
18. Pearce AI, Richards RG, Milz S, Schneider E, Pearce SG. Animal models for implant biomaterial research in bone: a review. *Eur Cells Mater*. 2007;13:1-10.
19. Donahue SW, McGee ME, Harvey KB, et al. Hibernating bears as a model for preventing disuse osteoporosis. *J Biomech*. 2006;39(8):1480-1488.
20. McGee-Lawrence ME, Wojda SJ, Barlow LN, et al. Grizzly bears (*Ursus arctos horribilis*) and black bears (*Ursus americanus*) prevent trabecular bone loss during disuse (hibernation). *Bone*. 2009;45:1186-1191.
21. Getty R. *Sisson and Grossman's the Anatomy of the Domestic Animals*. 5th ed. Philadelphia: W.B. Saunders; 1975:777.
22. National Osteoporosis Foundation. Fast facts on osteoporosis. http://www.nof.org/osteoporosis/diseasefacts.htm. Accessed October 10, 2009.
23. Morrow R, Deyhim F, Patil BS, et al. Feeding orange pulp improved bone quality in a rat model of male osteoporosis. *J Med Food*. 2009;12(2):298-303.
24. Sipos W, Rauner M, Skalicky M, et al. Running has a negative effect on bone metabolism and proinflammatory status in male aged rats. *Exp Gerontol*. 2008;43:578-583.
25. Egermann M, Goldhahn J, Schneider E. Animal models for fracture treatment in osteoporosis. *Osteoporos Int*. 2005; 16:S129-S138.
26. Watts ES. Skeletal development. In: Richard Dukelow W, Erwin J, eds. *Comparative Primate Biology: Reproduction and Development*, vol. 3. New York: A.R Liss; 1986: 415-439.
27. MacLeay JM, Olson JD, Enns RM, et al. Dietary induced metabolic acidosis decreases bone mineral density in mature ovariectomized ewes. *Calcif Tissue Int*. 2004;75:431-437.
28. MacLeay JM, Olson JD, Turner AS. Effect of dietary-induced metabolic acidosis and ovariectomy on bone mineral density and markers of bone turnover. *J Bone Miner Metab*. 2004;22:561-568.

29. Schorlemmer S, Ignatius A, Claes L, et al. Inhibition of cortical and cancellous bone formation in glucocorticoid-treated sheep. *Bone*. 2005;37:491-496.
30. Klopfenstein-Bregger MD, Schawalder P, Rahn B, et al. Optimization of corticosteroid induced osteoporosis in ovariectomized sheep. A bone histomorphometric study. *Vet Comp Orthop Traumatol*. 2007;20(1):18-23.
31. Aerssens J, Boonedn S, Lowet G, et al. Interspecies differences in bone composition, density, and quality: potential implications for in vivo bone research. *Endocrinology*. 1998;139:663-670.
32. Turner AS. Review: the sheep as a model for osteoporosis in humans. *Vet J*. 2002;163:1-8.
33. Turner AS, MacLeay JM. Osteoporosis: advantages and disadvantages of commonly used animal models. *Adv Osteoporotic Fract Manag*. 2002;1(3):80-86.
34. Turner AS. Seasonal changes in bone metabolism in sheep: further characterization of an animal model for human osteoporosis [Guest editorial]. *Vet J*. 2006;174(3):460-461.
35. Arens D, Sigrist I, Alini M, et al. Seasonal changes in bone metabolism in sheep. *Vet J*. 2007;174(3):585-591.
36. Kharode YP, Sharp MC, Bodine PV. Utility of the ovariectomized rat as a model for human osteoporosis in drug discovery. *Methods Mol Biol*. 2008;455:111-124.
37. Kennedy OD, Brennan O, Rackard SM, et al. Effects of ovariectomy on bone turnover, porosity, and biomechanical properties in ovine compact bone 12 months postsurgery. *J Orthop Res*. 2009;27(3):303-309.
38. Waarsing JH, Day JS, Verhaar JAN, et al. Bone loss dynamics result in trabecular alignment in aging and ovariectomized rats. *J Orthop Res*. 2006;24(5):926-935.
39. Norrdin RW, Histand MB, Sheahan HJ, et al. Effects of corticosteroids on mechanical strength of intervertebral joints and vertebrae in dogs. *Clin Orthop Relat Res*. 1990;259:68-76.
40. Egermann M, Goldhahn J, Holz R, et al. A sheep model for fracture treatment in osteoporosis: benefits of the model versus animal welfare. *Lab Anim*. 2008;42(4):453-464.
41. Leung KS, Siu WS, Li SF, et al. An in vitro optimized injectable calcium phosphate cement for augmenting screw fixation in osteopenic goats. *J Biomed Mater Res B*. 2006; 78B:153-160.
42. Kerstetter JE, O'Brien KO, Insogna KL. Dietary protein, calcium metabolism, and skeletal homeostasis revisted. *Am J Clin Nutr*. 2003;78(Suppl):584S-592S.
43. Lemann J, Bushinsky DA, Hamm LL. Bone buffering of acid and base in humans. *Am J Physiol Renal Physiol*. 2003;285:F811-F832.
44. Giannoudis PV, Schneider E. Principles of fixation of osteoporotic fractures. *J Bone Joint Surg Br*. 2006;88-B(10):1272-1278.
45. Goldhahn J, Reinhold M, Stauber M, et al. Improved anchorage in osteoporotic vertebrae with new implant designs. *J Orthop Res*. 2006;24(5):917-925.
46. Borsari V, Fini M, Giavaresi G, et al. Osteointegration of titanium and hydroxyapatite rough surfaces in healthy and compromised cortical and trabecular bone: in vivo comparative study on young, aged and estrogen deficient sheep. *J Orthop Res*. 2007;25(9):1250-1260.
47. Hayashi K, Fotovati A, Ali SA, et al. Prostaglandin EP4 receptor agonist augments fixation of hydroxyapatite-coated implants in a rat model of osteoporosis. *J Bone Joint Surg Br*. 2005;87-B:1150-1156.
48. McCann RM, Colleary G, Geddis C, et al. Effect of osteoporosis on bone mineral density and fracture repair in a rat femoral fracture model. *J Orthop Res*. 2008;26(3): 384-393.
49. Akbay A, Bozkurt G, Ilgaz O, et al. A demineralized calf vertebrae model as an alternative to classic osteoporotic vertebrae models for pedicle screw pullout studies. *Eur Spine J*. 2008;17(3):468-473.
50. Tranquilli WJ, Thurmon JC, Grimm KA. *Lumb and Jones' Veterinary Anesthesia and Analgesia*. 4th ed. Ames: Blackwell; 2007.
51. Gaynor JS, Muir WW III. *Handbook of Veterinary Pain Management*. Missouri: Mosby Elsevier; 2002.
52. Flecknell PA, Waterman-Pearson A, eds. *Pain Management in Animals*. Philadelphia: W.B. Saunders; 2000.
53. Wu ZX, Lei W, Hu YY, et al. Effect of ovariectomy on BMD, micro-architecture and biomechanics of cortical and cancellous bones in a sheep model. *Med Eng Phys*. 2008;30(9): 1112-1118.

2 Skeletal Phenotyping in Rodents: Tissue Isolation and Manipulation

Janet E. Henderson, Chan Gao, and Edward J. Harvey

2.1 Introduction

The pioneering work of Rudolph Jaenisch at the Whitehead Institute[1] and Mario Capecchi at the Howard Hughes Institute[2] used modification of the mouse genome to understand the etiology and pathogenesis of human disease. Their groundbreaking studies in the 1980s revealed the power of mouse genetic and genomic research and were the driving force behind the explosive growth of transgenic science as we know it today. Enormous resources have been expended in the academic and private sectors for vivaria to generate, breed, and house mice with targeted mutations in thousands of genes. Complicated breeding programs have been established to generate mice carrying compound mutations as well as recombinant congenic strains with known segments of one strain incorporated into the genome of another.[3] The success of these genetic-based approaches using animal models to predict susceptibility or resistance to human disease relies heavily on the ability to accurately and reliably characterize the phenotypic traits associated with that disease.

Like the vast majority of common pathologies that affect human populations, osteoporosis is a complex, polygenic, and multifactorial disease that is characterized by a reduction in bone strength that predisposes it to fracture.[4] Historically, bone mineral density (BMD) has been used as the principle surrogate marker of bone strength for the purpose of diagnosing osteoporosis in human[5] and mouse[6] populations. BMD remains an important diagnostic tool and an indicator of response to treatment. Additional tests including biochemical markers of bone metabolism[7] and noninvasive measurements of bone architecture using quantitative computed tomography (qCT) are also frequently used.[8] Although genetic profiling for bone disease is still at an early stage of development, it is widely accepted that genetic background plays a significant role in determining individual differences in bone development and the rate and extent to which bone metabolism changes over time.[9] Many of the genes that have been linked to osteopenic or osteoporotic phenotypes include components of growth factor, cytokine and steroid hormone-signaling pathways, and the major collagenous and non-collagenous bone matrix proteins.

Of primary importance in the selection of an appropriate animal model is its predictive value for use in the diagnosis or treatment of human disease. Mutations in osteoporosis-related genes in the mouse genome have produced remarkably similar phenotypes to those observed in humans, thus identifying these animals as a valuable resource to study the interplay between genetic and epigenetic factors in the pathogenesis of osteoporosis.[10] Among the many advantages that mice have over other animal models commonly used to study bone disease are preexisting disease with a well-documented progression, a program of skeletal development similar to that seen in humans, relatively low cost and wide accessibility, a rapid breeding cycle and defined genetics, and, above all, established protocols for the phenotypic and molecular analysis of their skeleton. For these reasons, genetically modified mice remain the model of choice for the functional analysis of osteoporosis as well as other diseases. The comprehensive skeletal phenotyping protocol described in this

J.E. Henderson (✉)
Department of Medicine and Surgery, McGill University Health Centre, Montreal General Hospital, Room A5.169, 1650 Cedar Ave., Montreal, Québec H3G 1A4, Canada
e-mail: janet.henderson@mcgill.ca

G. Duque and K. Watanabe (eds.), *Osteoporosis Research*,
DOI: 10.1007/978-0-85729-293-3_2,

chapter was developed for screening populations of mice arising from genetic recombination[3] and chemical mutagenesis,[11,12] and has been used with success to characterize the skeletons of mice with targeted genetic mutations.[13-21]

2.2 Primary Screen for a Skeletal Phenotype

The different steps in the primary skeletal screen can be performed rapidly and provide sufficient information to pinpoint heritable defects in trabecular and cortical bone that will impact on its functional properties. It is unlikely that the defects identified in a primary bone screen will resolve over time if the animals are phenotyped after 4 months of age when they are skeletally mature. The progressive nature of a comprehensive screen for a skeletal phenotype is illustrated in Fig. 2.1 along with examples of micro-computed tomography (μCT) and histological analyses performed in the primary (1°) and secondary (2°) screens.

2.2.1 Genetic Background

A skeletal phenotype analysis begins with documentation of the genetic background of the mice. Similar genetic and gender-determined differences in bone traits, such as size, shape, and BMD are seen in humans and in inbred strains of mice. The Jackson Laboratory maintains a Mouse Phenome Database (http://phenome.jax.org), which is an excellent source of information on inbred strain differences in body composition, skeletal morphology, BMD, bone strength, and other criteria that could potentially impact on the overall skeletal phenotype. These inter-strain differences in bone have been exploited as a mechanism to localize disease genes to specific segments of the genome. An example is the AcB/BcA gene discovery platform consisting of 36 recombinant congenic strains (RCS) that were generated from an intercross between A/J and C57BL6J mouse strains to study susceptibility to infection.[22] Subsequent backcross of the descendants for ten generations to one or the other original strain, designated the recipient, resulted in the RCS carrying 12.5% of the donor genome in the recipient genome. Using BMD and μCT as a screening tool, several RCS with 87.5% C57BL6J DNA exhibited reduced BMD compared with the parental strain. This indicated that low BMD, which is a characteristic of A/J mice, was conferred in the 12.5% of A/J DNA.[3] Genetic mapping of this segment can then identify novel molecular targets for diagnostic or therapeutic interventions.

2.2.2 Age and Sex

In addition to the genetic background, the age and sex of the mouse can impact heavily on the bone phenotype. Skeletal maturity is attained between 4 and 5 months of age in mice and in most strains there are significant differences between males and females. The parameters that are commonly used to characterize the bone phenotype, including BMD, cortical width, trabecular volume, and architecture, change over time in much the same way as they do in growing children. It is therefore difficult to draw conclusions regarding the impact of a specific gene mutation from phenotypic analyses performed before 4 months, for instance in strains that are neonatally or perinatally lethal. Even when dealing with adult mice it is always good practice to consult with the Mouse Phenome Database to familiarize oneself with the expected skeletal phenotype of wild-type mice in the genetic background on which a mutation is bred. Some examples of work performed by investigators in collaboration with the Jackson Labs include mapping of genetic variability in BMD,[23] bone strength,[24] biomechanical properties,[25] and IGF-1 status,[26,27] as well as genome-wide screening for mutations using advanced sequencing technologies.[28] Comparisons between C3H/HeJ and C57BL6J male and female mice revealed significantly greater BMD in the skull and lumbar vertebrae of C3H mice. The data came from five independent studies by four different investigators using two different technologies, dual x-ray absorptiometry (DXA) and peripheral quantitative computed tomography (pQCT). Striking differences in femoral cortical width and cross-sectional geometry were reflected in the differences in biomechanical strength, with the thinner cortex of C57BL6J mice conferring susceptibility

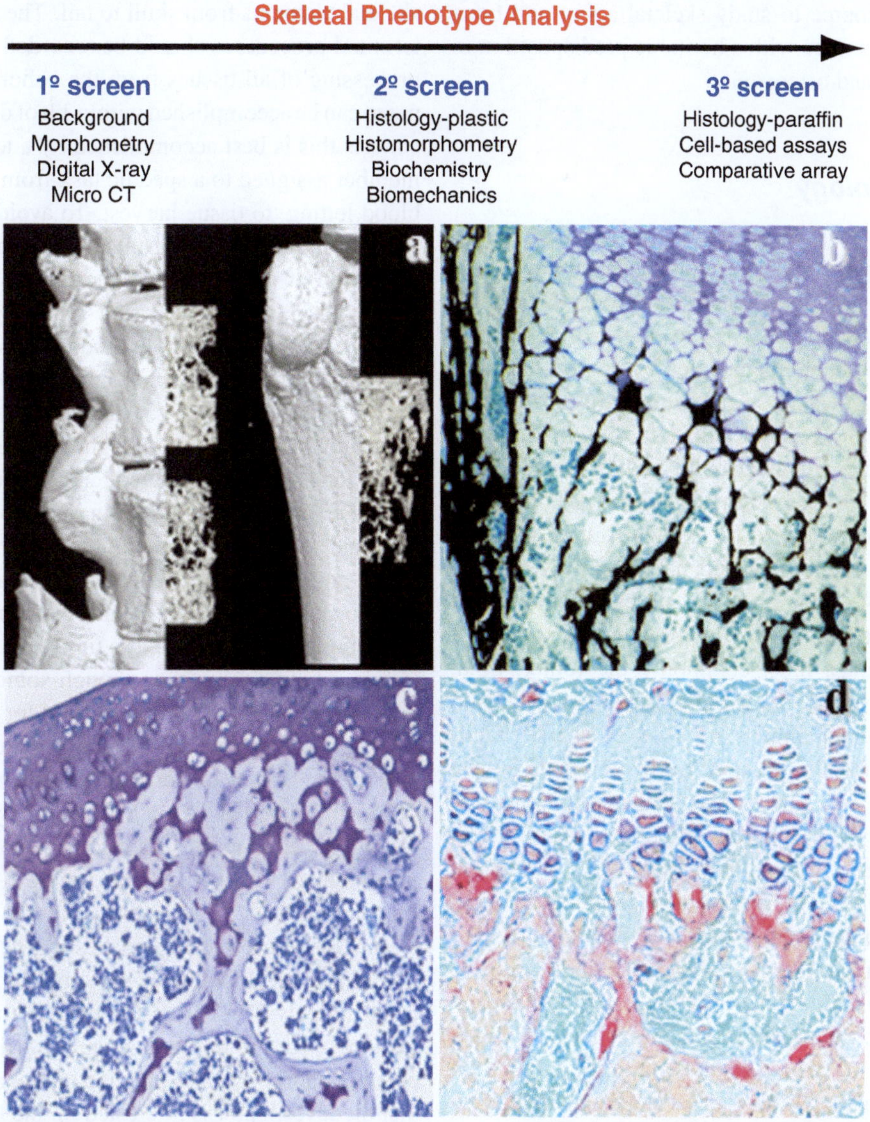

Fig. 2.1 Skeletal phenotype analysis through sequential screens. The skeleton is analyzed systematically and progressively for traits from the macroscopic to the molecular level through a series of screens. The primary (1°) screen provides information on the genetic background, the morphology of key skeletal elements, and analysis of bone architecture using μCT (**a**). The secondary (2°) screen involves detailed histological analyses of plastic-embedded bone for mineral, osteoid, osteoblast, and osteoclast activity. (**b**) Details of the deposition of mineral (black) at the chondro–osseous junction of the growth plate, and (**c**) the articular surface of a joint with metachromatic staining of mineralized cartilage cores (purple), and the bone that has been laid down by osteoblasts on top of them. (**d**) The chondro–osseous junction, with osteoblasts stained purple with ALP and osteoclasts stained red with TRAP. Immunochemical analyses of bone are not commonly performed and are thus placed in the tertiary (3°) screen along with detailed analyses of bone marrow–derived or limb bud MSC and gene- or protein-based comparative arrays to explore the molecular mechanisms

to fracture. Craniofacial morphology also differed, with the C3H mice exhibiting a shorter skull and nasal length and a deeper cranial vault than the C57BL6J strain. It is interesting to note that when mice homozygous for a null mutation of fibroblast growth factor receptor 3 (FGFR3) were bred onto a C3H background to improve longevity[15] the phenotype of the axial and appendicular skeleton was virtually identical to that seen on the C57BL/6 background.[29,30] The dramatic improvement in their viability identified these mice as a valuable resource to study skeletal aging and bone regeneration in mice with a heritable predisposition to osteomalacia and osteopenia.

2.2.3 Radiology

Once the pedigree and morphological features of the mouse have been documented it is time to perform radiological imaging of the skeleton. For a detailed discussion of animal imaging please refer to Chap. 5 of this book. A dedicated small animal x-ray instrument like the XPert 80 (Kubtek, Milford CT) with a 50 kV, 1 mA source and digital capability is best suited to this task. Imaging for longitudinal studies is performed on mice lightly anesthetized for immobilization and at a magnification of up to 5× depending on the region of interest (ROI). This provides an electronic record of the gross skeletal phenotype for the measurement of skeletal elements, most commonly the femur, tibia, vertebra, and skull. To avoid difficulties associated with the transfer of animals in and out of a barrier facility any instrument to be used on live animals is best placed inside the barrier. For skeletal imaging this might include a DXA, a μCT, and in rare cases a small animal magnetic resonance imaging MRI instrument for joint imaging. The gradual shift in emphasis from BMD alone in the clinical diagnosis of osteoporosis to a broader definition that involves bone architecture is reflected in a reduction in the use of DXA and an increase in μCT in preclinical animal models. This has been enabled in part by a reduction in the cost of the instruments over the past decade and by improved technology for data processing and storage capabilities. In keeping with the focus of this chapter, the following discussion of μCT imaging will be restricted to postmortem applications and from our experience using Skyscan (http://www.skyscan.be) instruments.

2.2.4 Terminal Procedures and Tissue Harvest

When euthanizing an animal for the purpose of characterizing its skeletal phenotype one should harvest body fluids for biochemical analyses along with the skeletal elements from skull to tail. The time taken for terminal procedures should be recorded to ensure that processing of all tissues from the cohort being euthanized can be accomplished within 1 h of death. For large cohorts this is best accomplished by a team with each member assigned to a specific task from anesthesia, to blood letting, to tissue harvest. To avoid using expensive and time-consuming metabolic protocols for the collection of urine samples, the mouse can be placed on a cold glass plate and spot urine aspirated with a sterile micropipette. Whole blood removed by cardiac puncture from anesthetized animals is processed to obtain serum or plasma for biochemical analyses and, if needed, high molecular weight DNA can be isolated for genetic studies. The selection of bones for analysis should ensure consistency from one experiment to the next and to obtain the maximum information from a single animal. Figure 2.2 shows an x-ray image with the allocation of different skeletal elements for a typical phenotyping experiment. It is time- and cost-effective to harvest everything even though some of the bones may not be used. All bones removed for μCT are fixed overnight at 4°C in fresh 4% paraformaldehyde, rinsed in three exchanges of sterile phosphate buffered saline (PBS) and stored at 4°C in PBS until they are scanned. Using the pelvic girdle as a reference point the lumbar vertebrae are removed en bloc for μCT and histological analysis and the thoracic vertebrae removed and frozen for micro-mechanical testing or RNA extraction if needed. Both femurs are carefully disarticulated from the pelvis and from the tibia at the knee, being extremely careful not to damage the articular surfaces or subchondral bone. Depending on the battery of tests that the investigator is interested in, the long bones are either fixed and scanned using μCT prior to histological processing (see below) or frozen for biomechanical testing or RNA analyses. The skull is usually frozen for future reference unless the investigator has a particular interest in its analysis.[18]

2.2.5 Microcomputed Tomographic Imaging

There are an increasing number of institutions using desktop μCT instruments for high-resolution three-dimensional

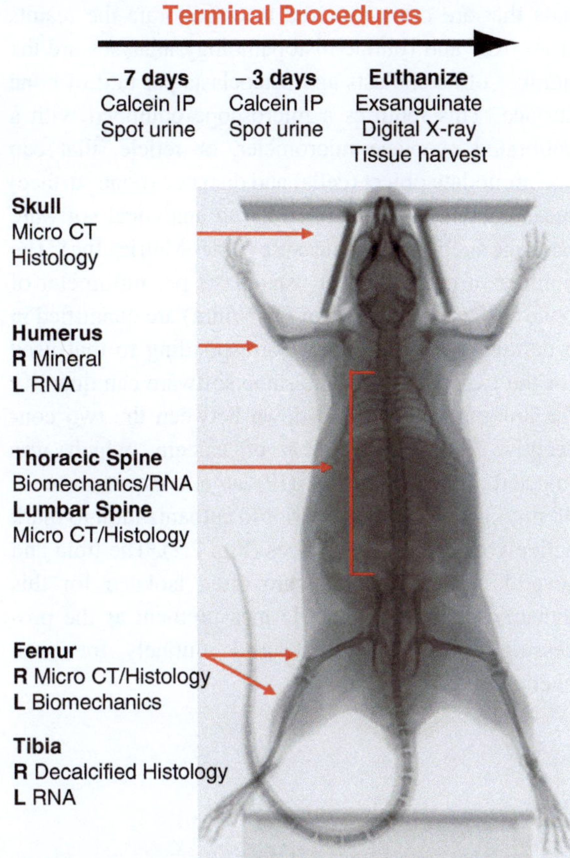

Fig. 2.2 Terminal procedures and bone harvest for skeletal phenotype. Seven days prior to euthanization young adult mice are first placed on a cold glass plate to induce voiding of the bladder and are then injected IP with 30 mg/kg calcein to label actively mineralizing bone. Four days later the same procedure is repeated. On the day of euthanization the mice are injected with a lethal dose of anesthetic, exsanguinated by cardiac puncture, and a contact x-ray captured before rigor mortis sets in. The skull, humeri, thoracic spine, and left femur and tibia are carefully disarticulated, placed in sterile polyethylene tubes, and frozen at –80°C along with the serum from separated blood to await analyses. The lumbar vertebrae and right femur and tibia are removed and placed immediately into cold 4% paraformaldehyde, fixed overnight at 4°C, rinsed thoroughly, and transferred to sterile PBS prior to μCT scanning on the Skyscan 1172 and processing for histology

(3D) imaging of rodent bones. The Skyscan 1172 currently in use at our institution is equipped with an x-ray source of maximum power 10 W and 100 kV. A 10 megapixel camera, micro-positioning stage, and NRecon software enable scanning and 3D reconstruction of specimens measuring approximately 7.0 × 3.5 cm at a resolution of up to 8,000 × 8,000 pixels and a detection limit of 0.7 μm isotropic detail. A typical ROI selected for quantitative μCT analysis is identified in reference to an anatomical landmark to ensure reproducibility from one specimen to the next. This is particularly relevant when comparing mice carrying mutations that affect the longitudinal growth of bones through the growth plates with their wild-type counterparts. A convenient landmark for the upper limit of the ROI in the distal femur is the lower edge of the femoral condyles as they appear in transverse sections. Typically, at a resolution of 5 μm the scan will be extended through a stack of 300 sections to generate a volumetric picture of trabecular bone in the proximal femur from which quantitative data can be generated. Many of the architectural parameters that were previously derived from histomorphometric analyses of serial two-dimensional (2D) sections can now be measured directly from these 3D CT reconstructions. The parameters most frequently used to describe bone architecture are the ratio of bone volume to tissue volume (BV/TV), trabecular thickness (Tr.Th), separation (Tr.Sp), and number (Tr.N), as well as measurements of their orientation (structure model index [SMI]) and connectivity (trabecular bone pattern factor [TbPf]). Additional measurements of cortical width at several different regions of the diaphysis as well as measuring BMD using an appropriate phantom are useful indices of the predicted biomechanical strength of the bone. If the primary interest is trabecular bone, then similar information can be captured from a defined ROI in vertebral bone.

2.3 Secondary Screen for Pathogenetic Mechanisms

When screening RCS or other populations of mice for skeletal defects, such as those that have undergone chemical mutagenesis, only those showing a distinct phenotype on the μCT analysis are subjected to a labor-intensive secondary screen. In contrast, investigators who have generated a single targeted mutation in a suspected bone active gene should always undertake this step, regardless of the outcome of the primary screen. While the primary screen provides quantitative data on the relative amount and micro-architecture of bone, it provides no information on non-mineralized tissue or cellular composition, both of which provide critical information on the pathogenetic mechanisms underlying a bone phenotype.

2.3.1 Undecalcified Histology

The same femur that was used for the μCT scan is trimmed and processed for embedding in polymethylmethacrylate (PMMA) at low temperature for preservation of enzyme activity and for undecalcified histological analysis.[31] Serial 2–5 μm sections are cut on a rotary microtome such as the Leica RM2265 (Leica Microsystems), which is equipped with a tungsten-carbide knife. Sections cut at intervals throughout the block and stained with Von Kossa and counterstained with toluidine blue can be accurately matched to 2D μCT images to corroborate the quantitative results. Von Kossa stains mineralized tissue black and distinguishes it from blue non-mineralized tissue, such as cartilage, osteoid, fibrous tissue, or bone marrow (Fig. 2.1b). Adjacent sections are stained with tartrate resistant acid phosphatase (TRAP) for multinucleate osteoclasts and their precursors, and with alkaline phosphatase (ALP) to identify osteoblasts and hypertrophic chondrocytes in the epiphyseal growth plates (Fig. 2.1d). Metachromatic staining with toluidine blue alone is also useful in immature bone specimens to distinguish the primary spongiosa bone that is deposited on cartilage cores (Fig. 2.1c). If the primary interest is growth plate or epiphyseal cartilage, then a Safranin O stain should also be used to identify proteoglycan. These histochemical stains provide valuable qualitative data on the cell and tissue composition of trabecular and cortical bone and the relationship between mineralized and non-mineralized tissues.

2.3.2 Histomorphometry

A detailed discussion of the applications and methodology for histomorphometry can be found in Chap. 4 of this book while this discussion will be restricted to those analyses that form an integral part of a secondary phenotypic screen. Quantitative histomorphometric data that are often required to corroborate the results from μCT and routine histopathology analyses are the number of osteoblasts and osteoclasts per unit of bone surface. This requires a microscope equipped with a calibrated eyepiece micrometer, or reticle, that can accommodate object (cells) and distance (bone surface) measurements accompanied by an analytical software package such as Osteomeasure (OsteoMetrics Inc). The number of osteoclasts or osteoblasts per millimeter of bone surface (Oc.N/mm or Ob.N/mm) are quantified in a defined ROI, preferably corresponding to that used for the μCT analyses. The same software can quantify the amount of bone laid down between the two consecutive fluorescent labels of calcein, which was injected intraperitoneally (IP) at a concentration of 30 mg/kg at 7 and 3 days prior to euthanization to mark actively mineralizing surfaces (Fig. 2.2). The tibia and several lumbar vertebrae are often isolated for this dynamic histomorphometric measurement as the processing differs from that used routinely for bone phenotyping.

2.3.3 Biochemistry

A more complete discussion of the applications and methodology for biochemical markers of bone disease can be found in Chap. 6 of this book. The similarities between human and murine bone growth and metabolism has facilitated the development of scaled-down rodent biomarker assays for serum and urine based on those used for screening human populations. Tests that are included in a secondary bone screen are calcium, phosphate, ALP, parathyroid hormone (PTH), vitamin D (VitD), markers of osteoblast and osteoclast activity and thype-1 collagen breakdown (CTX). Many of the early mutations exploring osteopenic bone disease were targeted directly or indirectly at components of the classic PTH/VitD axis and their effect on calcium and phosphate metabolism. It is therefore not surprising that PTH and VitD levels were the first to be analyzed along with calcium and phosphate in the systemic circulation of rodents undergoing a secondary bone screen. The anabolic action of PTH in bone, which led to its United States Food and Drug Administration (FDA) approval as a therapy for advanced osteoporosis, is believed to be mediated through the Wnt signaling pathway.[32] Abnormalities in histochemical staining of osteoblasts and osteoclasts in bone can be followed up with serum assays for many bone active growth factors and cytokines that are available commercially in kit form. These include FGFs, IGF-1, PDGF, EGF, VEGF, TGF beta, Interleukins 1 and 6, tumor necrosis factor alpha (TNF-α), osteoprotegerin (OPG), and RANK ligand. Needless to say, the number of assays performed is limited not only because of their high cost but also by the relatively small amount of serum from blood obtained by cardiac puncture at the time of euthanization.

2.3.4 Chemical Composition of Bone

Of increasing importance to the study of bone strength is its chemical composition. Historically the relationship between collagen and hydroxyapatite crystals has been examined at the ultrastructural level using electron microscopy[33,34] and the composition of the mineral phase quantified using a variety of biochemical assays including atomic absorption spectroscopy. Calcium, phosphate, magnesium, and various trace elements are measured in bone ash that is dissolved in acid and diluted in a solution, that is aspirated and burned in an acetylene air flame at a temperature of up to 2,800°C. This is a rapid, sensitive, and specific method for quantifying the ratio of calcium to phosphate or for determining the presence of elements such as magnesium, aluminum, strontium, zinc, or others that might influence bone strength.[35] Applications of alternative, nondestructive technology to examine the relationship between collagenous and non-collagenous components of bone in situ are gaining in popularity, including Fourier transform infrared (FT-IR)[36] and Raman spectroscopy.[37,38] Of particular interest is the development of methodology for transcutaneous Raman spectroscopy for use in live animals.[39]

2.3.5 Biomechanical Testing

Alterations in bone morphology, micro-architecture, composition, and turnover that are identified in the primary and secondary screens will ultimately impact on bone strength. A detailed discussion of the applications and methodology for biomechanical testing of trabecular and cortical bone strength is found in Chap. 3 of this book. These tests are best performed in specialized biomechanical engineering labs where the instruments have often been purpose-built and there is an acquired expertise. As a nonexpert it is reasonably easy to identify the need for expert advice and collaboration on testing the biomechanical strength of a mutant bone. For example, the thin femoral cortices demonstrated on a μCT screen of adult FGFR3$^{-/-}$ mice suggested the femoral diaphysis would be less resistant to loading and would fracture more readily in a three-point bending test.[15] The hypothesis was validated in collaboration with the Buschmann team at Ecole Polytechnique who had developed the Mach-1 micro-mechanical tester marketed through Biosyntech Inc. (Laval, Quebec). A similar micro-mechanical tester from Instron Corp. (Canton, MA) was used to determine the relative resistance to compressive force of trabecular bone in the vertebrae of inbred strains of mice with differing susceptibility to fluorosis.[40]

2.4 Tertiary Screen for Molecular Mechanisms

In situ analysis of bone cell function using immunohistochemical localization of proteins or in situ hybridization of RNA is technically challenging and labor-intensive and is therefore not commonly included in a secondary screen. The assays do, however, provide extremely valuable information on the identity of cells contributing to the bone phenotype. Protocols have been developed in specialized labs for immunochemical analysis of undecalcified tissue[41] while others prefer to perform immunostaining on decalcified specimens, which usually means processing another bone (Fig. 2.2).

2.4.1 Demineralization

To preserve the antigenicity of proteins and the integrity of RNA, bone should be demineralized slowly in suspension in 4% ethylenediaminetetraacetic acid (EDTA) over a period of a few weeks at 4°C. A simple, but time-consuming mechanism is to wrap individual specimens in a fine cheesecloth pouch with a dental-floss closure that is used to suspend the pouches in a 10× volume/specimen of EDTA that is slowly agitated on a stirring plate. The frequency of changes and length of time in the EDTA will depend on the number and size of specimens as well as the age and species of the donor. For example, adult mouse long bones take up to 4 weeks for complete demineralization whereas a 1 cm core from an equine carpal bone takes up to 12 weeks before it yields to a needle-prick test for malleability. A variety of rapid demineralization protocols that use up to 20% EDTA with microwave treatment or 8% hydrochloric/formic acid have been developed for specific applications including clinical diagnostics using in situ hybridization and immunochemical analyses. While the rapid demineralization protocols are more convenient and less tedious they tend to compromise certain histochemical stains and also result in some loss of resolution in cellular structure. To maintain the full range of options for high-resolution histochemical, in situ hybridization and apoptosis labeling, and immunochemical staining that are needed to characterize a skeletal phenotype both plastic and paraffin embedding should be performed. Once the specimens are adequately demineralized, they can be embedded in paraffin using automated equipment in any high-quality fee-for-service facility located in most academic departments and centers.

2.4.2 Immunohistochemistry

The focus of a tertiary immunochemical screen for anabolic or catabolic markers will depend largely on the outcome of the initial histological screen on undecalcified specimens. For example, an apparent decrease in ALP staining along trabecular bone surfaces in association with a decrease in mineralized tissue and no change in TRAP staining suggests a primary defect in osteogenic cells. On the other hand, a similar osteopenic phenotype in association with no apparent change in ALP but increased TRAP staining warrants further examination of osteoclasts and their precursors. Of course these clear-cut discrepancies are the exception rather than the rule and an extensive analysis involving several markers is usually required. The antibodies used in an immunochemical screen of histological sections of bone should be selected carefully on the basis of the role of target antigens and the protocols should contain adequate controls, such as pre-adsorbed antisera, to avoid false-positive results. With the current widespread access to commercial facilities for the rapid and cost-effective production of high-quality antisera to novel proteins, the use of in situ hybridization is often restricted to cases where the protein is extremely low in abundance due to low production levels or rapid turnover.

2.4.3 Bone Cell Culture Ex Vivo

The second arm of a tertiary bone screen involves *ex vivo* investigation of the cells that manufacture and maintain *in vivo* mineralized tissue in order to identify potential alterations in their growth, differentiation, and activity. These assays can be performed in any wet lab with tissue culture facilities and molecular biology expertise. However, the knowledge required for the isolation of primary cells from whole bone or bone marrow is best learned from a lab that specializes in these techniques. There are a few labs that are focused primarily on the isolation, *ex vivo* differentiation, and activity of osteoclasts and their precursors. If the primary bone phenotype is one of osteopetrosis rather than osteoporosis, then a lab specializing in the isolation and functional characterization of osteoclasts should be consulted. Given the current interest in regenerative and reconstructive medicine (see below) there are a growing number of labs in the engineering, health sciences, and the private sectors that are developing techniques for the isolation and *ex vivo* expansion of cells of the osteogenic lineage. Although there is no consensus on the best source of cells to study the process of bone formation *ex vivo*, one promising approach appears to be the use of bone marrow stromal cells (MSCs).[42] MSCs are accessible in relatively large numbers from the long bones of mice and rats, have some capacity for self-renewal, and can be induced to differentiate down the osteogenic lineage. Their capacity for self-renewal renders them conducive to gene transfer *ex vivo*, for the purpose of controlled release of critical factors necessary to induce or maintain the differentiated phenotype when transplanted *in vivo* (www.cshprotocols.org August 2009). An alternative approach has been to use mature cells although this is frequently hampered by their limited proliferative capacity and the tendency to dedifferentiate in culture.[43]

Protocols for the harvest, culture, and *ex vivo* phenotypic analysis of cells of the osteogenic lineage were established in the 1960s, well in advance of the 1980s explosion in transgenic science. The ability to make direct comparisons between primary osteogenic cells harvested from wild-type mice and their genetically modified litter-mates has been largely responsible for the shift away from the use of immortalized and transformed cell lines such as MC3T3 and UMR. A comprehensive discussion of the characteristics of multi-potent bone marrow–derived MSCs and their stepwise transition to fully functional osteoblasts can be found in Aubin et al.[44] Two-dimensional cultures and the "bone nodule" assay have been used extensively to explore the molecular mechanisms that give rise to a particular *in vivo* bone phenotype. The skeletally mature FGFR3-deficient mouse is a good example, where the *in vivo* phenotype is primarily one of osteomalacia and osteopenia.[15] The absence of any obvious alterations in circulating levels of PTH or VitD suggested a problem in the bone micro-environment, most probably at the level of the osteoblast. Whole bone marrow harvested from the femora and tibia was filtered to remove debris and obtain a single cell solution that was plated on tissue culture plastic to select for adherent MSCs, which were plated at high density to perform a classic "bone nodule" assay. The commitment of MSCs to mature bone-forming osteoblasts is monitored *ex vivo* using similar techniques as those for *in vivo* histological analyses including ALP staining as an early marker of osteoblast differentiation and von Kossa stain to identify the mineralized matrix. In the absence of FGFR3 the population of MSCs grew faster, as demonstrated by MTT assay and ALP staining, but failed to form as many mineralized nodules as the wild-type cells. This *ex vivo* assay effectively demonstrated that there was a fundamental flaw in the capacity of isolated FGFR3-deficient osteoblasts to deposit mineral in the matrix they produced, which correlated with the *in vivo* observations of osteomalacia and osteopenia. Subsequent experiments would typically involve comparative microarray to identify differentially expressed genes and the use of analytical software such as Ingenuity Pathways® to identify biologically relevant gene networks. A more detailed description of the use of 3D culture of MSCs for *ex vivo* studies of bone formation follows under the heading of bone regeneration and repair.

2.5 Phenotyping Skeletal Regeneration and Repair

In developed countries, the average age of the population will continue to rise over the next two decades as the "baby boomers" currently in their fifth to seventh decades continue to age and their average life expectancy continues to increase with technological advancements in the health-care industry.[45] Bone mass normally declines in the fourth decade, thus placing individuals at increased risk to sustain a fracture, but they also become susceptible to failed union of those fractures as a consequence of an age-related decline in the capacity of tissue to repair itself.[46,47] The reader is referred to Chap. 11 of this book for a detailed discussion of the mechanisms that have been proposed to account for age-related changes in bone regeneration which include a decrease in the availability of progenitor cells and in their ability to differentiate into bone-forming osteoblasts. As a consequence, the surgical reconstruction of fractures with hardware and the fixation of implants used in joint replacement are severely compromised in elderly patients. The result is an increase in patient morbidity and mortality, an escalation of the economic, personal, and social burdens associated with prolonged hospitalization and assisted homecare, as well as reduced mobility and access to public spaces by our increasingly aged population.[48] These alarming facts emphasize the need to expedite research into regenerative medicine for the skeleton, to improve the quality of life of the aging population, and to decrease the economic burden associated with skeletal disease.

2.6 Bone Reconstruction in Clinical Practice

Therapeutic options for bone reconstruction are currently limited to rudimentary bone-grafting techniques with autogenous or allograft bone and single-dose intra-operative protein-based therapies.[49] Autogenous bone harvest from a remote site at the time of surgery that contains functional cells and matrix is preferred for grafting due to its superior osteo-inductive capability. Major drawbacks to this approach are the limited tissue supply and the high incidence of morbidity associated with bone harvest. An alternative approach is to use sterilized, devitalized allograft bone harvested from cadaveric sources Allograft bone is more readily available but it has poor osteo-inductive capability, which leads to graft failure. Augmentation of allograft bone with vascularized fibular grafts[50] and adjuvant bone morphogenetic proteins (BMPs), to stimulate the recruitment and differentiation of endogenous osteogenic cells, have met with limited success in promoting integration of the graft with host bone.[49] Although these approaches can work well in some younger individuals, they are certainly not suitable for older patients who have structurally weak bones and a limited availability of endogenous MSCs and biologic factors for tissue repair.[51] A promising approach for the "assisted" repair of bones under these and other poor healing conditions is transplantation of scaffolds pre-seeded with bone-forming cells and carrying bone anabolic agents, all of which require *in vivo* validation in an appropriate animal model.[52,53]

2.7 Preclinical Animal Models

One approach that is gaining momentum is to use genetically defined mice, previously characterized with age-related bone phenotypes, to examine the efficacy of tissue-engineering strategies to induce regeneration and repair of surgically induced defects. However, mice are often too small to perform the surgical procedures such as an osteotomy with rigid fixation with any degree of consistency even when the hardware is custom-made. Rats are more than ten times the size of mice and can therefore be used for these complex orthopedic interventions to model fracture nonunion using instruments and hardware similar to that used for clinical applications. Like inbred mice, inbred rats offer the combined advantages of low cost, ease of access, extensive characterization, and genetic uniformity. Recent advances in rat genetics and genomics, together with a vast literature accumulated over a century on the physiology and pharmacology of the laboratory rat, predict that these animals will be used with increasing frequency for *in vivo* proof-of-concept studies.[54] In this context, the FDA guidelines recommend the use of the ovariectomized (OVX) rat model for the evaluation of new therapeutic agents for postmenopausal osteoporosis.[55] Surgically induced defects in the long bones of rats are gaining wide popularity to model bone healing under a variety of circumstances.[56-58]

2.8 Bone Tissue Engineering

2.8.1 Smart Scaffolds

Native bone is a nanocomposite material with a 3D hierarchical structure. It is composed of a largely inorganic phase dispersed in an oriented collagen matrix. Bone serves not only as a functional skeletal unit but also as an innate bio-incubator for cells that produce both matrix proteins and soluble factors required for renewal and repair of the scaffold.[34] The organic and inorganic components of bone exhibit nano- and microscale features believed to be important for the healing cascade.[59] It is thought that these features should be incorporated into implantable materials in order to control biological activity at the implant–bone interface. Controlling the interface, as well as the composition of the core scaffold structure itself, will result in improved mechanical strength and enhanced osteogenic function of the cellular component.[60] Advances in materials fabrication processes have enabled the manufacture of synthetic scaffolds that resemble bone in their structural hierarchy of nano- and microscale features. Synthetic bone analogues with useful mechanical properties and reproducible micro- and nanosized features are relatively easy to fabricate from calcium phosphate and porous coralline ceramics for use in orthopedic applications. They can be used to deliver exogenous MSCs to the site of bone injury and their surfaces can be further functionalized with proteins that are conducive to the replication and differentiation of these cells into bone-forming osteoblasts. These microporous scaffolds made from biologic substrates, as well as those derived synthetically from degradable polymers or glass (Bioglass®), are easy to fabricate with reproducible structure and mechanical properties[52] and have been approved for clinical use. However, their early promise for clinical applications has been limited by their resistance to degradation and replacement over time with mechanically and biologically functional, mineralized tissue, which is the primary objective of bone tissue engineering. In an attempt to overcome this shortcoming, porous ceramics loaded with bioactive agents for subsequent controlled release *in vivo* have been developed to allow for controlled resorption and replacement by native bone.[61] These bone substitutes have significant advantages over bio-inert allografts, which include the capacity for neo-vascularization and an extended surface area arising from their nanocrystallinity that is available for modification. Incorporation of microsensors into the 3D macroporous scaffolds would enable real-time monitoring of biological information such as pH, protein binding, oxygen, and growth factor availability.[62] All of these factors will impact on the differentiation of precursor cells into osteoblasts and their subsequent capacity to manufacture new bone matrix. "Sense and Response Systems" can be programmed to record this biological information from the micro-environment and respond with the automated delivery of drugs and therapeutic agents to expedite bone healing.

Native collagen gels represent an alternative, biologically relevant scaffold that can be reconstituted *ex vivo* to encase viable cells for subsequent implantation in a bone defect. Dilute solutions of type-I collagen produce gels within minutes by the process of "fibrillogenesis" to form 3D lattices of collagen fibrils that self-assemble into a mesh that entraps cells and a large volume of fluid (>99%). To overcome the mechanical weakness of the hydrated gel, a novel process was developed that exploits the inherent property of collagen to release fluid when subjected to unconfined compression.[63] The end result of this compression yields a 3D tissue-like construct with useful mechanical properties and viable osteogenic cells[64] that can be implanted *in vivo*.[65] This scaffold has the obvious advantages of ultrarapid engineering compared with conventional cell-seeded collagen gels and, unlike synthetic polymers, will be resorbed and replaced with native bone.[66] Their ultimate success will be dependent on their physical properties, on "contingency" factors required to drive osteogenesis, and on robust phenotyping protocols, such as those described above, to evaluate their functional impact on bone formation *in vivo*.

2.8.2 Surgical Models to Study Bone Healing

A variety of surgical modifications of the bones of mice, rats, and rabbits have been developed in the laboratory to model fracture repair relying on the generation of a critical-sized defect, fixed internally or externally, which will not heal in the absence of adjunct therapy.[67-69] This critical-sized osteotomy to model fracture nonunion is technically challenging in the rat. A 15 mm lateral incision is made and the subcutaneous tissue carefully separated to expose the femur from the lateral femoral condyle proximally to the third trochanter. A custom polyethylene plate manufactured at the McGill Institute for Advanced Materials is aligned to span the mid-femoral diaphysis and attached to the bone using four 1.2 mm threaded Kirshner wires. A segment of bone measuring 1–5 mm, depending on the application, is then removed using an oscillating saw. Although attempts have been made to generate this nonunion with stable fixation model in mice, it is difficult to generate consistently and reproducibly. For this reason smaller drill-hole and window defects, which will eventually heal spontaneously over time, have been developed to study both trabecular and cortical bone regeneration.[70,71] A small incision is made in the skin on the anterior aspect of the femur at the mid-diaphysis and the muscles splayed to expose the bone surface. One or two (window) overlapping full-thickness defects per femur are drilled through the cortex into the bone marrow cavity using a 1 mm dental burr with continuous saline irrigation to prevent thermal necrosis of the bone margins, and a jig to ensure a consistent depth. Depending on the objective of the experiment to study early or late events in bone healing the animals are maintained for up to 4 weeks post operation. Another model that is reasonably simple to generate in mouse femurs to investigate implant fixation under adverse conditions such as osteopenia is a modification of a classic technique used originally in 30 kg dogs. A 3 mm incision is made from the dorsal aspect where the femoral head joins the pelvic bone. The muscle insertion on the greater trochanter is then dissected free and the hip adducted to expose the piriformis fossa. A 25 gauge needle is inserted into the femoral canal immediately medial to the greater trochanter. Therapeutic agents are then injected into the femoral canal prior to insertion of a biocompatible orthopedic device. This model has been modified as illustrated in Fig. 2.3 to examine the potential of MSC transplantation for assisted bone repair in patients with poor-quality bone.

2.8.3 Phenotyping Bone Regeneration and Repair

The terminal procedures and quantitative analyses of bone regeneration and repair are essentially the same as

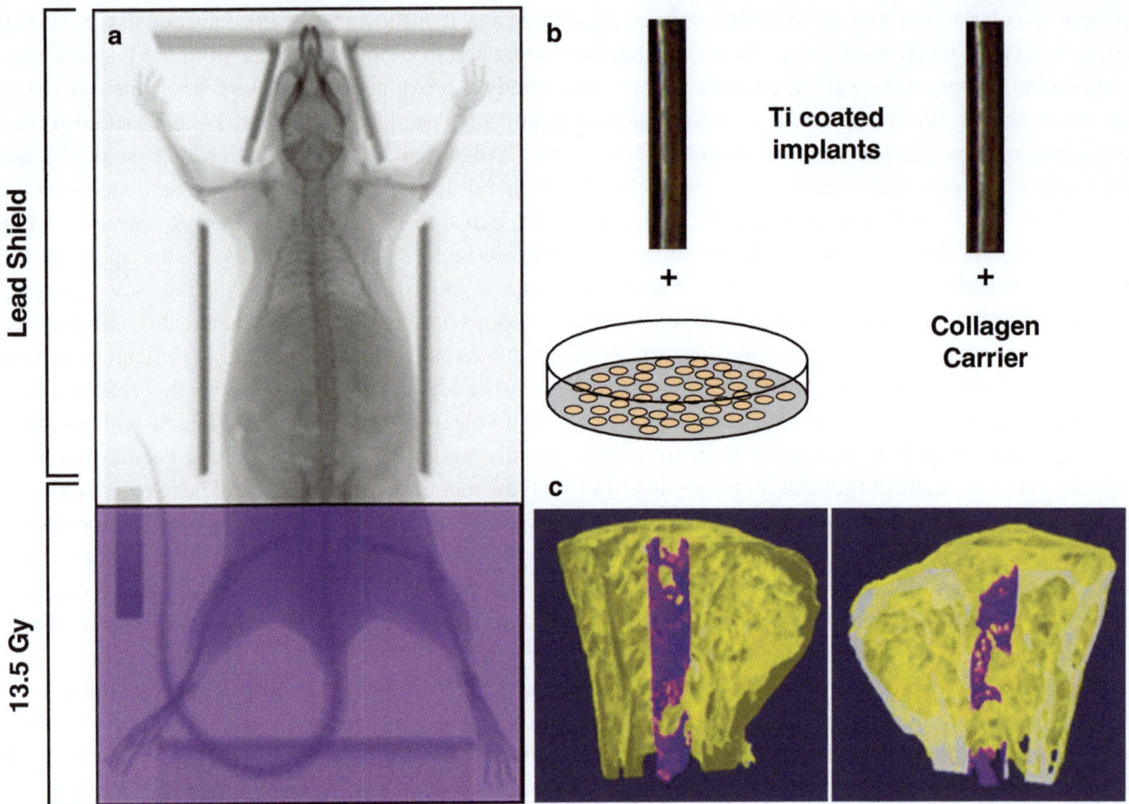

Fig. 2.3 Adult mouse sublethal irradiation and stem cell transplantation. Mice that have been characterized with defects in bone development or metabolism can be surgically modified to examine a variety of therapeutic interventions to promote bone regeneration. In this example, an osteopenic mouse was given a sublethal 13.5 Gy dose of irradiation to the lower limbs to kill endogenous bone marrow cells while a lead shield spared the depots in the upper body for hematopoiesis (**a**). MSCs from a young healthy donor were transplanted into the right femur with a Ti-coated implant but only the implant with a collagen carrier was inserted into the left femur (**b**). The femurs were harvested after 6 weeks and the bones subjected to μCT analysis, which showed that MSC transplantation stimulated significantly more new bone formation around the implant than was seen in the femur that received collagen alone (**c**)

those outlined above for the primary and secondary screens, with minor modifications. The animals are anesthetized with isoflurane, exsanguinated by cardiac puncture, and the serum separated and stored at −80°C for the biomarker assays. In contrast to a comprehensive screen where the entire axial and appendicular skeleton is harvested, only the surgically modified bones are removed for analysis in bone regeneration experiments. An x-ray instrument inside the pathogen-free zone is highly recommended in order to monitor the repair process over time, which can extend over 12 weeks for the rat critical-sized defects. Selection of the area of interest for μCT analyses is difficult in the drill-hole and window defects due to their irregularity and slight inter-animal variation in shape. BMD around implants and in cortical defects can be assessed by comparing the μCT scans with those of standard hydroxyapatite "phantoms" of known density. The quantitative microstructural data obtained from μCT can be correlated with FT-IR analysis of its elemental composition and the ratio of matrix to mineral, and with the mechanical properties evaluated by micro-indentation.

The histological analysis of bone regeneration is frequently complicated by the difference in composition between the trabecular bone surrounding intrafemoral implants and the implant itself, or between bone in a window defect and the surrounding femoral diaphysis. These specimens should be embedded in a more rigid resin such as LR White, Spurr, or Epon in order to minimize tissue damage at the implant–bone interface or between dense cortical and fine trabecular bone. The downside to these procedures, which are normally reserved for electron microscopy applications, is that the stringent processing and curing often destroy enzyme activity and the resin must be removed from the sections before performing immunohistochemistry. Calcein labeling in the region of bone repair is evaluated on unstained sections and bone, osteoid, and fibrous tissue on von Kossa/toluidine blue–stained sections. Residual cartilage in bone undergoing endochondral ossification is identified by Safranin O/fast green staining. Bone-forming surfaces are identified by ALP activity and type-I collagen immunoreactivity in osteoblasts, while active areas of resorption are identified by TRAP activity in osteoclasts. It is also important to determine the relative rates of cell proliferation, using BrdU or proliferating cell nuclear antigen (PCNA) immunohistochemistry, and apoptotic cell death using ApopTag or an equivalent assay. These assays are particularly relevant when using animal models in which heritable defects are linked to excessive or insufficient apoptosis in endochondral bone development.

2.8.4 Ex Vivo Culture of MSCs in Scaffolds

For tissue-engineering applications, MSCs are most commonly grown in 3D culture on biocompatible, biodegradable scaffolds that mimic the composition and architecture of bone tissue to more closely simulate the *in vivo* environment. However, adherent cells can also be cultured under conditions that simulate the micro-mechanical forces and fluid flow dynamics of the *in vivo* environment.[72] Thus, critical factors that will influence the replication and differentiation of the cells, such as load duration, magnitude, and cycle, as well as the fluid flow rate and fluid composition, can be precisely controlled. Much of the work aimed at developing effective scaffolds to promote bone formation *in vivo* has been driven by *ex vivo* studies that examine the response of isolated anabolic and catabolic cells to different chemical formulations.[61,73-75] In addition to their chemical composition, an extensive literature documents the critical importance of surface topography in guiding the attachment, movement, and differentiation of osteogenic cells to scaffold materials during bone formation. It has been demonstrated that surface morphology is more important than surface chemistry in promoting bone formation *in vivo*[76,77] and inducing MSC differentiation *in vitro*.[78] In fact, it could be argued that the culture of stem cells can theoretically be optimized simply through modification of the nano- and micro-topography of the surface on which they are grown. These studies have been facilitated by the development of nondestructive assays such as AlamarBlue® to monitor the metabolic activity of cells growing in 3D scaffolds in the presence or absence of soluble factors over extended periods of time. At the termination of the experiment, the cell-seeded scaffolds are fixed in 4% paraformaldehyde and subjected to similar phenotyping protocols as have been described for native bone in the preceding sections. The process starts with μCT quantification of mineral content followed by histological and ultrastructural assessment of the cells and matrix. The composite material generated by the *in vitro* culture system can also be subjected to FT-IR combined with x-ray diffraction to provide critical chemical and structural information on the calcium phosphate mineral deposited by the cells in the scaffold. Nano-indentation with the Mach-1 micro-mechanical tester can be used to measure the properties of the cell-seeded dense collagen scaffolds in much the same way as shown previously for articular cartilage. These data complement ultrastructural, chemical, and gene expression studies as they are performed in tissue samples.

2.9 Summary

Most academic institutions with extensive translational research programs that rely on the use of animal models of human disease have developed comprehensive services for biochemical analysis of body fluids, live animal imaging, soft tissue harvest, and processing and microscopic analysis. In parallel with the growth in transgenic science over the past two decades there has been a parallel increase in core facilities with the instrumentation and technical support for mineralized tissue analyses. These cores have enabled researchers with expertise in bone development and metabolism and an interest in bone phenotyping to develop customized protocols for the research community at large. The preceding paragraphs have described in detail a comprehensive phenotyping platform that was developed from experience accumulated over a decade characterizing the skeletons of mice with targeted gene mutations and those generated through mutagenesis screens. The knowledge gained from this skeletal phenotyping platform is now being applied to address the changing needs of the research community for assessment of bone regeneration, fracture repair, and implant fixation.

Acknowledgments This work was supported in part by grants from the Canadian Institutes of Health Research, Genome Québec, the Fonds de la recherche en sante Quebec sponsored Réseau de recherché en transgenèse du Québec, and the Réseau de recherche en santé buccodentaire et osseuse. Dr. C. Gao is a scholar of the MENTOR Strategic Training in Health Research program. The authors thank Ailian Li, Wei Li, and Huifen Wang for their invaluable assistance with the mouse phenotyping work and Dr. J. Seuntjens of the Medical Physics Unit, McGill University, for collaboration with the mouse irradiation studies.

References

1. Jaenisch R. Mammalian neural crest cells participate in normal embryonic development on microinjection into post-implantation mouse embryos. *Nature.* 1985;318:181-183.
2. Thomas K, Capecchi M. Site-directed mutagenesis by gene targeting in mouse embryo-derived stem cells. *Cell.* 1987; 51:503-512.
3. Fortin A, Diez E, Henderson J, Mogil J, Gros P, Skamene E. The AcB/BcA recombinant congenic strains of mice: strategies for phenotype dissection, mapping and cloning of quantitative trait genes. *Novartis Found Symp.* 2007;281: 141-153.
4. Rivadeneira F, Consortium GFfO. Twenty bone mineral-density loci identified by large-scal meta-analysis of genome-wide association studies. *Nat Genet.* 2009;41:1199-1206.
5. Miller P, Zapalowski C. Bone mineral density measurements. In: Goltzman D, ed. *The Osteoporosis Primer.* Cambridge: Cambridge University Press; 2000:262-276.
6. Klein R, Mitchell S, Phillips T, Belknap J, Orwoll E. Quantitative trait loci affecting peak bone mineral density in mice. *J Bone Miner Res.* 1998;13:1648-1656.
7. Lim L, Hoeksema L, Sherin K, Committee APP. Screening for osteoporosis in the adult US population: ACPM position statement on preventative practice. *Am J Prev Med.* 2009;36: 366-375.
8. Griffith J, Genant H. Bone mass and architecture determination: state of the art. *Best Pract Res Clin Endocrinol Metab.* 2008;22:737-764.
9. Richards J, Kavvoura F, Rivadeneira F, GFfO Consortium. Collaborative meta-analysis: association of 150 candidate genes with osteoporosis and osteoporotic fractures. *Ann Int Med.* 2009;151:528-537.
10. Karsenty G. Transcriptional control of skeletogenesis. *Annu Rev Genomics Hum Genet.* 2008;9:183-196.
11. Flenniken AM, Osborne L, Anderson N, Disease CfMH. A Gja1 missense mutation in a mouse model of oculodentodigital dysplasia (ODDD). *Development.* 2005;132:4375-4386.
12. Ochotny N, Flenniken A, Owen C, et al. A point mutation in the V-ATPase subunit a3, R740S, uncouples ATP hydrolysis from proton transport and results in a dominant osteopetrosis phenotype. *J Bone Miner Res.* 2011 in press Feb 8. doi: 10.1002/.
13. Amizuka N, Davidson D, Liu H, et al. Signaling by fibroblast growth factor receptor 3 (FGFR3) and parathyroid hormone related protein (PTHrP) coordinate cartilage and bone development. *Bone.* 2003;34:13-25.
14. Miao D, Liu H, Plut P, et al. Impaired endochondral bone development and osteopenia in Gli2 deficient mice. *Exp Cell Res.* 2003;294:210-222.
15. Valverde-Franco G, Liu H, Davidson D, et al. Defective bone mineralization and osteopenia in young adult FGFR3-/- mice. *Hum Mol Genet.* 2004;13:271-284.
16. Richard S, Valverde-Franco G, Tremblay GA, et al. Ablation of the Sam68 RNA-binding protein protects mice from age-related bone loss. *PLoS Genet.* 2005;1:e74-e84.
17. Valverde-Franco G, Binette JS, Li W, et al. Defects in articular cartilage and early arthritis in fibroblast growth factor receptor 3 deficient mice. *Hum Mol Genet.* 2006;15:1783-1792.
18. Deckelbaum RA, Majithia A, Booker T, Henderson JE, Loomis CA. The homeoprotein Engrailed-1 has pleiotropic functions in calvarial intramembranous bone formation and remodeling. *Development.* 2006;133:63-74.
19. Lengner CJ, Steinman HA, Gagnon J, et al. Osteoblast differentiation and skeletal development are regulated by Mdm2-p53 signaling. *J Cell Biol.* 2006;172:909-921.
20. Haston CK, Li W, Li A, Lafleur M, Henderson JE. Persistent osteopenia in adult Cftr-deficient mice. *Am J Respir Crit Care Med.* 2008;177:309-315.
21. Rivas D, Li W, Akter R, Henderson J, Duque G. Accelerated features of age-related bone loss in Zmpste24 metalloproteinase-deficient mice. *J Gerontol.* 2009;10:1015-1024.
22. Marquis J, Gros P. Genetic analysis of resistance to infections in mice: A/J meets C57BL6/J. *Curr Top Microbiol Immunol.* 2008;321:27-57.
23. Beamer W, Donahue L, Rosen C, Baylink D. Genetic variability in adult bone density among inbred strains of mice. *Bone.* 1996;18:397-403.
24. Turner C, Hsieh Y, Muller R, et al. Genetic regulation of cortical and trabecular bone strength and microstructure in inbred strains of mice. *J Bone Miner Res.* 2000;15:1126-1131.
25. Turner C, Hsieh Y, Muller R, et al. Variation in bone biomechanical properties, microstructure, and density in BXH recombinant inbred mice. *J Bone Miner Res.* 2001;16:206-213.
26. Rosen CJ, Dimal HP, Veraeault D, et al. Circulating and skeletal insulin like growth factor 1 (IGF-1) concentrations in two inbred strains of mice with different bone mineral densities. *Bone.* 1997;21:217-223.
27. Delahunty K, Shultz K, Gronowicz G, et al. Congenic mice provide *in vivo* evidence for a genetic locus that modulates serum insulin-like growth factor-1 and bone acquisition. *Endocrinology.* 2006;147:3915-3923.
28. D'Ascenzo M, Meacham C, Kirzman J, et al. Mutation discovery in the mouse using genetically guided array capture and resequencing. *Mamm Genome.* 2009;20:424-436.
29. Colvin JS, Bohne BA, Harding GW, McEwen DG, Ornitz DM. Skeletal overgrowth and deafness in mice lacking fibroblast growth factor receptor 3. *Nat Genet.* 1996;12:390-397.

30. Deng C, Wynshaw-Boris A, Zhou F, Kuo A, Leder P. Fibroblast growth factor receptor 3 is a negative regulator of bone growth. *Cell*. 1996;84:911-921.
31. Chappard D, Palle S, Alexandre C, Vico L, Riffat G. Bone embedding in pure methyl methacrylate at low temperature preserves enzyme activities. *Acta Histochem*. 1987;81:183-190.
32. Williams B, Insogna K. Where Wnts went: the exploding field of Lrp5 and Lrp6 signaling in bone. *J Bone Miner Res*. 2009;24:171-178.
33. Boyde A, Jones S. Scanning electron microscopy of bone: instrument, specimen ans issues. *Microsc Res Tech*. 1996; 33:92-120.
34. Marks S, Odgren P. Structure and development of the skeleton. In: Bilezekian J, Raisz L, Rodan G, eds. *Principles of Bone Biology*. San Diego: Academic; 2002:3-16.
35. Lvov B. Fifty years of atomic absorption spectrometry. *J Anal Chem*. 2005;60:382-392.
36. Boskey A, Camacho N. FT-IR imaging of native and tissue-engineered bone and cartilage. *Biomaterials*. 2006;28:2465-2478.
37. Gentleman E, Swain R, Evans N, et al. Comparative materials differences revealed in engineered bone as a function of cell-specific differentiation. *Nat Mater*. 2009;8:763-770.
38. Goodyear S, Gibson I, Skakle J, Wells R, Aspden R. A comparison of cortical and trabecular bone from C57 Black 6 mice using Raman spectroscopy. *Bone*. 2009;44:899-907.
39. Schulmerich M, Cole J, Kreider J, et al. Transcutaneous Raman spectroscopy of murine bone *in vivo*. *Appl Spectrosc*. 2009;63:286-295.
40. Mousny M, Banse X, Wise L, et al. The genetic influence on bone susceptibility to fluoride. *Bone*. 2006;39:1283-1289.
41. Yang R, Davies C, Archer C, Richards R. Immunohistochemistry of matrix markers in Technovit 9100 New-embedded undecalcified bone sections. *Eur Cell Mater*. 2003;6:57-71.
42. Tamer E, Reis R. Progenitor and stem cells for bone and cartilage regeneration. *J Tissue Eng Regen Med*. 2009;3: 327-337.
43. Hasegawa T, Oizumi K, Yoshiko Y, Tanne K, Maeda N, Aubin J. The PPARgamma-selective ligand BRL-49653 differentially regulates the fate choices of rat calvaria versus rat bone marrow stromal cell populations. *BMC Dev Biol*. 2008;8:1-12.
44. Aubin JE, Triffitt J. Mesenchymal stem cells and the osteoblast lineage. In: Bilezikian JP, Raisz LG, Rodan GA, eds. *Principles of Bone Biology*. 2nd ed. New York: Academic; 2002:59-81.
45. Johnell O, Kanis J. An estimate of the worldwide prevalence and disability associated with osteoporotic fractures. *Osteoporos Int*. 2006;17:1726-1733.
46. Shapiro F. Bone development and its relation to fracture repair. The role mesenchymal osteoblasts and surface osteoblasts. *Eur Cells Mater*. 2008;15:53-76.
47. Duque D. Bone and fat connection in aging bone. *Curr Opin Rheumatol*. 2008;20:429-434.
48. Pasco J, Sanders KM, Hoekstra FM, Henry MJ, Nicholson GC, Kotowicz MA. The human cost of fracture. *Osteoporos Int*. 2005;16:2046-2052.
49. Jones A, Bucholz R, Bosse M, et al. Recombinant BMP-2 and allograft compared with autogenous bone graft for reconstruction of diaphyseal tibial fractures with cortical defects. A randomized controlled trial. *J Bone Joint Surg Am*. 2006;88:1431-1441.
50. Friedrich J, Moran S, Bishop A, Wood C, Shin A. Free vascularized fubular graft salvage of complications of long-bone allograft after tumor reconstruction. *J Bone Joint Surg Am*. 2008;90:93-100.
51. Gruber R, Koch H, Doll B, Tegtmeier F, Einhorn T, Hollinger J. Fracture healing in the elderly patient. *Exp Gernotol*. 2006;41:1080-1093.
52. Khan Y, Yaszemski M, Mikos A, Laurencin C. Tissue engineering of bone: material and matrix considerations. *J Bone Joint Surg Am*. 2008;90:36-42.
53. Lee K, Chan C, Patil N, Goodman S. Cell therapy for bone regeneration: bench to bedside. *J Biomed Mater Res B Appl Biomater*. 2009;89:252-263.
54. Mashimo T, Serikawa T. Rat resources in biomedical research. *Curr Pharm Biotechnol*. 2009;10:214-220.
55. Whitfield J, Morley P, Willick G. Parathyroid hormone, its fragments and their analogs for the treatment of osteoporosis. *Treat Endocrinol*. 2002;1:175-190.
56. Herbenick M, Sprott D, Still H, Lawless M. Effects of a cyclooxygenase 2 inhibitor on fracture healing in a rat model. *Am J Orthop*. 2008;37:133-137.
57. Miettinen S, Jaatinen J, Pelttari A, et al. Effect of locally administered zoledronic acid on injury-induced intramembranous bone regeneration and osseointegration of a titanium implant in rats. *J Orthop Sci*. 2009;14:431-436.
58. Boerckel J, Dupont K, Kolambkar Y, Lin A, Guldberg R. *In vivo* model for evaluating the effects of mechanical stimulation on tissue-engineered bone repair. *J Biomech Eng*. 2009;131:084502:1-5.
59. Ma D, Guan J, Normandin F, et al. Multifunctional nanoarchitecture for biomedical applications. *Chem Mater*. 2006; 18:1920-1927.
60. Dalby M, Gadegaard N, Tare R, et al. The control of human mesenchymal cell differentiation using nanoscale symmetry and disorder. *Nat Mater*. 2007;6:997-1003.
61. Ibasco S, Tamimi F, Meszaros R, et al. Magnesium-sputtered titanium for the formation of bioactive coatings. *Acta Biomater*. 2009;5:2338-2347.
62. Harvey E, Henderson J, Vengallatore S. Nanotechnology and bone healing. *J Ortho Trauma*. 2010;24:S25-S30.
63. Brown R, Wiseman M, Chuo C, Cheema U, Nazhat S. Ultrarapid engineering of biomimetic materials and tissues: fabrication of nano- and microstructures by plastic compression. *Adv Funct Mater*. 2005;15:1762-1770.
64. Bitar M, Brown R, Salih V, Kidane A, Knowles J, Nazhat S. Effect of cell density on osteoblastic differentiation and matrix degradation of biomimetic dense collagen scaffolds. *Biomacromolecules*. 2008;9:129-135.
65. Mudera V, Morgan M, Cheema U, Nazhat S, Brown R. Ultra-rapid engineered collagen constructs tested in an *in vivo* nursery site. *J Tissue Eng Regen Med*. 2007;1: 192-198.
66. Buxton P, Bitar M, Gellynck K, et al. Dense collagen matrix accelerates osteogenic differentiation and rescues the apoptotic response to MMP inhibition. *Bone*. 2008;43:377-385.
67. Bonnarens F, Einhorn T. Production of a standard closed fracture in laboratory animal bone. *J Orthop Res*. 1984;2: 97-101.

68. Palomares K, Gleason R, Mason Z, et al. Mechanical stimulation alters tissue differentiation and molecular expression during bone healing. *J Orthop Res*. 2009;27:1123-1132.
69. Fu L, Tang T, Miao Y, Hao Y, Dai K. Effect of 1, 25-dihydroxy vitamin D3 on fracture healing and bone remodeling in ovariectomized rat femora. *Bone*. 2009;44:893-898.
70. Karp J, Sarraf F, Shoichet M, Davies J. Fibrin-filled scaffolds for bone-tissue engineering: an *in vivo* study. *J Biomed Mater Res A*. 2004;71:162-171.
71. Nagashima M, Sakai A, Uchida S, Tanaka S, Tanaka M, Nakamura T. Bisphosphonate (YM520) delays the repair of cortical bone defect after drill-hole injury by reducing terminal differentiation of osteoblasts in the mouse femur. *Bone*. 2005;36:502-511.
72. Majd H, Wipff P, Buscemi L, et al. A novel method of dynamic culture surface expansion improvesmesenchymal stem cell proliferation and phenotype. *Stem Cells*. 2009; 27:200-209.
73. Jabbarzadeh E, Starnes T, Khan Y, et al. Induction of angiogenesis in tissue-engineered scaffolds designed for bone repair: a combined gene therapy transplantation approach. *Proc Natl Acad Sci USA*. 2008;105:11099-11104.
74. Rosa A, de Oliveira P, Beloti M. Macroporous scaffolds associated with cells to construct a hybrid biomaterial for bone tissue engineering. *Expert Rev Med Devices*. 2008; 5:719-728.
75. LeNihouannen D, Komarova S, Gbureck U, Barralet J. Bioactivity of bone resorptive factor loaded on osteoconductive matrices: stability post-dehydration. *Eur J Pharm Biopharm*. 2008;70:813-818.
76. Hacking S, Zuraw M, Harvey E, Tanzer M, Krygier J, Bobyn J. A physical vapor deposition method for controlled evaluation of biological response to biomaterial chemistry and topography. *J Biomed Mater Res A*. 2007;82:179-187.
77. Hacking SA, Tanzer M, Harvey EJ, Krygier JJ, Bobyn JD. Relative contributions of chemistry and topography to the osseointegration of hydroxyapatite coatings. *Clin Orthop Relat Res*. 2002;405:24-38.
78. Hacking S, Harvey E, Roughly P, Tanzer M, Bobyn J. The response of mineralizing culture systems to microtextured and polished titanium surfaces. *J Orthop Res*. 2008;26: 1347-1354.

3 Methods in Bone Biology in Animals: Biomechanics

José B. Volpon and Antonio C. Shimano

3.1 Introduction

The locomotor system has important mechanical functions that are concerned with the production, conduction, and modification of forces. This intimate relationship is seen in the adaptive changes of bones, muscles, tendons, and joints to increased or decreased mechanical solicitations. In bones, the relationship between structure and function is known as Wolff's law, but the concept can be expanded to other components of the locomotor system.

Reduction of mechanical demands, such as those occurring during orthopedic immobilization, prolonged bed rest, or time spent in a microgravity environment (as experienced by astronauts), may affect all the components of the locomotor system, leading to joint stiffness, muscular wasting, and osteopenia.[1–4] Muscles become hypotrophic with interstitial proliferation of connective tissue, less resistant to fatigue,[5] and mechanically weakened.[6] The opposite effect is also true: increased mechanical demands cause reinforcement of the structures. The system seems to recognize the necessity to adapt its mass to maintain structural integrity and, as a consequence, hypotrophy or hypertrophy results with modification not only of the whole mass but also of the microstructure.[7]

The study of the mechanical behavior of the components of the locomotor system, in particular of bones, is thus an important tool to characterize the functional changes that occur at macroscopic and microscopic levels. Techniques of study, mainly those associated with histomorphometry, give information about the changes in the microstructure, but mechanical testing provides information about the functional impact of such changes. Consequently, both techniques are complementary.

3.2 Basic Concepts

The skeleton is a mechanical system continuously submitted to an association of forces that cause deformation of its parts. The direction and the amount of deformations depend on the direction and the magnitude of the applied forces, on the structural geometry of bone, on the geometry of the cross section, and on the properties of the osseous tissue. Forces acting on the locomotor system are usually complex but can be distinguished into four basic components: compression, traction, torsion, and bending. Compressive force causes a shortening of the length of the structure, while traction elongates it. Torsion causes a twisting of the structure around its long axis and bending causes it to bow at the center. When such forces are applied, they may generate three kinds of internal stresses: tension, compression, and shear. Stress is represented by the internal resistance that a material displays to being deformed, and it is defined as the force divided by the area over which it acts (stress = force/area; N/m^2). This is an important concept because it represents a way of normalizing data. For example, when comparing two different bodies submitted to the same force but one of them with a half cross-sectional area of the other, the stress will be twice as great in the smaller body. When the applied force is perpendicular to the surface,

J.B. Volpon (✉)
Department of Biomechanics, Medicine and Rehabilitation of the Locomotor System, University of São Paulo, Ribeirão Preto School of Medicine,
Avenida dos Bandeirantes, 3900, Ribeirão Preto, São Paulo, Brazil
e-mail: jbvolpon@fmrp.usp.br

G. Duque and K. Watanabe (eds.), *Osteoporosis Research*,
DOI: 10.1007/978-0-85729-293-3_3, © Springer-Verlag London Limited 2011

compression or traction occurs, but when the applied force is tangential to the surface, there is shearing generation. Strain is the measure of deformation and, during loading, can be obtained by the length of an object after force application divided by its original length.

3.3 Mechanical Properties of Bones

Mechanical properties of bones can be studied by the same methodology used in engineering, but some limitations and restrictions should be kept in mind in interpreting the results. The osseous tissue is anisotropic, that is, its mechanical properties depend on the direction and orientation of the force,[8] while the bone is a viscoelastic material, meaning that deformation is time-dependent, that is, the structure exhibits both viscous and elastic characteristics when undergoing deformation. A typical elastic behavior is represented by the deformation that occurs in a spring. When a compression force is applied, the spring immediately shortens in proportion to the force. The viscous behavior is exemplified by a fluid compressed in a syringe: the stronger the compression, the greater the fluid resistance. Therefore, bone deformation is not exclusively linear, but depends on the rate of force application.[8]

Moreover, the osseous tissue does not have a homogeneous structure, but exhibits microscopic inhomogeneities represented by a tunnel of vessels, osteocytic lacunae, porosity, different collagen fiber orientation, and internal cracks in different stages of healing. These irregularities act as local points of stress concentration and influence the bone deformation, fracture line, and breaking point.

The following concepts are important in understanding bone biomechanics.

(a) Mechanical resistance is the material capacity of resisting a certain demand (static or dynamic) without breaking. It measures the tension that the material supports.
(b) Elasticity is the capacity of the material to deform and recover its original shape, once the external force is released, that is, there is no permanent deformation.
(c) Plasticity is the capacity of the material to be permanently deformed without failure. Malleability is the material ability to deform under compression, for example, forming blades, and ductility is the mechanical property used to describe the extent to which materials can be deformed plastically in a direction without fracture (as occurs in wiring).
(d) Fragility is a property that is opposed to the ductility and indicates the material capacity's resistance to permanent deformation without failure and shows low permanent deformations before fracturing (as occurs in ceramic).
(e) Hardness is the capacity of one solid to penetrate or scratch another solid or to be penetrated or scratched.
(f) Stiffness is a measure of the resistance offered by an elastic body to deformation in the elastic phase (bending, stretching, torsion, or compression). It is defined by Young's modulus (E).
(g) Resistance to fatigue is the material capacity to support cyclic tensions without breaking.

3.4 Mechanical Testing

Mechanical testing is generally classified as destructive and nondestructive. In the former, there is permanent damage to the structure of the material (breaking, fissures, etc.) as seen in bending, torsion, fatigue, etc. Conversely, the nondestructive tests preserve the integrity of the material structure (ultrasound, magnetic resonance, etc.).

The mechanical tests are called *static* when force is applied slowly and gradually, with a short loading time so that the load speed is considered not to be important. Bending, compression, traction, torsion, and combined tests are some examples of static tests. On the other hand, a *dynamic test* occurs when the force is applied quickly (impact). Another modality is the *fatigue test* in which cyclic loads are a function of time. This kind of test is important when implants are investigated; however, they will not be addressed in this article. Static tests are used to study the mechanical properties in bone samples, whole bones, and experimental models. However, fractures occur at high speeds and are better studied dynamically.

Whole-bone tests express the behavior of the bone as an organ and are the result of a combination of bone dimensions, shape, and osseous material, and the tests give information about the structural properties.

Therefore, whole-bone tests are mostly used in long bones and vertebral body of small animals (mice, rats, rabbits). On the other hand, samples of bones provide information about the osseous material and results can be more precise as the sample can be machined, with dimensions chosen previously. Material properties describe the mechanical behavior of a given substance independent of its shape and dimension. However, some precautionary measures should be taken on harvesting the samples, that is, the location of the bone must be carefully chosen and standardized because of the inhomogeneities, viscoelasticity, variation of the internal architecture, and piezoelectricity of bone. In addition, the cranial and caudal extremities of the sample should be recorded and taken into consideration during positioning in the testing machine.

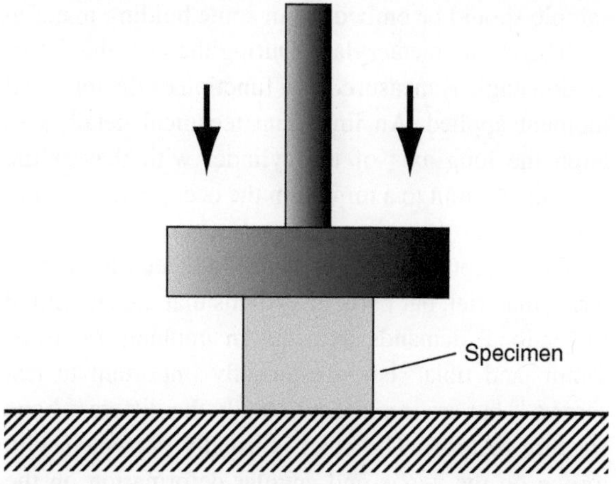

Fig. 3.1 Schematic representation of a compression test. The upper and lower surfaces of the specimen should be parallel and an axial force is vertically and homogeneously applied on the surface

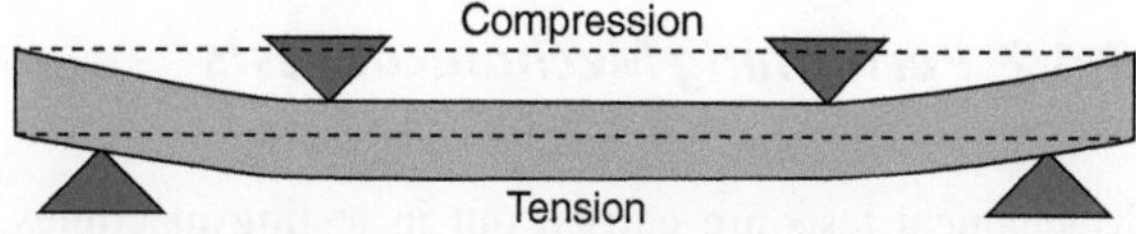

Fig. 3.2 In the four-bending test, the extremities of the sample lie on two metallic supports and a vertical force is applied in two points of its center, causing a bending with a compression stress (concave) and tension stress (convex) surfaces

3.4.1 Main Mechanical Tests

3.4.1.1 Compression Test

The compression testing consists of applying compression force on a specimen or a sample previously standardized. In general, this test is more frequently used to study fragile materials and the following suggestions are recommended:

(a) The axial force should be applied vertical to the object surface to avoid occurrence of other kinds of force. To achieve this, both surfaces of the extremities should be parallel and the force applied should be vertically and homogeneously distributed over the surface (Fig. 3.1).
(b) The specimen should have a cylindrical shape, with its length being up to twice its width. When the specimen is too long, bending stress may appear with a tendency to flex the sample. For ductile materials, the relationship of length × diameter should stay between 1:2 and 1:6.

3.4.1.2 Bending Test

The bending test is one of the commonest and simplest tests performed in bones. Basically, it consists of laying the extremities of the specimen on two metallic supports and applying a progressive vertical force in its center, so that the displacement can be recorded. This test is recommended when the main physiological forces supported by the specimen are in flexion. When force is applied, the bending of the sample gives rise to the formation of compression stress on the concave surface and traction stress on the convex surface (Fig. 3.2). Likewise, in the interface between the two opposite tensions, there is no stress (neutral line). Common bending tests are flexion at two points, three points, and four points. For biological purposes the three-point and four-point tests are more used. The difference between them is that in a four-point bending test the stresses are more evenly distributed in the specimen.

3.4.1.3 Torsion Test

Torsion test applies torsional force on cylindrical or almost cylindrical bodies. Usually, the ends of the sample should be embedded in some holding material such as methylmetacrylate. During the test, the deformation angle is measured as a function of the torsional moment applied. An important technical detail is to align the long axis of the cylinder with that of the machine to limit to a minimum the occurrence of other stresses.

The torsion test usually is not indicated to characterize material, but parts of systems that are submitted to torsional demands as occur in implants in spine, femur, and tibia,[9] being especially important to test screws,[10] but are important to study the different bone fracture patterns. The chart is usually presented with torque on the *y*-axis and angular deformation on the *x*-axis. The types of fractures that result from loading a cylindrical structure in torsion display either an oblique or a spiral configuration.

3.4.2 Performing Mechanical Tests

Mechanical tests are carried out in testing machines that apply controlled traction, compression, bending, or torsion forces to the construct and measure the displacement occurred. Figure 3.3 depicts the schematic drawing of a typical assembly to test a whole bone in bending. The basic parts of a testing machine are two vertical parallel supports that permit the sliding of a crosshead that moves upward or downward at a chosen speed, thereby applying force to the sample whose displacement (deformation) is recorded. Load is recorded by an interposed load cell. The specimen to be tested lies on metallic supports for bending, but for compression or torsion it can be embedded in acrylic cement and special accessories must be made to hold the testing body in case of traction. Usually, the test is carried out until failure occurs (fracture). As the test is being performed, software plots displacement versus force (load) in real time and, for most biological materials, a typical curve is obtained (Fig. 3.4), with a graphic line that presents five well-defined regions:

(a) An initial straight line known as *elastic deformation* because there is a linear correspondence between force and displacement, so that if the load is removed, the construct will return to its original shape. The slope of the curve in the elastic phase,

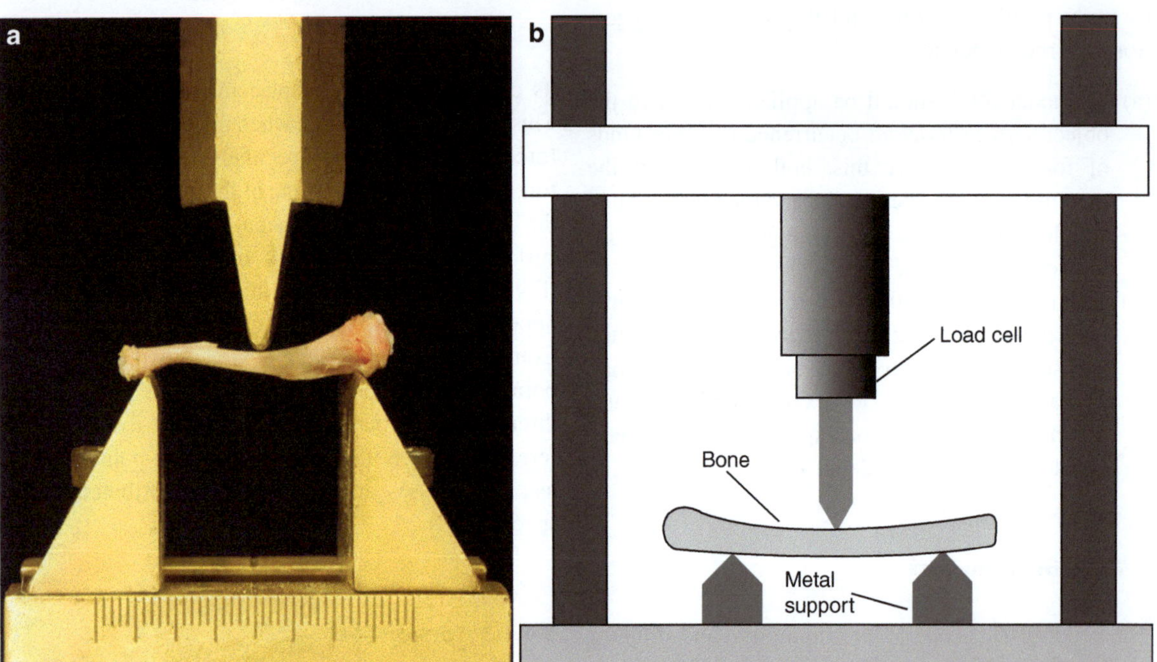

Fig. 3.3 Real testing (**a**) and the schematic drawing (**b**) of a typical assembly to submit a whole bone in three-bending test. The specimen lies on two metallic supports and a vertical force is driven onto its middle part as displacement is being recorded

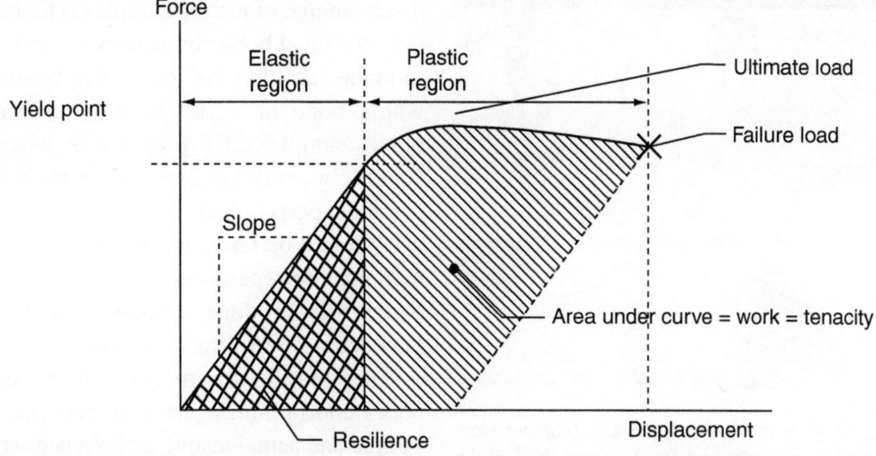

Fig. 3.4 Illustration of a theoretical curve generated during a mechanical test, correlating load versus displacement. The elastic deformation is characterized by a straight line showing a linear correspondence between force and displacement. The slope of this curve represents stiffness and the area under it represents resilience. As testing progresses, the material deformation changes to plastic and the shape of the curve changes. The total area under the curve until material failure represents tenacity (work)

which is the tangent of force and deformation at a given point, is called *stiffness*.

(b) Yield point, yield limit, or proportional limit is a turning point at which the plastic behavior changes to plastic. For some kinds of bones, the passage from elastic to plastic is not sharp, thus leading to difficulties in establishing the real limit between both curves. The factors that govern stiffness and yield point are the material and the shape of the construct. The yield point depicts the working or safe range.

(c) The plastic region is the next segment of the line and when it is reached, if the load is released, some permanent deformation in the construct will remain.

(d) Ultimate load is defined as the maximum load that a material can support before breaking.

(e) Failure load is the load that causes the failure of the material and it is represented by the end of the curve.

If, instead of force and displacement, a tension (force/area) versus displacement graph is built, it is possible to obtain the elastic (or Young's) modulus, which is determined by dividing the stress applied by the resulting strain (plastic slope). However, when whole bones are tested, it is not easy to obtain the cross-sectional area at the breaking point. This can be done noninvasively by previously computed tomography (CT) images, or after testing, by reducing and gluing the fragments together and performing cross cuts in the failure region. On the other hand, when samples are used, the tension can be easily calculated because the dimensions were previously established.

From the load versus deformation curve, it is still possible to define resilience, meaning the material capacity to absorb energy in the elastic phase of deformation that is represented by the area under the curve (linear phase to the yield point). In addition, the whole area under the curve (elastic plus plastic deformations) represents the work generated until failure.

3.5 Technical Notes on Mechanical Testing of Bones

3.5.1 Choice of the Test

As bones are usually subjected to a wide variety of forces, they should be resolved in basic components that express the main mechanical demands. Therefore, the most adequate mechanical testing should mimic the major mechanical solicitations that a particular bone is submitted to. Long bones are better tested in compression,

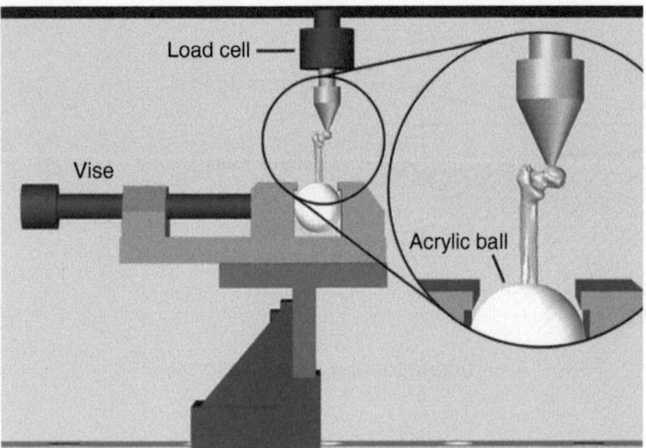

Fig. 3.5 Illustration of a combined force test (compression, bending, and shearing) performed on the proximal third of the rat femur to simulate the mechanical solicitations experienced by the region in the living animal. The distal end of the femur in embedded in an acrylic ball to facilitate the correct positioning of the bone in the vertical position. A vertical force is applied to the top of the femoral head (detail) generating a combination of mechanical solicitations

bending, and torsion, whereas vertebral bodies are tested in compression.

The proximal femur is best tested in flexion–compression–shearing, which can be obtained with the application of vertical force on the top of the femoral head. In this case, proper positioning of the bone in the vertical position can be facilitated with inclusion of its distal extremity in an acrylic bone sphere, thus allowing mobilization of the entire specimen until the adequate positioning is achieved. Forces applied to the top of the femoral head mimic the mechanical solicitation that takes place on the region and that may explain the femoral neck or trochanteric fracture that occurs in older people[3] (Fig. 3.5).

When fatigue is the main interest, for example, in cases of certain bone implants and joint prostheses, the cyclic test should be chosen. Mechanical tests can be performed even at submicroscopic level[11] and even in single osteons.[12]

3.5.2 Whole Bone Versus Bone Samples

As mentioned earlier, samples are chosen when the principal interest is to study the bone as a tissue. This kind of test has the advantage of being more standardized as its dimensions can be chosen beforehand, according to the study interest. The main disadvantage of testing samples is that they represent only the local bone characteristics and it is necessary to make sure that the results can be extensive to the whole bone or skeleton. Another limitation is to obtain samples of a proper size when the bone is small (e.g., vertebra of mice) or when it is necessary to collect parts of bone for other studies. Furthermore, care should be taken not to damage the sample with methods of preparation such as sawing and grinding, which may produce scratches, cracks, or holes that may act as concentration of stresses.

The study of the mechanical properties of intact bones can minimize the time between obtaining the sample and actual testing and obviates some questions that arise from the use of small samples, for example, if the properties are affected by removal from its original location and how representative the samples are in relation to the whole bone. However, the main advantage of testing the intact bone is to reproduce more real conditions as the whole bone test reflects not only characteristics of the osseous tissue, but also the size and shape influences. Nevertheless, a drawback with this kind of test is that bones can vary greatly in their dimensions with resultant changes in some physical constants (e.g., moment of inertia) with the result that it becomes difficult to reduce data to a standard basis for comparison of results.[13] Therefore, efforts should be made to minimize bone morphological variations with standardization of animal gender, age, and weight, in addition to the selection of bones with measurements of their length, weight, and shaft diameter within an interval of ±1.0 standard variation.

3.5.3 Bone Preservation Methods

After harvesting, the bone specimens should be cleaned of soft tissues taking care not to scratch the surface. During harvesting, temporary maintenance in saline is recommended.

In general, drying or any other chemical method used in the fixation of biological samples, such as alcohol and formaldehyde, alters mechanical parameters of the bone and should be proscribed. Bones should be packed separately and stored at −20°C until testing. A day before testing, it is recommended to transfer the specimens to an ordinary refrigerator and, on the day of testing, the bone should be kept in thermal equilibrium with the environment (20–22°C) and in saline or

Ringer lactate solution. During testing, the samples should be moistened with saline spray.[14]

3.5.4 Specimen Positioning

For compression, the specimen should be placed parallel to the force direction to avoid the influence of other kinds of stress that may arise after the formation of lever arm or twisting. To obtain control of positioning, one or two sample extremities can be embedded in acrylic cement. For three- or four-bending tests, the specimen ends are placed on two metal supports and force is applied to the middle part of the segment.

3.5.5 Load Cell

The choice of the load cell capacity is related to the maximum load that will be applied to the system. Usually, the load cell capacity should not be greater than 90% of the maximum load.

3.5.6 Load Speed

After assembling the bone in the testing machine, a preload can be applied for 10–30 s to allow accommodation of the system. Preloading should be 5% of the maximum force. The speed of load application should be chosen according to the material tested and the study interest. For bones, usually a speed of 1 mm/min is adequate for traction, compression, and bending. Usually, force is applied until sample failure, unless there is a specific interest in studying the deformation in the plastic phase, as occurs in the study of the hysteresis loops.

3.6 Final Remarks

Mechanical testing of bones is a useful methodology to characterize the functional status of bone as it provides objective data on the bone strength, characteristics of deformation, and may mimic bone failure and deformities observed in clinical practice. Furthermore, in experimental research, the method may produce fast and reliable information about therapeutic methods, as well as genetic and bone diseases.[15]

However, many important variables should be taken into account in relation to bone biomechanics such as the storage method, physical conditions, sample preparation, testing procedures, and individual variation. In addition, differences may exist among animal species and man and a careful selection of bones and test variables are needed to achieve reliable and accurate results.[15] When the whole bone is mechanically tested, rats and mice are the most used animals, and it should be borne in mind that they are quadrupeds and that the internal bone architecture corresponds to stress conditions that are different from those in man, mainly for the femur and spine. Another point is the choice of which bone of an animal species is more adequate for testing. This, of course, depends on the purpose of the investigation and how the bone fulfills the necessary conditions to be tested (size, shape, type of force, whole bone, machined specimens, etc.). In order to achieve all the necessary information, anatomical details obtained by more sophisticated methods such as microcomputerized tomography (μCT) may be necessary. Using this method, Schriefer et al. tested different long bones of mice and found that the radius demonstrated more consistent results.[16]

Finally, bones are complex geometric structures that are subjected to unknown multiple indeterminate loads, and samples should be loaded under well-defined conditions in the laboratory in such a manner as to produce uniform, known stresses throughout the specimen.[17]

References

1. Turner RT. Physiology of a microgravity environment. What do we know about the effects of spaceflight on bone? *J Appl Physiol*. 2000;89:840-848.
2. Bloomfield SA, Allen MR, Hogan HA, Delp MD. Site-and compartment-specific changes in bone with hindlimb unloading in mature adult rats. *Bone*. 2002;31:149-157.
3. Shimano MM, Volpon JB. Biomechanics and structural adaptations of the rat femur after hindlimb suspension and treadmill running. *Braz J Med Biol Res*. 2009;42:330-338.
4. Milani JGPO, Matheus JPC, Gomide LB, Volpon JB, Shimano AC. Biomechanical effects of immobilization and

rehabilitation on the skeletal muscle of trained and sedentary rats. *Ann Biomed Eng*. 2008;36:1641-1648.
5. Jarvinen M. Immobilization effect on the tensile properties of striated muscle: an experimental study in the rat. *Arch Phys Med Rehabil*. 1977;58:123-127.
6. Jarvinen MJ, Einola SA, Virtanen EO. Effect of the position of immobilization upon the tensile properties of the rat gastrocnêmios muscle. *Arch Phys Med Rehabil*. 1992;73: 253-257.
7. Ohira Y, Kawano F, Wang XD, et al. Irreversible morphological changes in leg bone following chronic gravitational unloading of growing rats. *Life Sci*. 2006;79:686-694.
8. Evans FG. *Mechanical Properties of Bone*. 1st ed. Springfield: Charles C Thomas; 1973.
9. Volpon JB, Batista LC, Shimano MM, Moro CA. Tension band wire fixation for valgus osteotomies of the proximal femur: a biomechanical study of three configurations of fixation. *Clin Biomech*. 2008;23(4):395-401.
10. Haje DP, Moro CA, Volpon JB. Bovine bone screws: metrology and effects of chemical processing and ethylene oxide sterilization on bone surface and mechanical properties. *J Biomater Appl*. 2008;23:453-471.
11. Vashishth D. Small animal bone biomechanics. *Bone*. 2008;43:794-797.
12. Ascenzi A, Bonucci E. The compressive force of single osteons. *Anat Rec*. 1968;161:377-392.
13. Sedlin ED. A rheologic model for cortical bone. *Acta Orthop Scand Suppl*. 1965;83:1-77.
14. Sedlin ED, Hirsch C. Factors affecting the determination of the physical properties of femoral cortical bone. *Acta Orthop Scand*. 1966;37(1):29-48.
15. Turner CH, Burr DB. Basic biomechanical measurements of bone: a tutorial. *Bone*. 1993;14:595-608.
16. Schriefer JL, Robling AG, Warden SJ, Fourier AJ, Mason JJ, Turner CH. A comparison of mechanical properties derived from multiple skeletal sites in mice. *J Biomech*. 2005;38: 467-475.
17. Hayes WC, Carter DR. Skeletal research. An experimental approach. In: Simmons DJ, Kunin AS, eds. *Biomechanics of Bone*. New York: Academic; 1979:263-300.

4 Methods in Bone Histomorphometry for Animal Models

Natalie Dion, Audray Fortin, and Louis-Georges Ste-Marie

4.1 Animal Models for Bone Research

Animal models are essential for preclinical skeletal research, notably in the study of physiopathology of metabolic bone diseases as well as in the evaluation of a test agent for the prevention and treatment of bone diseases such as osteoporosis. However, rat or mouse models do not completely reflect human bone disorders and therapeutic responses, but they provide insight into the understanding of bone pathologies and their treatments. The adult ovariectomized (OVX) rat is certainly the model mostly used as an archetype of human postmenopausal osteoporosis. Although the OVX rat model has no fragility fractures associated with osteopenia induced by estrogen deficiency, the translation of serum biochemistry, bone densitometry, and histomorphometry between preclinical and clinical findings has been validated and readily used.[1] In recent years, the development of genetically modified mouse models (GM mouse) has certainly enhanced the opportunity to produce new models for the study of physiopathology of bone diseases and for the evaluation of new therapeutic agents. The GM mouse is the gold standard model for the study of hereditary bone pathologies or for identifying important factors involved in bone turnover via gene knockout. However, the poor survival rate of GM mice limits the investigator to perform bone histology in embryonic or younger animals. This is a problem for gene impact studies in growing or mature bone.[1] In 1986, a mouse model identified as a strain of senescence-accelerated mouse (SAM) was described by Matsushita et al. The SAM-P/6 strain is a model of senile osteoporosis characterized by spontaneous leg fractures and a low peak bone mass resulting from a decrease in bone formation and an increase in bone resorption.[2]

4.2 Bone Histomorphometry

Bone histomorphometry is a valuable tool in the diagnosis of metabolic bone diseases, in preclinical and clinical research in the field of bone metabolism, and in the evaluation of the efficacy and safety of a pharmaceutical agent. It provides information that is not currently available from bone densitometry and biochemical markers of bone turnover. The histological examination of undecalcified bone specimens allows the evaluation of the "quality" of bone as well as its quantity, which both contribute to the biomechanical performance of the skeleton. Moreover, bone histomorphometry enables one to determine the kinetics of bone turnover and to quantify the changes in bone balance at the tissue and cellular levels.

4.3 Remodeling Versus Modeling

In adult man, most of bone turnover activity consists of remodeling. Bone remodeling is the process of turnover by which, in response to various stimuli, bone cellular activities follow a precise sequence in the same site. There is, first, osteoclastic resorption, which is followed

L.-G. Ste-Marie (✉)
Laboratory of Metabolic Bone Diseases,
CRCHUM – Hôpital Saint-Luc,
Montréal, Québec, Canada
e-mail: lg.ste-marie@umontreal.ca

G. Duque and K. Watanabe (eds.), *Osteoporosis Research*,
DOI: 10.1007/978-0-85729-293-3_4, © Springer-Verlag London Limited 2011

by osteoblastic formation. So the bone remodeling sequence is activation–resorption–formation in a specific site. Without changing bone shape, it allows the maintenance of bone strength and mineral homeostasis. In contrast, bone formation and bone resorption activities are not coupled to each other in the same site during bone modeling. So in modeling, the cycles of activity are activation–formation and activation–resorption, which can occur over long periods of time. This process occurs during growth and will induce bone shape changes in response to biomechanical stress or physiological influences.

In small animals, both bone modeling and remodeling occur but their ratio will differ according to skeletal site and age. In young growing animals, modeling is the prevailing activity in trabecular bone. With age, there is a slowing down of longitudinal growth and bone modeling will gradually yield its place to remodeling according to the bone site. For example, in rats, this transition will be observed in lumbar vertebrae from the age of 3 months, whereas in the proximal tibial metaphysis it will occur between 6 and 9 months of age.[3]

4.4 Bone Sites

Because bone modeling and remodeling are closely related to the bone site and the age of the animal, it is important to consider these two variables in the experimental design before carrying out studies in animals as models of metabolic bone disease in humans. Therefore, to investigate the effects of therapeutic interventions, the bone site and the age of the animal must be at a point where bone remodeling is the prevailing activity.[3–5] For example, in mature animals, specimens adequate for histomorphometric study of trabecular bone mass, structure, and turnover can be best obtained from the proximal tibial metaphysis in rat and the distal femoral metaphysis in mouse.[1]

It has been demonstrated that rodent cortical bone lacks true Haversian cortical bone remodeling. Moreover, the loss of cortical bone is very slow in osteoporotic rat models. This can be overcome by selecting diaphyseal tibia, which is known to be a site where cortical bone mass adaptation occurs in response to certain stimuli.[5]

Proximal tibia metaphysis, distal femur metaphysis, and lumbar vertebral body are the most common sites selected to perform histomorphometric analysis in small animal models. As suggested,[3] it is judicious to study more than one bone site in the same animal. For example, in addition to the tibia metaphysis, the vertebral body of L4 is frequently analyzed in an OVX rat model. Moreover, to accelerate cortical and trabecular bone loss, ovariectomy and immobilization could be combined in the same animal model.[5]

In addition to age and bone site, interspecies differences in bone histology are related to strain and gender of the animal. So when rodents are selected as a model for bone research, these parameters have to be carefully determined. Moreover, the age at which they attain their peak bone mass has to be considered. It takes 6–10 months for a female rat to reach its peak bone mass and to undergo trabecular bone remodeling whereas in a mouse, peak bone mass is attained at 4–6 months of age.[1,6] Compared to rats, the bone turnover rate is quite high in healthy mice and their small amount of trabecular bone contributes to the difficulty of studying bone modeling or remodeling in this model. It was demonstrated that trabecular bone loss and high bone turnover induced by OVX in the rat is a relatively good model of postmenopausal bone loss in women. However, it was shown that bone effects of OVX in the mouse are strain-dependent and vary according to skeletal site. Thus, these factors are important to consider in osteoporosis research using the mouse model.[7] On the other hand, in rat, the very low level of Haversian remodeling makes this model not the best one for the study of cortical bone behavior.[5]

4.5 Histological Processing

In order to process undecalcified bone, it is important to use a tissue fixative that will not decalcify the sample or alter fluorochrome labeling. In addition, it should allow the performance of a large selection of histochemical stainings. In bone histology, the most commonly used fixatives are formalin and ethanol.

Formalin is a non-precipitant fixative. It acts by binding the aminic groups of proteins, inducing a modification of the tertiary structure leading to the formation of a proteic network. By forming this network, the enzymatic activity of bone phosphatases (Fig. 4.4) revealed by histochemical reactions is drastically reduced. In order to break down this network, formalin-fixed tissues may by treated by heating or enzymatic digestion but this will not assure the complete activity recovery. Formalin diffuses rapidly in tissue but is light-sensitive and carcinogenic. After fixation, specimen fixed with formalin must be completely washed with buffered saline because the fixative could affect staining. However, because it does not dissolve lipids as ethanol would, it could be advantageous to use formalin fixation in the aim of performing immunohistochemistry for lipoprotein detection.

Ethanol is a precipitant fixative that acts by coagulation and precipitation of proteins. It dissolves lipids and has a weak penetrating strength. In addition, if specimens stay in ethanol for a long period of time, it can induce brittleness and hardness of the tissue and will tend to shrink the cells, altering their morphology. On the other hand, ethanol promotes methylmetacrylate infiltration and has a low toxicity potential. Because it does not alter enzymatic activities, ethanol is the selected fixative used for the detection of bone phosphatases.

Due to its enzymatic activity preservation, our laboratory uses ethanol fixative for bone histomorphometry. The regular procedure used in our laboratory is as follows: Bone specimens are fixed by immersion in 70% ethanol for at least 10 days. Then, they are dehydrated in gradual passages to 100% ethanol for an additional 2 days. Samples are infiltrated at 4°C with a mixture of 80% methylmethacrylate from which hydroquinone was removed,[8] 20% *N*-dibutylphtalate, and 0.4% (weight) benzoyl peroxide. The resin polymerizes at 4°C by adding 0.1% *N*,*N*-dimethylaniline to the methylmethacrylate mixture. In addition, to exclude the oxygen contained in ambient air, which interferes with resin polymerization, nitrogen gas is applied to flush out air from the glass vial before sealing[9,10] (see Table 4.1 for the detailed procedure).

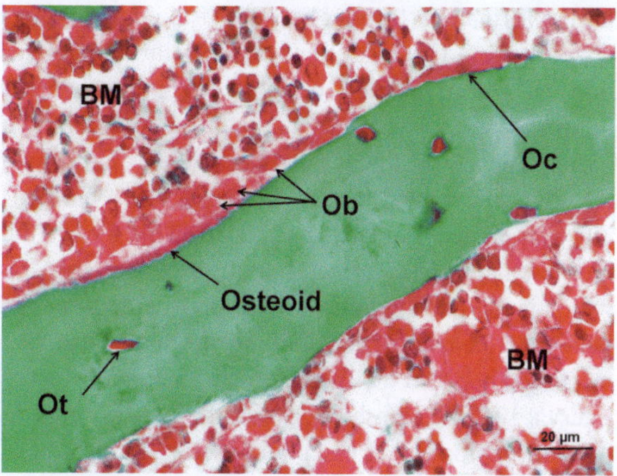

Fig. 4.1 Goldner trichrome staining of trabecular bone from rat proximal tibia. Mineralized bone is colored in green. Osteoid (non-mineralized bone), osteocyte (*Ot*), osteoblast (*Ob*), osteoclast (*Oc*), and bone marrow cells (*BM*) are colored in *red* (*pink* to *red* gradient). Five micrometer thick section

Undecalcified bone specimens are cut longitudinally. At 50 µm intervals, serial 5 and 10 µm thick sections are obtained by using a polycut-E microtome (Reichert-Jung, Leica, Heerbrugg, Switzerland), and they are mounted on gelatin-coated or superfrost (permanent positive charge; VWR International) glass slides. Sections of 5 µm thickness are stained with Goldner's trichrome method[11,12] and used for the structural and static parameters of bone remodeling. Goldner's trichrome stain allows a good differentiation between osteoid (colored in red) and mineralized (colored in green) bone matrix. In addition, bone cell morphologies are well defined with this stain, which is particularly important for the assessment of cellular activity (Fig. 4.1).

4.6 Fluorochrome Labeling

Fluorochromes, such as tetracycline (TC), calcein, and alizarin red, are calcium-seeking agents that integrate the bone matrix at the mineralization front

Table 4.1 Histological procedure

	Fixation[b] (ETOH 70%)	Dehydration[b] (ETOH 95%; 100%)	Impregnation[b] (#1–#2 passage)	Embedding Third passage
Rat tibia/vertebra	10 Days	4–24 h;12–48 h	2–3 Days; 2 days	2–3 Days
Mouse femur/vertebra[a]	7 Days	3–24 h;12–48 h	2–3 Days; 2 days	1–3 Days

[a]Same procedure for rats younger than 2 months of age
[b]Slight vaccum can be applied to accelerate the procedure

during formation (frontier between osteoid and mineralized bone). These substances allow the quantification of the dynamics of bone formation. Their fluorescence is visualized under ultraviolet or blue lights. They form linear bands (or labels) laid down into the mineralized matrix. Fluorochromes are usually administered in two doses apart. This allows the measurement of the mineral apposition rate (MAR), which is the rate at which new bone is being mineralized. It is calculated by dividing the mean distance measured between the two fluorochrome bands by the interval of time elapsed between the two dosings of the fluorochrome. It is essential to select an interval of time that allows the assessment of bone formation. Consequently, to adequately quantify the MAR, the two labels have to be incorporated into the same site of forming bone which corresponds to an individual bone structural unit (BSU). Therefore, it is important to precisely determine a dosing interval that is not longer than the formation period to avoid the risk of underestimating mineralizing surfaces. This phenomenon has been defined and called the "label escape error" by Frost.[13] It was suggested that, to minimize the labeling escape error, the fluorochrome dosing interval should be less than one-fifth of the formation period.[14] For the purpose of measuring dynamic bone formation parameters, we recommend testing different labeling intervals in a preliminary feasibility study before starting the main research protocol. In our laboratory, we have determined that for adult rats and mice, intervals of 6 days and 4 days, respectively, permit the avoidance of the label escape error.[15,16] Fluorochromes are injected intraperitoneally (IP) at doses of 20 mg/kg demeclocycline or 10 mg/kg calcein dissolved in physiological saline. Rats or mice are sacrificed 4 days or 36–48 h, respectively, after the second labeling. Unstained 10 μm thick sections mounted with a medium suitable for fluorescent microscopy are used for the observation of fluorochrome epifluorescence (Fig. 4.2).

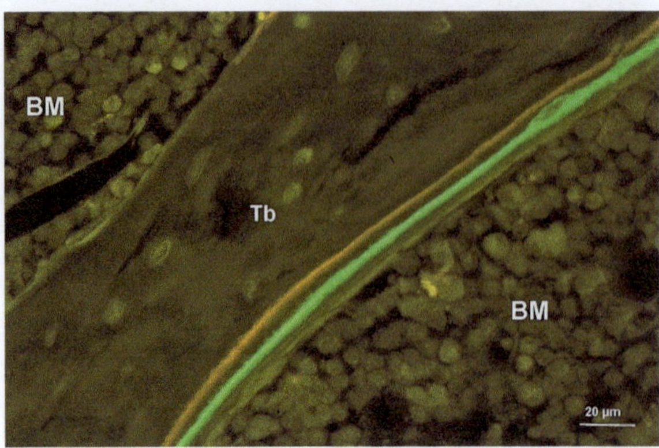

Fig. 4.2 Fluorochrome labeling of trabecular bone from rat proximal tibia. The *orange* fluorescence corresponds to demeclocycline label and the *green* fluorescence corresponds to calcein label. *BM*: Bone marrow, *Tb*: Trabecular bone. Ten micrometer thick section. Ultraviolet (UV)/blue-violet excitation

4.7 Bone Histomorphometric Method

Classical histomorphometry is achieved in cancellous bone tissue. However, before performing histomorphometric measurements, it is important to precisely delimit the tissue area where remodeling activity is predominant. For long bone specimens, this area is in the metaphyseal region but at some distance from the growth plate–metaphyseal junction in order to exclude the primary spongiosa. This distance is around 0.7–1 mm for rat proximal tibia[15] and 0.2–0.4 mm for mouse distal femur.[16] In addition, it is approximately 0.15–0.2 mm distant from the endocortical bone (for rat and mouse specimens) excluding the dysphasic zone, which corresponds to cortical parallelism. For lumbar vertebral bone, this area is delimited by caudal and proximal growth plates at a distance from the endocortical bone (Fig. 4.3).

Measurements are carried out on at least two nonconsecutive sections containing a minimum total of 40 mm of trabecular bone perimeter. Histomorphometry can be done with different semiautomated systems. In our laboratory, we use a semi-automated image-analyzing system combining a microscope equipped with a camera lucida and digitizing tablet linked to a computer using the OsteoMeasure Software (Osteometrics Inc., Decatur, GA, USA). Nomenclature and abbreviations of histomorphometric parameters follow the recommendations of the American Society for Bone and Mineral Research.[17]

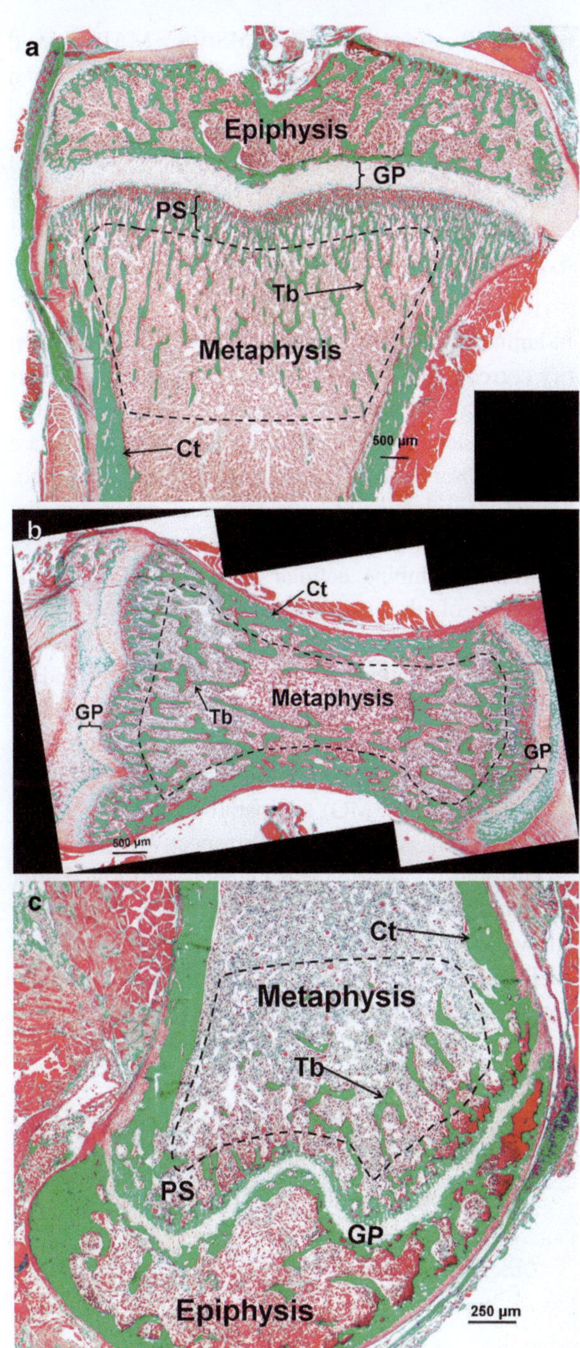

Fig. 4.3 Tissue area delimitations for bone histomorphometric measurements: (**a**) Rat proximal tibia. (**b**) Rat lumbar vertebra. (**c**) Mouse distal femur. *GP*: growth plate, *PS*: primary spongiosa, *Tb*: trabecular bone, *Ct*: cortical bone; *dashed lines* delimit the tissue area where histomorphometric measurements are usually performed. Five micrometer thick section

4.8 Histomorphometric Parameters

4.8.1 Structural Parameters

- Cancellous Bone
  - *Trabecular bone volume (BV/TV;%)*: Percentage of trabecular bone volume per tissue volume.

    This parameter is derived from the measurements of trabecular bone area (B.Ar; mineralized and nonmineralized) and the total area of tissue examined corresponding to the medullary cavity (T.Ar; bone, marrow and associated tissue): BV/TV = 100 × B.Ar/T.Ar.
  - *Trabecular thickness (Tb.Th; µm)**: Mean thickness of the trabeculae.
  - *Trabecular separation (Tb.Sp; µm)**: Derived parameter from (BV/TV)/Tb.Th.
  - *Trabecular number (Tb.N;/mm)**: Mean distance between individual trabeculae.
- Cortical Bone
  - *Cortical thickness (Ct.Th; µm)*: Mean thickness of the cortices.
  - *Cortical porosity (Ct.Po)*: The percentage of the cortical bone that contains pores without osteocyte lacunae.

4.8.2 Static Parameters

- *Osteoid surfaces (OS/BS;%)*: Percentage of surfaces covered by osteoid seams.
  - Under normal conditions, OS/BS is directly proportional to activation frequency (Ac.f or "birth rate") of the bone remodeling unit (BRU) and the duration of formative phase of the basic multicellular unit (BMU).
- *Osteoid volume (OV/BV;%)*: Percentage of a given amount of bone (bone + osteoid) that is osteoid.

*Tb.Th; Tb.Sp; and Tb.N are derived from measurements of trabecular perimeter (B.Pm) and B.Ar according to Parfitt's formulae.[17]

- OV/BV depends upon mean osteoid thickness (O.Th) and OS/BS.

- *Osteoid thickness (O.Th; μm)*: Mean thickness of osteoid seams.
  - O.Th is directly proportionnal to osteoblastic appositional rate and mineral lag time.
- *Osteoblastic surfaces (Ob.S/BS;%)*: Percentage of total trabecular bone surface covered by plump (cuboidal) osteoblasts.
  - In rodents, it is difficult to observe plump osteoblasts. Consequently, the flat shape is frequently considered for this parameter. Ob.S/BS is directly proportional to the bone turnover and new bone formation.
- *Eroded surfaces (ES/BS;%)*: Percentage of trabecular bone surface that shows current or prior osteoclastic activity (Howship's lacunae).
  - ES/BS is directly proportional to activation frequency of new bone remodeling units and lifespan of Howship's lacunae on the trabecular surface.
- *Osteoclast surfaces (Oc.S/BS;%)*: Percentage of trabecular bone surface covered by mono- and multinucleated osteoclasts (ideally identified as tartrate resistant acid phosphatase (TRAP)-positive by enzymo-histochemistry).
- *Osteoclast number (N.Oc/T.Ar; N.Oc/B.Pm; N. Oc/E.Pm)*: The number of osteoclasts per area (millimeters squared) of medullary cavity (T.Ar) or the number of osteoclasts per length (in millimeters) of the trabecular bone (B.Pm and E.Pm).

4.8.3 Dynamic Parameters of Bone Formation

- *Mineralizing surfaces (MS/BS;%)*: Percentage of total trabecular bone surface that exhibits double-labeled surfaces + half of single-labeled surfaces.
- *Mineral Appositional rate (MAR; μm/d)*: Mean distance between the two labels divided by the time interval between the dosing of TC. So, in order to be assessed, it needs double-labeled surfaces to be present.
- *Bone Formation Rate (BFR)*: MS/BS × MAR. It could be expressed as BFR volume referent, as the fraction of total bone formed per year, expressed per year and calculated as BFR/BV: MS/BS × MAR × BS/BV.

4.9 Enzymo-Histochemistry

In animal specimens, it is sometimes difficult to identify correctly the type of bone cells based only on their morphology by routine stainings. This is particularly true for osteoclasts because their numerous nuclei are often unobservable or hidden.[5] Moreover, the morphological identification of bone cells does not ensure that they are potentially active. Consequently, it is very helpful to combine cellular morphologies with the detection of the osteoblastic alkaline phosphatase (ALP) and the osteoclastic TRAP by an enzymo-histochemistry technique. These activities are revealed on unstained 5 μm thick sections according to the method of Liu.[18] Naphthol-AS-TR is used as a substrate for both enzymes, while Fast Blue BB salt (SIGMA-Aldrich, St. Louis, MO) and pararosaniline were used as couplers for ALP and TRAP, respectively (Fig. 4.4).

Histomorphometric measurements performed after phosphatase detections by enzymo-histochemistry allow the quantification of bone surfaces covered with ALP-positive osteoblasts (Ob.S ALP+/BS), the number of osteoclast TRAP-positive cells (N.Oc TRAP+/T. AR or/B.Pm or E.Pm), and the bone surfaces covered

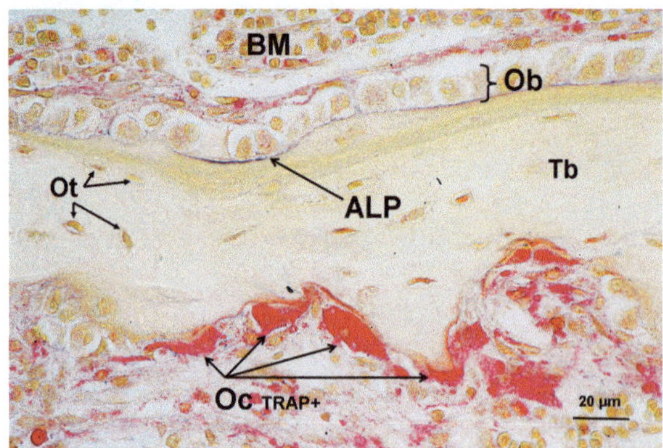

Fig. 4.4 Enzymo-histochemistry with ALP reaction shown in *violet* and TRAP reaction shown in *red*. Mineralized bone appears *light beige* (no counter stain used). *BM*: bone marrow, *Ob*: osteoblast, *Oc*: osteoclas, *Ot*: osteocyte, *Tb*: trabecular bone. Eight micrometer thick section

by TRAP-positive osteoclast (Oc.S TRAP+/BS). These histomorphometric parameters help for the evaluation of bone cell activities, notably during modeling or remodeling.[10,15,16]

4.10 Limitations

Although bone histomorphometry is a powerful tool to directly assess bone cell activity, bone turnover on the different bone envelopes (trabecular, endosteal, cortical, perisoteal), and can lead to the assessment of bone quality, it has some limitations. Obviously, as it needs the sacrifice of the animal, it cannot perform longitudinal assessment of the parameters in the same animal. In addition, it is not the best way to assess bone mass. Bone densitometry and peripheral quantitative computed tomography (QCT) are most likely more precise tools to follow bone mass evolution in animals. As for the evaluation of micro-architecture, bone histomorphometry provides a two-dimensional (2D) assessment whereas microcomputerized tomography (μCT) study of the bone specimen allows a three-dimensional (3D) evaluation which can be considered more global although it cannot distinguish osteoid from mineralized bone. Finally, analysis of a small portion of the skeleton should not be generalized to the entire skeleton.

Acknowledgment We are grateful to Claire Deschênes for her excellent technical assistance.

References

1. Kimmel DB. Animal models in osteoporosis. In: Bilezikian JP, Raisz LG, Rodan GA, eds. *Principles of Bone Biology*, vol. 2. 2nd ed. San Diego: Academic; 2002:1635-1655.
2. Matsushita M, Tsuboyama T, Kasai R, et al. Age-related changes in bone mass in the senescence-accelerated mouse (SAM). SAM-R/3 and SAM-P/6 as new murine models for senile osteoporosis. *Am J Pathol*. 1986;125(2): 276-283.
3. Erben RG. Trabecular and endocortical bone surfaces in the rat: modeling or remodeling? *Anat Rec*. 1996;246(1):39-46.
4. Lelovas PP, Xanthos TT, Thoma SE, et al. The laboratory rat as an animal model for osteoporosis research. *Comp Med*. 2008;58(5):424-430.
5. Jee WS, Yao W. Overview: animal models of osteopenia and osteoporosis. *J Musculoskelet Neuronal Interact*. 2001;1(3): 193-207.
6. Li M, Jee WSS. Models of predlinical skeletal research. ICHTS-CSBME 2nd APBM workshop on bone histomorphometry and imaging Beijng, China; 2008:14-15.
7. Iwaniec UT, Yuan D, Power RA, et al. Strain-dependent variations in the response of cancellous bone to ovariectomy in mice. *J Bone Miner Res*. 2006;21(7):1068-1074.
8. Chappard D, Alexandre C, Camps M, et al. Embedding iliac bone biopsies at low temperature using glycol and methyl methacrylates. *Stain Technol*. 1983;58(5):299-308.
9. Erben RG. Embedding of bone samples in methylmethacrylate: an improved method suitable for bone histomorphometry, histochemistry, and immunohistochemistry. *J Histochem Cytochem*. 1997;45(2):307-313.
10. Laboux O, Dion N, Arana-Chavez V, et al. Microwave irradiation of ethanol-fixed bone improves preservation, reduces processing time, and allows both light and electron microscopy on the same sample. *J Histochem Cytochem*. 2004;52(10):1267-1275.
11. Hall D. *The Methodology of Connective Tissue Research*. Oxford: Joynson-Bruvvers; 1976:130.
12. Gruber HE. Adaptations of Goldner's Masson trichrome stain for the study of undecalcified plastic embedded bone. *Biotech Histochem*. 1992;67(1):30-34.
13. Frost HM. Bone hostomorphometry: correction of labeling "escape error". In: Recker RR, ed. *Bone Histomorphometry: Techniques and Interpretation*. Boca Raton: CRC; 1983: 133-142.
14. Erben RG. Bone-labeling techniques. In: An YH, Martin KL, eds. *Handbook of Histology Methods for Bone and Cartilage*. Totowa: Humana Press; 2003:99-117.
15. Mailhot G, Petit JL, Dion N, et al. Endocrine and bone consequences of cyclic nutritional changes in the calcium, phosphate and vitamin D status in the rat: an in vivo depletion-repletion-redepletion study. *Bone*. 2007;41(3):422-436.
16. Duque G, Macoritto M, Dion N, et al. 1, 25(OH)2D3 acts as a bone-forming agent in the hormone-independent senescence-accelerated mouse (SAM-P/6). *Am J Physiol Endocrinol Metab*. 2005;288(4):E723-E730.
17. Parfitt AM, Drezner MK, Glorieux FH, et al. Bone histomorphometry: standardization of nomenclature, symbols, and units. Report of the ASBMR Histomorphometry Nomenclature Committee. *J Bone Miner Res*. 1987;2(6):595-610.
18. Liu C, Sanghvi R, Burnell BM, et al. Simultaneous demonstration of bone alkaline and acid phosphatase activities in plastic-embedded sections and differential inhibition of the activities. *Histochemistry*. 1987;86:559-565.

5 Methods in Bone Biology in Animals: Imaging

Blaine A. Christiansen and Mary L. Bouxsein

5.1 Introduction

Animal models are essential research tools for investigating the musculoskeletal system. Analysis of bone morphology and bone density can provide information about skeletal phenotypes, including characterization of the skeletal effects of aging, disease, and dietary, genetic, pharmacologic, or mechanical interventions. Until recently, quantitative histology was the standard technique used for assessing trabecular and cortical bone architecture. Although histological analyses provide unique information on cellularity and dynamic indices of bone remodeling, they are destructive and have limitations with respect to assessment of bone micro-architecture since structural parameters are derived from stereologic analysis of a few two-dimensional (2D) sections, usually assuming that the underlying structure is plate-like.[1] In comparison, three-dimensional (3D) imaging techniques can directly measure bone micro-architecture without relying on stereologic models.

Several imaging modalities are available for the assessment of skeletal morphology in animal models (Table 5.1). Some of these techniques, such as radiographs and peripheral dual energy x-ray absorptiometry (pDEXA), provide relatively inexpensive and fast assessments of bone mass and gross morphology *in vivo*, but have poor resolution and are limited to planar (2D) images. In comparison, high-resolution 3D imaging techniques, such as microcomputed tomography (μCT), can directly measure bone micro-architecture. Likewise, some imaging techniques can be used in live animals (*in vivo*), while others are restricted for use in excised specimens (*ex vivo*). In this chapter, we review the imaging techniques commonly used to assess bone mass and micro-architecture in animal models.

B.A. Christiansen (✉)
University of California-Davis Medical Center, Department of Orthopaedics, 4635, 2nd Ave., Suite 2000 Sacramento, CA 95817
e-mail: bchristiansen@ucdavis.edu

5.2 Imaging Modalities

5.2.1 Radiographs

Though often overlooked in favor of higher-resolution imaging techniques, whole-body radiographs are an important tool for evaluating gross skeletal morphology *in vivo* and *ex vivo*. Radiographs are produced by the summation of attenuation along a single scan direction (Fig. 5.1). The advantage of planar radiographs is the rapid, relatively inexpensive visualization of skeletal morphology; however, they are limited to 2D (typically qualitative) evaluations.

5.2.2 Peripheral Dual Energy X-Ray Absorptiometry

pDEXA is a method for planar (2D) assessment of bone mineral content (BMC, g), areal bone mineral density (BMD, g/cm^2), and body composition (% fat, lean tissue mass) of small animals, both *in vivo* and *ex vivo* (Fig. 5.2). DEXA imaging uses two x-ray beams with different energy levels. The ratio of attenuation of the high- and low-energy beams allows the separation of bone from soft tissue, as well as lean tissue from fat. A typical pixel size for pDEXA mea-

G. Duque and K. Watanabe (eds.), *Osteoporosis Research*,
DOI: 10.1007/978-0-85729-293-3_5, © Springer-Verlag London Limited 2011

Table 5.1 Summary of skeletal imaging modalities

Imaging modality	Approximate resolution	2D or 3D	*In vivo*	Benefits and typical uses
Planar radiography	10 lp/mm	2D	x	Rapid, inexpensive visualization of skeletal morphology
Peripheral DEXA	180 μm	2D	x	Rapid, highly reproducible measures of bone mass and body composition
Peripheral QCT	70 μm	3D	x	Assessment of bone geometry, bone mass, and vBMD
Ex vivo μCT	6–90 μm	3D		High-resolution imaging of bone micro-architecture and vBMD
In vivo μCT	10–150 μm	3D	x	High-resolution *in vivo* imaging of bone micro-architecture and vBMD
SR-CT	<1 μm	3D	x	Extremely high-resolution imaging of bone micro-architecture or ultrastructure, highly accurate vBMD measurement

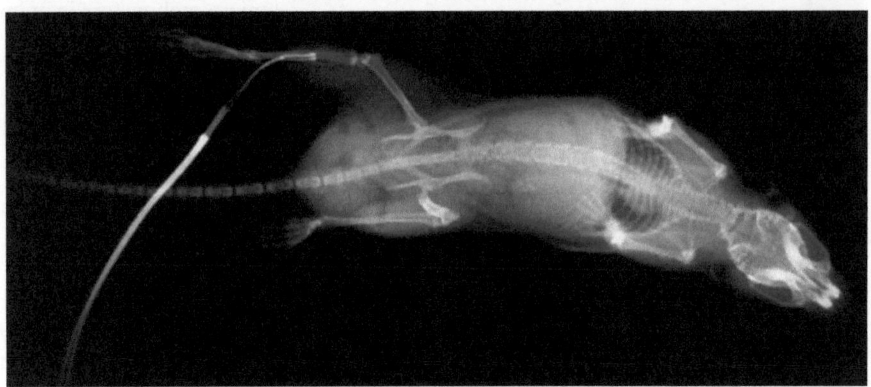

Fig. 5.1 Radiograph image of a mouse skeleton with an attached strain gage. Radiographs are an important tool for evaluating gross skeletal morphology *in vivo* and *ex vivo*

surement in mice and rats is 180 μm per side. *In vivo* pDEXA measurements have been used to demonstrate the skeletal changes following estrogen deficiency,[2] dietary and pharmacologic interventions,[3,4] as well as mouse strain–related differences in bone mass and body composition.[5,6]

Generally, pDEXA provides highly reproducible measures of bone mass and body composition, with precision errors for whole-body measurements less than 2%[7,8] and relatively short scan times (~5 min). Precision of bone measurements at individual skeletal sites, such as the lumbar spine or distal femur, are slightly worse (up to 8%) due to the challenges in consistently identifying the region of interest (ROI).[8] Additionally, measurements of body composition suffer from poor accuracy, with general underestimation of lean tissue mass and overestimation of fat mass.[7,9,10] These errors can largely be eliminated with careful calibration of the DEXA system to body fat content measured independently, such as by carcass analysis,[9,10] though few investigators take the time to do this. In summary, pDEXA has relatively limited spatial resolution, assesses areal BMD rather than volumetric BMD, and cannot distinguish cortical and trabecular bone compartments. Despite these limitations, the technique is highly reproducible and thus very useful for rapid, relatively low-cost measures of longitudinal changes in BMD.

5.2.3 Peripheral Quantitative Computed Tomography

Peripheral quantitative computed tomography (pQCT) is a quantitative imaging method used for 3D assessment of bone geometry, BMC, and volumetric bone

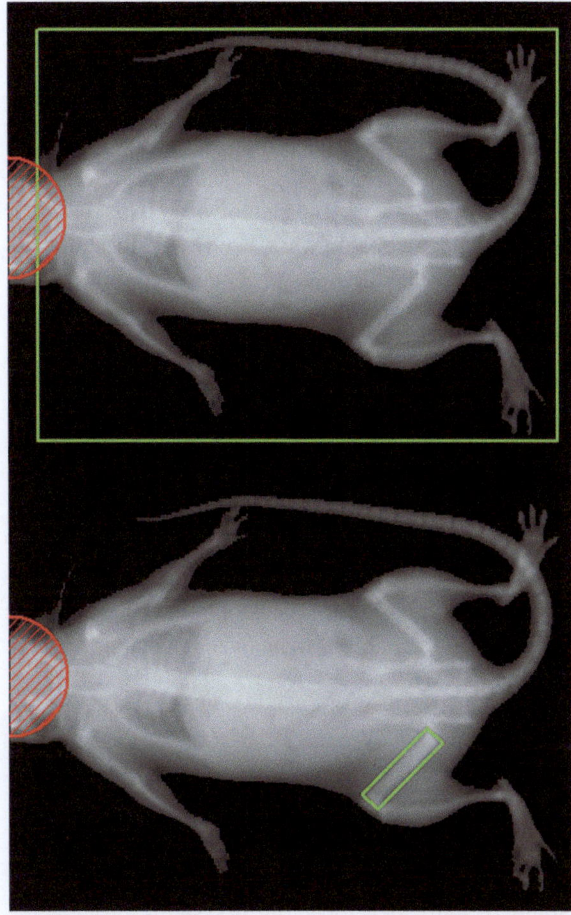

Fig. 5.2 Image of a mouse scanned with peripheral DEXA. The head is typically excluded from measurements of body composition or bone mineral content. The *boxes* represent areas of interest for analyzing BMC or BMD of the whole body or femur

mineral density (vBMD) in animal models, both *in vivo* and *ex vivo*. pQCT uses x-ray attenuation data acquired at multiple viewing angles to reconstruct a 3D representation of the specimen that characterizes the spatial distribution of material density. Commercially available pQCT scanners can achieve an in-plane voxel size of approximately 70 μm. The ability to measure bone mass and morphology *in vivo* makes pQCT useful for longitudinal assessment of the skeletal response to aging, disease, and/or interventions. However, the resolution of commercially available pQCT scanners does not allow for effective imaging of trabecular architecture.

Many studies have used pQCT in rats to monitor changes in cortical bone geometry along with cortical and trabecular vBMD following pharmacologic[11,12] or mechanical[13] interventions, and to monitor fracture healing.[14] pQCT has also been used to quantify bone density and geometry in mice.[15,16] It has been suggested that this imaging method yields satisfactory *in vivo* precision and accuracy in skeletal characterization of mice[17]; however, the voxel size of pQCT is relatively large compared to the cortical thickness of a mouse femur (typically 100–300 μm). This may introduce errors due to partial volume averaging (see Sect. 5.7.1.1). This issue can be partially addressed with the careful selection of an analysis threshold that yields physiologically accurate results; however, due to these concerns, the accuracy of pQCT for assessment of trabecular bone parameters in mice is questionable. Regardless, pQCT is an effective method of measuring cortical bone morphology in larger animal models *in vivo*.

5.2.4 Microcomputed Tomography

In recent years, μCT has become the gold standard for *ex vivo* evaluation of bone morphology in mice and other small animal models. Similar to pQCT, μCT relies on x-ray attenuation data acquired at multiple angles, which are then reconstructed into 3D images of bone morphology (Fig. 5.3). Currently available desktop μCT scanners can achieve an isotropic voxel size of as low as a few microns, which is sufficient resolution for investigating structures such as mouse trabeculae that have widths of approximately 30–50 μm.[18]

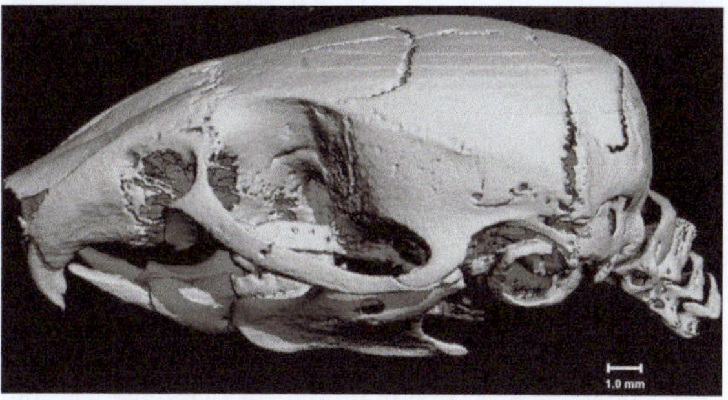

Fig. 5.3 Three-dimensional reconstruction of a mouse skull scanned by μCT. μCT uses x-ray attenuation data acquired at multiple viewing angles to reconstruct a 3D representation of the specimen that characterizes the spatial distribution of material density

Assessment of bone microarchitecture with μCT provides several distinct advantages compared to 2D histology and histomorphometry techniques: (1) it allows for direct 3D measurement of trabecular morphology such as trabecular thickness and separation, rather than computing these values based on 2D stereological models, as is done with standard histological evaluations; (2) compared to 2D histology, a much larger volume of interest can be analyzed; (3) measurements can be performed with a much faster throughput than typical histomorphometric analyses of undecalcified bone specimens; (4) assessment of bone morphology by μCT scanning is nondestructive, thus samples can subsequently be used for other assays, such as histology or mechanical testing; and (5) μCT scans may be used to provide an estimate of bone tissue mineralization by comparing x-ray attenuation in the bone to that of hydroxyapatite standards, though this must be done with care given the constraints of the polychromatic x-ray source (see Sect. 5.7.1).[19]

Several studies have reported excellent reproducibility and accuracy of μCT measurements of bone morphology. μCT measurements have been compared to traditional measures from 2D histomorphometry, both in animal[20-23] and human specimens.[24-26] These studies have consistently shown that morphology measurements by μCT are highly correlated to those from 2D histomorphometry. For example, Müller et al. reported very high correlations ($r = 0.84$–0.92) and low percent differences between the two methods.[24] Some studies have reported that μCT measures overestimate trabecular thickness relative to histomorphometric measures[26]; however, it is likely that this disparity could be eliminated by adjusting the image resolution and segmentation threshold in order to achieve more consistent results. Regardless, high correlation between the two techniques provides strong rationale for the continued use of μCT for assessing skeletal morphometry.

μCT has been used for a wide range of studies of bone mass and bone morphology, including the analysis of growth and development,[27] skeletal phenotypes in genetically altered mice, and animal models of disease states such as postmenopausal osteoporosis and renal osteodystrophy. Additionally, μCT has been used to assess the effects of pharmacologic interventions,[28] as well as mechanical loading[29] and unloading,[30] to image macrocracks in cortical bone,[31] and to evaluate fracture healing.[32-37]

μCT imaging combined with a perfused contrast agent can been used to evaluate the morphology of soft tissue structures. Duvall et al. demonstrated the ability of contrast-enhanced μCT analysis to quantify 3D vascular network morphology.[38,39] This vascular μCT imaging technique has been used to study the response to ischemic injury,[38,39] phenotypic characterization of tissue repair and remodeling,[39] therapeutic angiogenesis,[40] postnatal growth and development,[41,42] cerebral circulation,[43] vascular biomechanics and disease,[44] and tissue engineering.[45,46] Palmer et al. have also introduced a technique to quantify morphology and proteoglycan content in cartilage by imaging the equilibrium partitioning of an ionic contrast agent via μCT.[47] Contrast-enhanced regions of cartilage can be segmented from subchondral bone, providing a detailed thickness map of the articular cartilage and the ability to analyze bone and cartilage simultaneously.

5.2.5 In Vivo Microcomputed Tomography

Some recently developed μCT systems provide the ability to measure bone morphology in small animal models *in vivo*. This technique provides a high resolution of μCT while allowing for longitudinal studies of morphological changes. Current *in vivo* μCT systems provide a slightly lower resolution than *ex vivo* systems (typical voxel size for *in vivo* μCT systems: 10–150 μm), but they still have scanning resolutions high enough to measure trabecular bone morphology in small animal models. *In vivo* μCT is an ideal method for tracking bone changes that occur on a timescale of weeks or months, such as bone loss associated with disuse or ovariectomy, or increased bone mass due to pharmacological or mechanical intervention. By registering 3D images against images from previous time points, it is possible to determine the precise locations of bone formation or resorption[48,49] (Fig. 5.4). However, users should be careful when attempting to register scans taken at different time points, as the accuracy and reproducibility of this technique has not been fully

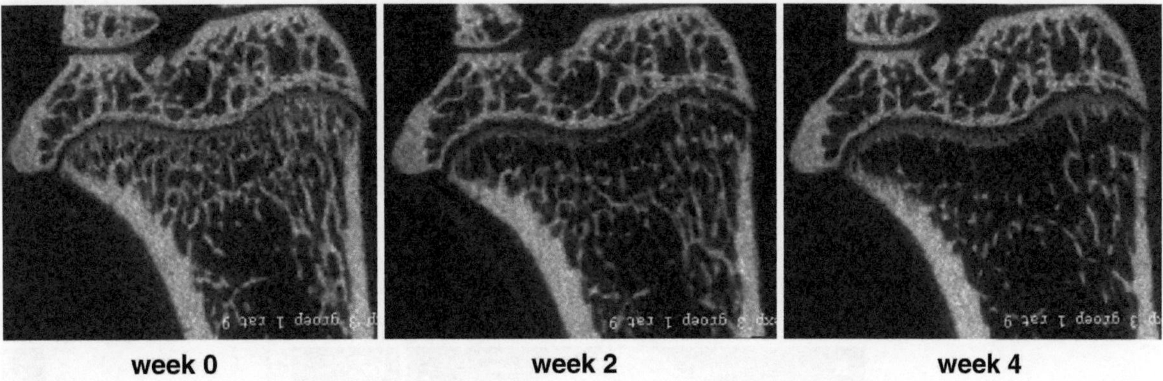

Fig. 5.4 Images showing typical trabecular bone loss at the proximal tibia of a 30-week-old Wistar rat after OVX, assessed by *in vivo* μCT at weeks 0, 2, and 4 (Images courtesy of J.E.M. Brouwers, Eindhoven University of Technology)

characterized. The ability to perform longitudinal assessments of bone microstructure has the potential to reduce the number of animals needed in a given study, and provide novel information about skeletal development, adaptation, repair, and response to disease or therapeutic interventions. *In vivo* μCT has been used to follow the rapid trabecular bone loss in rats in the weeks immediately following ovariectomy,[50,51] to study the effects of aging,[52] and of zoledronic acid or parathyroid hormone (PTH) treatment on bone in ovariectomized (OVX) rats,[53,54] as well as changes in the epiphyseal bone of rats following either surgical destabilization of the knee[55] or intra-articular injection of an inhibitor of glycolysis that promotes loss of articular cartilage.[56]

Despite the clear advantages of *in vivo* μCT, there are also several potential limitations associated with this method of imaging. In particular, there are concerns about the amount of ionizing radiation delivered during the scan, especially when animals are scanned multiple times throughout an experimental period. It is possible that this radiation may introduce unwanted effects on the tissues or processes of interest, or on the animals in general. Young, growing animals and proliferative biologic processes, such as fracture healing or tumor growth, may be particularly susceptible to radiation exposure. The radiation exposure reported by Waarsing et al.,[48] 0.4 Gy for a single 20 min μCT scan (10 μm voxel size) of a rat hindlimb, is not predicted to have significant deleterious effects on bone cells,[57] but the effect of multiple exposures has not been thoroughly investigated. Klinck et al.[58] performed weekly *in vivo* μCT scans on the proximal tibia of OVX and SHAM-OVX rats beginning at 12 weeks of age. They found no observable effects of radiation on the animals' health; however, trabecular bone volume was decreased by 8–20% in the irradiated limbs compared to the contralateral nonirradiated limbs. These observations confirm that additional studies are needed to determine the potential effects of repeated *in vivo* μCT scans, and provide strong rationale for the inclusion of measurements of an internal nonirradiated control limb in the study design.

5.2.6 Synchrotron Radiation Computed Tomography

Synchrotron radiation-based computed tomography (SR-CT or nano-computed tomography) is an imaging technique that allows for extremely high-resolution imaging of bone tissue, with resolution of less than 1 μm. SR-CT uses a high photon flux monochromatic x-ray beam that is extracted from a synchrotron source, rather than the polychromatic x-ray source used for standard desktop μCT imaging systems. This monochromatic x-ray beam eliminates beam-hardening artifacts, allowing for accurate assessment of tissue mineral density (TMD).[59] The high spatial resolution associated with SR-CT affords extremely precise assessment of trabecular bone architecture,[18] and may be particularly useful for assessment of small-scale bone structures in the cortical bone of animal models.[60,61] SR-CT has been used to investigate genetic variations in the mineral density and ultrastructural properties of murine cortical bone, including the vascular canals and osteocyte lacunae (Fig. 5.5).[62,63] Although studies with SR-CT are generally performed on excised specimens, Kinney et al. used SR-CT *in vivo* to show the early deterioration in trabecular architecture in the rat proximal tibia following estrogen deficiency.[64] SR-CT is limited by the fact that it has extremely limited availability (requires access to synchrotron source), and may be limited to analysis of relatively small volumes of interest.

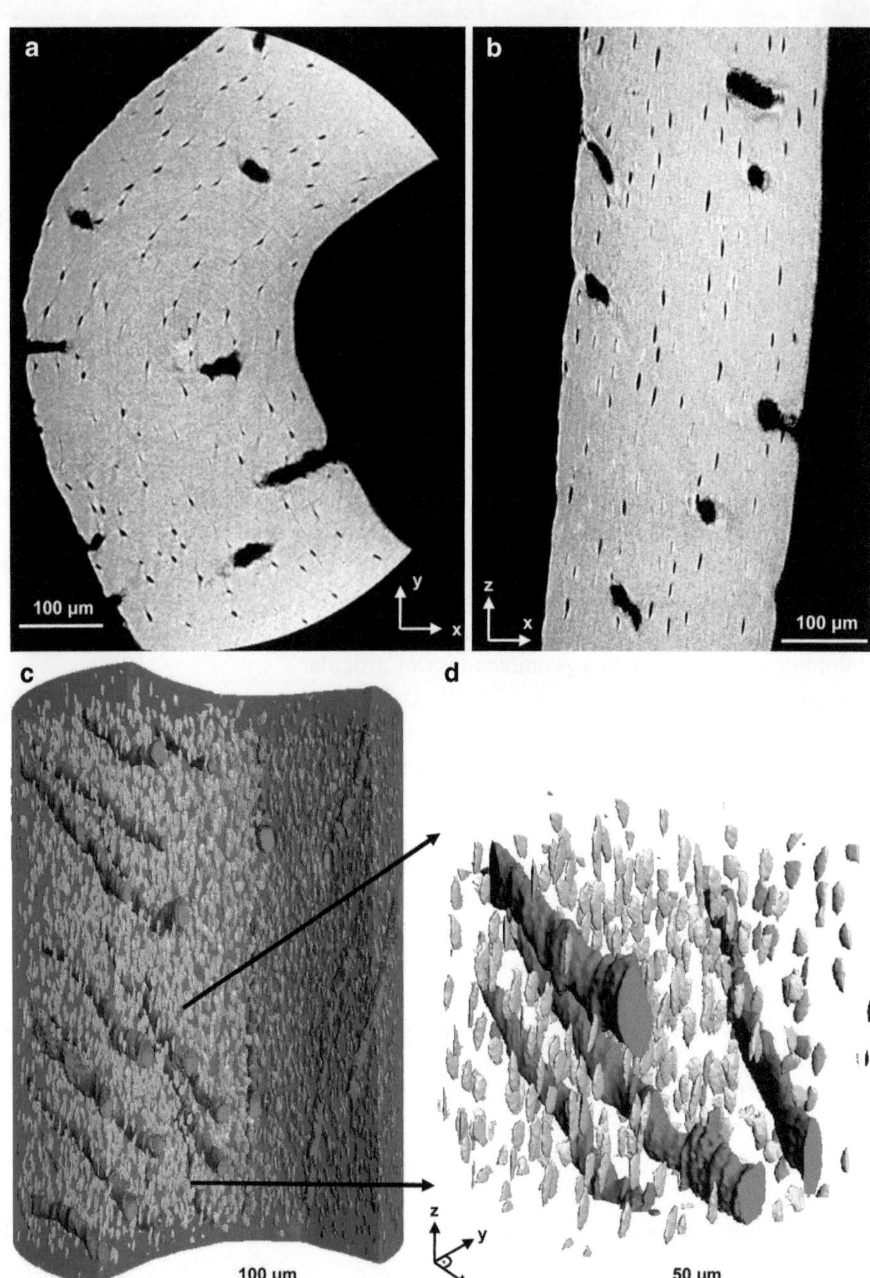

Fig. 5.5 Cortical bone from the femoral mid-diaphysis of mice measured with SR-CT at 700 nm nominal resolution. The *top* row shows the lateral cortical mid-diaphysis of a mouse femur in a transversal (**a**) and sagittal (**b**) view. The *bottom* row ((**c**) and (**d**)) is a reconstruction of the canal network and osteocyte lacunae within the same lateral cortical bone (Figure originally published in Schneider et al.[63] Reproduced with permission)

5.3 Special Considerations for Skeletal Imaging of Animal Models

There are a number of issues that must be carefully considered in order to achieve accurate measurement of bone morphometry and density from skeletal scans of small animal models. In this section, these issues are described in the context of μCT scanning, but these considerations can be applied to other imaging methods as well.

5.3.1 Density Calibration

If results from a QCT scan are to be used to report an estimate of the TMD of a sample, it is necessary for the scanning system to be properly calibrated using solid-state phantoms of known densities. If a scanner is properly calibrated using these phantoms, it is then possible to convert CT pixel brightness values to a measure of mineral density (typically mg/cm^3 of calcium hydroxyapatite). Many manufacturers provide phantoms that should be measured on a regular basis to ensure proper calibration.

However, density readings can also be strongly affected by beam hardening artifacts if a polychromatic x-ray source is used (as in nearly all μCT systems). Beam hardening refers to the changes that occur in a polychromatic beam as it passes through a sample – the lower-energy portion of the beam is preferentially absorbed by the sample, while the high-energy portion passes through more easily. This differential absorption of low- and high-energy photons leads to beam hardening, whereby the average energy of the x-ray beam is increased (Fig. 5.6). Beam hardening can result in a different density reading in the middle of a sample compared to the edges, even in a homogeneous sample. Possible errors in measuring TMD due to beam hardening are particularly important when measuring specimens of unequal sizes or structures.[19] In general, a higher-energy scan is needed for thicker and denser samples. Optimizing the absorption contrast can be achieved by experimenting with varying x-ray energies and beam-hardening reduction methods (filters, software). However, density measurements of specimens of unequal size or quantities of bone mineral must be interpreted with caution unless appropriate steps are taken to minimize these potential artifacts.

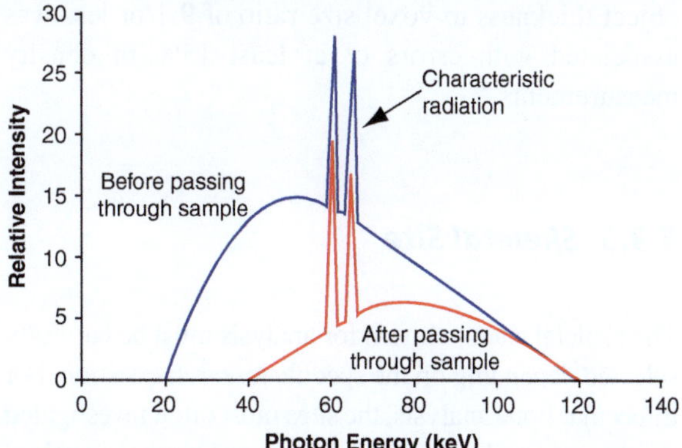

Fig. 5.6 The energy spectrum of a polychromatic beam before and after passing through a sample. The characteristic radiation of the beam will remain at the same photon energy. Lower-energy components of the beam will be absorbed more readily than high-energy components, causing an effective energy to shift toward higher-energy values (beam hardening)

5.3.2 Voxel Size and Image Resolution

A voxel is a discrete unit of the scan volume resulting from tomographic reconstruction of the scan data. It is a 3D volume representing two dimensions within the slice, and the slice thickness. Ideally, the smallest voxel size (highest scan resolution) available would be used for all scans; however, higher-resolution scans require longer acquisition and reconstruction times, and generate large data sets. Therefore, the trade-off between scan resolution and scan time must be carefully considered. Differences in voxel size have only a small effect on the evaluation of structures with relatively high thickness (i.e., 100–200 μm), such as cortical bone or trabeculae in humans or large animal models. However, when analyzing smaller structures such as mouse or rat trabeculae (20–60 μm), voxel size can significantly affect the results.[65] Scanning with low resolution (large voxel size) relative to the size of the structure of interest may introduce errors due to partial volume averaging, in which a CT voxel samples a region containing two materials with different densities (i.e., bone and soft tissue). In this case, the voxel would return a density value that is the mean of all tissue in the voxel volume. Partial volume averaging may cause cortical bone or trabeculae to appear thicker and less dense than they actually are. This has been confirmed in mouse femoral cortical bone as well as similarly sized aluminum tubes, where an object thickness to voxel size ratio of 9:1 or less was associated with errors of at least 15% in density measurements.[66]

5.3.3 Skeletal Site

The skeletal site(s) chosen for analysis must be carefully selected depending on the specific research question. For trabecular bone analysis, the sites most often investigated are the proximal tibia, distal femur, and lumbar vertebral body. If possible, it is desirable to analyze more than one skeletal site, since there can be significant heterogeneity among skeletal sites.[67-69] Age-related trabecular bone loss in mice begins at a relatively young age in the metaphyseal regions of the long bones, and continues into old age, such that bone volume fraction can be extremely low in aged animals.[68] This very low bone volume fraction makes it challenging to detect differences between groups, and makes it particularly difficult to detect bone loss or inhibition of bone loss. In comparison, age-related trabecular bone loss in the vertebral body begins at a later age and is not as dramatic.[68]

5.3.4 Region of Interest

Careful selection of an appropriate ROI at a particular skeletal site is also necessary for obtaining optimal bone morphology results. In mice especially, trabecular bone in the metaphyseal region is largely confined to a few millimeters adjacent to the metaphyseal growth plate. Extending a volume of interest beyond this region would include more "empty space," thereby reducing the mean values for BV/TV at that skeletal site and possibly masking relevant differences between study groups (Fig. 5.7). For consistency between samples, the ROI should be defined based on the location of the start point of the scan and the size of the scan region. The starting point should be defined as an absolute (mm) or relative distance (%) from a reproducible landmark, such as the proximal tibial plateau, the

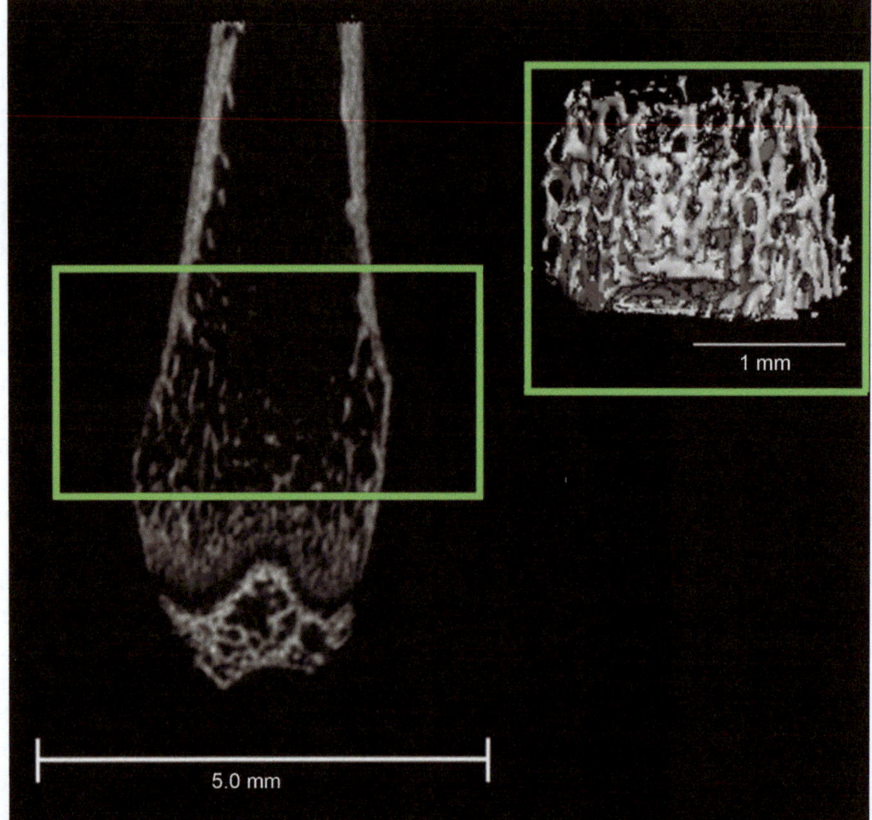

Fig. 5.7 Volume of interest of a distal mouse femur. Trabecular bone in the metaphyseal region is largely confined to a few millimeters adjacent to the growth plate. Extending a volume of interest beyond this region would include more "empty space," thereby reducing the mean values for BV/TV at that skeletal site and possibly masking relevant differences between groups

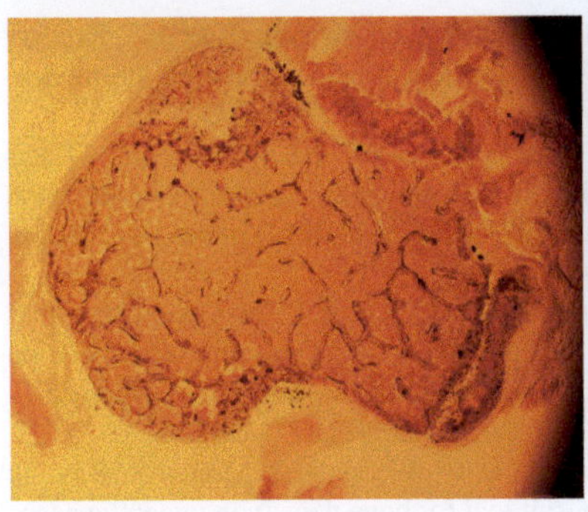
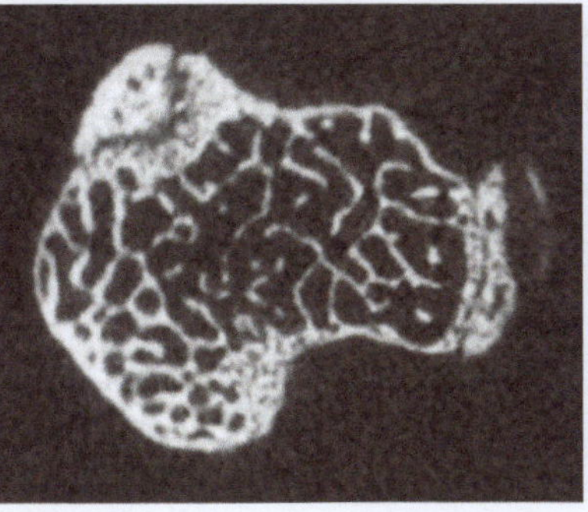
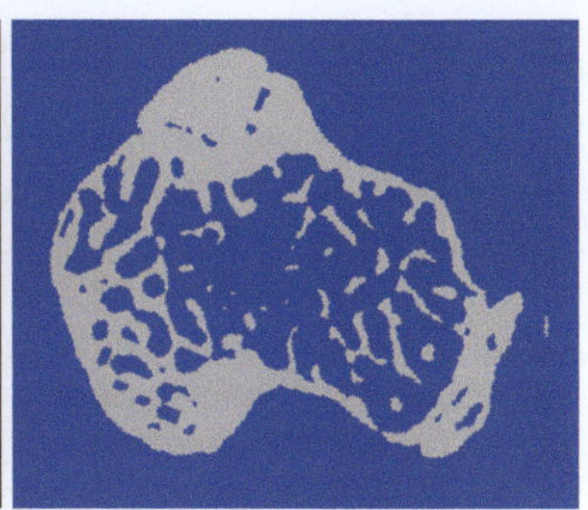

Fig. 5.8 Transverse histological section of a mouse proximal tibial metaphysis (*left*), with corresponding 2D image obtained with μCT (*center*), and segmented μCT image (*right*) designating bone from non-bone. It is important to visually compare the original and segmented 2D images to ensure accuracy of the segmentation

metaphyseal growth plate, the mid-diaphysis, or another suitable anatomical site.

5.3.5 Segmentation

Segmentation is the process of differentiating bone from non-bone from a scan. There are several methods of performing segmentation, all of which seek to extract a "physiologically accurate" representation of the bone tissue (i.e., similar to histology). The simplest approach is to use a global threshold, defining all voxels exceeding a given CT value (density) as bone and all voxels below this threshold as non-bone. The advantage of using a global threshold is that it is easy and efficient, since it only requires setting one parameter. However, care must be taken when using a global threshold, since bone mineralization may not be constant for all samples or all groups (i.e., during growth and development). More sophisticated segmentation methods include specimen-specific thresholds[70,71] and/or local segmentation methods,[22] where the inclusion of each voxel is based on its local neighborhood. At high scan resolutions, global and local segmentation methods will both provide accurate representations of trabecular bone structure; however, when samples are not homogeneous (e.g., thick cortices and thin trabeculae) or when scan resolution is relatively low, a local segmentation method may provide more accurate results than a global threshold.[22] No matter what segmentation routine is applied, it is important to visually compare the original and segmented 2D images to ensure accuracy of the segmentation (Fig. 5.8). If a study design requires the analysis of both cortical and trabecular bone at the same site (e.g., vertebral body), it may be preferable to segment the two tissue types separately.[72]

5.3.6 Animal Models

There are several factors to consider when selecting an animal model for skeletal imaging, including animal size and bone structure. Mice and rats are by far the most commonly used animal models for imaging studies of the skeletal system. Mice in particular are heavily used for studies of skeletal biology, as their genome can be readily manipulated to generate animals with global or tissue-specific deletion or over-expression of specific genes.[73] However, despite their common use, mice have disadvantages for imaging studies relative to larger animal models. Larger animals have bigger regions of trabecular bone, and larger structures that may allow for more accurate and consistent analyses of bone density and morphometry. It is desirable to have a large region of trabecular bone, as it is unclear how changes in trabeculae near the trabecular/cortical interface may affect trabecular morphology results. In addition, certain strains of mice have few trabeculae at some skeletal sites (e.g., proximal tibia of C57BL/6J), particularly in older animals,[68] which may lead to exaggerated conclusions (e.g., trabecular thickness averaged for only a small number of trabeculae may not provide an accurate mean value). Additionally, skeletal structures are larger in large animal models, so scanner resolution becomes less of an issue. When using mice, it is also important to consider the background strain, as trabecular and cortical bone morphology vary widely by strain. Genetically manipulated mice with mixed genetic backgrounds often have higher variability in bone morphology than mice with pure genetic backgrounds, leading to difficulties in interpretation of experimental findings.

In addition to animal size, the composition of cortical bone in mice and rats is fundamentally different from that of humans or large animal models. In particular, cortical bone of large animals form lamella, while that of mice does not. In this way, the porosity and composition of cortical bones from large animal models is more comparable to that of humans. In addition, rodent cortical bone rarely undergoes intracortical remodeling, unlike that of higher mammals. For this reason, direct comparison between the canal network and porosity in mice cortices and that in human bone might be misleading. In the mouse, cortical bone is considered to be unchanged since the time the bone was originally formed, whereas in humans cortical bone is extensively remodeled over time.

5.4 Conclusions

Assessment of skeletal mass and morphology in animal models via nondestructive imaging is an important component of current investigations aimed at improving our understanding of musculoskeletal development, growth, adaptation, and disease. Currently, several different imaging modalities aimed at whole-animal, organ, tissue, and cellular levels are available, and will be increasingly used to study the hierarchy of bone structure.

Acknowledgments The authors acknowledge funding from NIH (AR053986, AR057522, AR058389 and AG023480). The authors would like to thank Alison Cloutier and Rajaram Manoharan for assistance with preparation of figures.

References

1. Parfitt AM, Drezner MK, Glorieux FH, et al. Bone histomorphometry: standardization of nomenclature, symbols, and units. Report of the ASBMR Histomorphometry Nomenclature Committee. *J Bone Miner Res*. 1987;2(6):595-610.
2. Binkley N, Dahl DB, Engelke J, Kawahara-Baccus T, Krueger D, Colman RJ. Bone loss detection in rats using a mouse densitometer. *J Bone Miner Res*. 2003;18(2):370-375.
3. Brochmann EJ, Duarte ME, Zaidi HA, Murray SS. Effects of dietary restriction on total body, femoral, and vertebral bone in SENCAR, C57BL/6, and DBA/2 mice. *Metabolism*. 2003;52(10):1265-1273.
4. Iida-Klein A, Hughes C, Lu SS, et al. Effects of cyclic versus daily hPTH(1-34) regimens on bone strength in association with BMD, biochemical markers, and bone structure in mice. *J Bone Miner Res*. 2006;21(2):274-282.
5. Masinde GL, Li X, Gu W, Wergedal J, Mohan S, Baylink DJ. Quantitative trait loci for bone density in mice: the genes determining total skeletal density and femur density show little overlap in F2 mice. *Calcif Tissue Int*. 2002;71(5): 421-428.
6. Reed DR, Bachmanov AA, Tordoff MG. Forty mouse strain survey of body composition. *Physiol Behav*. 2007;91(5): 593-600.
7. Nagy TR, Clair AL. Precision and accuracy of dual-energy X-ray absorptiometry for determining *in vivo* body composition of mice. *Obes Res*. 2000;8(5):392-398.
8. Kolta S, De Vernejoul MC, Meneton P, Fechtenbaum J, Roux C. Bone mineral measurements in mice: comparison of two devices. *J Clin Densitom*. 2003;6(3):251-258.
9. Brommage R. Validation and calibration of DEXA body composition in mice. *Am J Physiol Endocrinol Metab*. 2003;285(3):E454-E459.
10. Johnston SL, Peacock WL, Bell LM, Lonchampt M, Speakman JR. PIXImus DXA with different software needs individual calibration to accurately predict fat mass. *Obes Res*. 2005;13(9):1558-1565.
11. Gasser JA, Ingold P, Venturiere A, Shen V, Green JR. Long-term protective effects of zoledronic acid on cancellous and cortical bone in the ovariectomized rat. *J Bone Miner Res*. 2008;23(4):544-551.
12. Armamento-Villareal R, Sheikh S, Nawaz A, et al. A new selective estrogen receptor modulator, CHF 4227.01, preserves bone mass and microarchitecture in ovariectomized rats. *J Bone Miner Res*. 2005;20(12):2178-2188.
13. Silva MJ, Touhey DC. Bone formation after damaging *in vivo* fatigue loading results in recovery of whole-bone monotonic strength and increased fatigue life. *J Orthop Res*. 2007;25(2):252-261.
14. McCann RM, Colleary G, Geddis C, et al. Effect of osteoporosis on bone mineral density and fracture repair in a rat femoral fracture model. *J Orthop Res*. 2008;26(3):384-393.
15. Beamer WG, Donahue LR, Rosen CJ, Baylink DJ. Genetic variability in adult bone density among inbred strains of mice. *Bone*. 1996;18(5):397-403.
16. Breen SA, Loveday BE, Millest AJ, Waterton JC. Stimulation and inhibition of bone formation: use of peripheral quantitative computed tomography in the mouse *in vivo*. *Lab Anim*. 1998;32(4):467-476.
17. Schmidt C, Priemel M, Kohler T, et al. Precision and accuracy of peripheral quantitative computed tomography (pQCT) in the mouse skeleton compared with histology and microcomputed tomography (microCT). *J Bone Miner Res*. 2003;18(8):1486-1496.
18. Martin-Badosa E, Amblard D, Nuzzo S, Elmoutaouakkil A, Vico L, Peyrin F. Excised bone structures in mice: imaging

at three-dimensional synchrotron radiation micro CT. *Radiology*. 2003;229(3):921-928.

19. Fajardo RJ, Cory E, Patel ND, et al. Specimen size and porosity can introduce error into microCT-based tissue mineral density measurements. *Bone*. 2009;44(1):176-184.
20. Kapadia RD, Stroup GB, Badger AM, et al. Applications of micro-CT and MR microscopy to study pre-clinical models of osteoporosis and osteoarthritis. *Technol Health Care*. 1998;6(5–6):361-372.
21. Bonnet N, Laroche N, Vico L, Dolleans E, Courteix D, Benhamou CL. Assessment of trabecular bone microarchitecture by two different x-ray microcomputed tomographs: a comparative study of the rat distal tibia using Skyscan and Scanco devices. *Med Phys*. 2009;36(4):1286-1297.
22. Waarsing JH, Day JS, Weinans H. An improved segmentation method for *in vivo* microCT imaging. *J Bone Miner Res*. 2004;19(10):1640-1650.
23. Alexander JM, Bab I, Fish S, et al. Human parathyroid hormone 1-34 reverses bone loss in ovariectomized mice. *J Bone Miner Res*. 2001;16(9):1665-1673.
24. Muller R, Van Campenhout H, Van Damme B, et al. Morphometric analysis of human bone biopsies: a quantitative structural comparison of histological sections and micro-computed tomography. *Bone*. 1998;23(1):59-66.
25. Fanuscu MI, Chang TL. Three-dimensional morphometric analysis of human cadaver bone: microstructural data from maxilla and mandible. *Clin Oral Implants Res*. 2004;15(2): 213-218.
26. Chappard D, Retailleau-Gaborit N, Legrand E, Basle MF, Audran M. Comparison insight bone measurements by histomorphometry and microCT. *J Bone Miner Res*. 2005;20(7): 1177-1184.
27. Hankenson KD, Hormuzdi SG, Meganck JA, Bornstein P. Mice with a disruption of the thrombospondin 3 gene differ in geometric and biomechanical properties of bone and have accelerated development of the femoral head. *Mol Cell Biol*. 2005;25(13):5599-5606.
28. von Stechow D, Zurakowski D, Pettit AR, et al. Differential transcriptional effects of PTH and estrogen during anabolic bone formation. *J Cell Biochem*. 2004;93(3):476-490.
29. Christiansen BA, Silva MJ. The effect of varying magnitudes of whole-body vibration on several skeletal sites in mice. *Ann Biomed Eng*. 2006;34(7):1149-1156.
30. Squire M, Donahue LR, Rubin C, Judex S. Genetic variations that regulate bone morphology in the male mouse skeleton do not define its susceptibility to mechanical unloading. *Bone*. 2004;35(6):1353-1360.
31. Uthgenannt BA, Silva MJ. Use of the rat forelimb compression model to create discrete levels of bone damage *in vivo*. *J Biomech*. 2007;40(2):317-324.
32. Naik AA, Xie C, Zuscik MJ, et al. Reduced COX-2 expression in aged mice is associated with impaired fracture healing. *J Bone Miner Res*. 2009;24(2):251-264.
33. Gardner MJ, Ricciardi BF, Wright TM, Bostrom MP, van der Meulen MC. Pause insertions during cyclic *in vivo* loading affect bone healing. *Clin Orthop Relat Res*. 2008;466(5): 1232-1238.
34. Duvall CL, Taylor WR, Weiss D, Wojtowicz AM, Guldberg RE. Impaired angiogenesis, early callus formation, and late stage remodeling in fracture healing of osteopontin-deficient mice. *J Bone Miner Res*. 2007;22(2):286-297.
35. Shen X, Wan C, Ramaswamy G, et al. Prolyl hydroxylase inhibitors increase neoangiogenesis and callus formation following femur fracture in mice. *J Orthop Res*. 2009;27(10): 1298-1305.
36. Gerstenfeld LC, Sacks DJ, Pelis M, et al. Comparison of effects of the bisphosphonate alendronate versus the RANKL inhibitor denosumab on murine fracture healing. *J Bone Miner Res*. 2009;24(2):196-208.
37. Morgan EF, Mason ZD, Chien KB, et al. Micro-computed tomography assessment of fracture healing: relationships among callus structure, composition, and mechanical function. *Bone*. 2009;44(2):335-344.
38. Duvall CL, Taylor WR, Weiss D, Guldberg RE. Quantitative microcomputed tomography analysis of collateral vessel development after ischemic injury. *Am J Physiol Heart Circ Physiol*. 2004;287(1):H302-H310.
39. Duvall CL, Weiss D, Robinson ST, Alameddine FM, Guldberg RE, Taylor WR. The role of osteopontin in recovery from hind limb ischemia. *Arterioscler Thromb Vasc Biol*. 2008;28(2):290-295.
40. Chen RR, Snow JK, Palmer JP, et al. Host immune competence and local ischemia affects the functionality of engineered vasculature. *Microcirculation*. 2007;14(2):77-88.
41. Guldberg RE, Lin AS, Coleman R, Robertson G, Duvall C. Microcomputed tomography imaging of skeletal development and growth. *Birth Defects Res C Embryo Today*. 2004;72(3):250-259.
42. Wang Y, Wan C, Deng L, et al. The hypoxia-inducible factor alpha pathway couples angiogenesis to osteogenesis during skeletal development. *J Clin Invest*. 2007;117(6):1616-1626.
43. Abruzzo T, Tumialan L, Chaalala C, et al. Microscopic computed tomography imaging of the cerebral circulation in mice: feasibility and pitfalls. *Synapse*. 2008;62(8):557-565.
44. Suo J, Ferrara DE, Sorescu D, Guldberg RE, Taylor WR, Giddens DP. Hemodynamic shear stresses in mouse aortas: implications for atherogenesis. *Arterioscler Thromb Vasc Biol*. 2007;27(2):346-351.
45. Awad HA, Zhang X, Reynolds DG, Guldberg RE, O'Keefe RJ, Schwarz EM. Recent advances in gene delivery for structural bone allografts. *Tissue Eng*. 2007;13(8):1973-1985.
46. Rai B, Oest ME, Dupont KM, Ho KH, Teoh SH, Guldberg RE. Combination of platelet-rich plasma with polycaprolactone-tricalcium phosphate scaffolds for segmental bone defect repair. *J Biomed Mater Res A*. 2007;81(4): 888-899.
47. Palmer AW, Guldberg RE, Levenston ME. Analysis of cartilage matrix fixed charge density and three-dimensional morphology via contrast-enhanced microcomputed tomography. *Proc Natl Acad Sci USA*. 2006;103(51):19255-19260.
48. Waarsing JH, Day JS, van der Linden JC, et al. Detecting and tracking local changes in the tibiae of individual rats: a novel method to analyse longitudinal *in vivo* micro-CT data. *Bone*. 2004;34(1):163-169.
49. Boyd SK, Moser S, Kuhn M, et al. Evaluation of three-dimensional image registration methodologies for *in vivo* micro-computed tomography. *Ann Biomed Eng*. 2006;34(10): 1587-1599.
50. Boyd SK, Davison P, Muller R, Gasser JA. Monitoring individual morphological changes over time in ovariectomized rats by *in vivo* micro-computed tomography. *Bone*. 2006; 39(4):854-862.

51. Campbell GM, Buie HR, Boyd SK. Signs of irreversible architectural changes occur early in the development of experimental osteoporosis as assessed by *in vivo* micro-CT. *Osteoporos Int*. 2008;19(10):1409-1419.
52. Buie HR, Moore CP, Boyd SK. Postpubertal architectural developmental patterns differ between the L3 vertebra and proximal tibia in three inbred strains of mice. *J Bone Miner Res*. 2008;23(12):2048-2059.
53. Brouwers JE, Lambers FM, Gasser JA, van Rietbergen B, Huiskes R. Bone degeneration and recovery after early and late bisphosphonate treatment of ovariectomized wistar rats assessed by *in vivo* micro-computed tomography. *Calcif Tissue Int*. 2008;82(3):202-211.
54. Brouwers JE, van Rietbergen B, Huiskes R, Ito K. Effects of PTH treatment on tibial bone of ovariectomized rats assessed by *in vivo* micro-CT. *Osteoporos Int*. 2009;20(11): 1823-1835.
55. McErlain DD, Appleton CT, Litchfield RB, et al. Study of subchondral bone adaptations in a rodent surgical model of OA using *in vivo* micro-computed tomography. *Osteoarthritis Cartilage*. 2008;16(4):458-469.
56. Morenko BJ, Bove SE, Chen L, et al. *In vivo* micro computed tomography of subchondral bone in the rat after intra-articular administration of monosodium iodoacetate. *Contemp Top Lab Anim Sci*. 2004;43(1):39-43.
57. Dare A, Hachisu R, Yamaguchi A, Yokose S, Yoshiki S, Okano T. Effects of ionizing radiation on proliferation and differentiation of osteoblast-like cells. *J Dent Res*. 1997;76(2):658-664.
58. Klinck RJ, Campbell GM, Boyd SK. Radiation effects on bone architecture in mice and rats resulting from *in vivo* micro-computed tomography scanning. *Med Eng Phys*. 2008;30(7):888-895.
59. Nuzzo S, Lafage-Proust MH, Martin-Badosa E, et al. Synchrotron radiation microtomography allows the analysis of three-dimensional microarchitecture and degree of mineralization of human iliac crest biopsy specimens: effects of etidronate treatment. *J Bone Miner Res*. 2002;17(8):1372-1382.
60. Burghardt AJ, Wang Y, Elalieh H, et al. Evaluation of fetal bone structure and mineralization in IGF-I deficient mice using synchrotron radiation microtomography and Fourier transform infrared spectroscopy. *Bone*. 2007;40(1): 160-168.
61. Matsumoto T, Yoshino M, Asano T, Uesugi K, Todoh M, Tanaka M. Monochromatic synchrotron radiation muCT reveals disuse-mediated canal network rarefaction in cortical bone of growing rat tibiae. *J Appl Physiol*. 2006;100(1): 274-280.
62. Raum K, Hofmann T, Leguerney I, et al. Variations of microstructure, mineral density and tissue elasticity in B6/C3H mice. *Bone*. 2007;41(6):1017-1024.
63. Schneider P, Stauber M, Voide R, Stampanoni M, Donahue LR, Muller R. Ultrastructural properties in cortical bone vary greatly in two inbred strains of mice as assessed by synchrotron light based micro- and nano-CT. *J Bone Miner Res*. 2007;22(10):1557-1570.
64. Kinney JH, Ryaby JT, Haupt DL, Lane NE. Three-dimensional *in vivo* morphometry of trabecular bone in the OVX rat model of osteoporosis. *Technol Health Care*. 1998;6(5–6):339-350.
65. Muller R, Koller B, Hildebrand T, Laib A, Gianolini S, Ruegsegger P. Resolution dependency of microstructural properties of cancellous bone based on three-dimensional mu-tomography. *Technol Health Care*. 1996;4(1):113-119.
66. Brodt MD, Pelz GB, Taniguchi J, Silva MJ. Accuracy of peripheral quantitative computed tomography (pQCT) for assessing area and density of mouse cortical bone. *Calcif Tissue Int*. 2003;73(4):411-418.
67. Hamrick MW, Pennington C, Newton D, Xie D, Isales C. Leptin deficiency produces contrasting phenotypes in bones of the limb and spine. *Bone*. 2004;34(3):376-383.
68. Glatt V, Canalis E, Stadmeyer L, Bouxsein ML. Age-related changes in trabecular architecture differ in female and male C57BL/6J mice. *J Bone Miner Res*. 2007;22(8):1197-1207.
69. Judex S, Garman R, Squire M, Donahue LR, Rubin C. Genetically based influences on the site-specific regulation of trabecular and cortical bone morphology. *J Bone Miner Res*. 2004;19(4):600-606.
70. Ridler T, Calvard S. Picture thresholding using an iterative selection method. *IEEE Trans Syst Man Cybern*. 1978;SMC-8(8):630-632.
71. Meinel L, Fajardo R, Hofmann S, et al. Silk implants for the healing of critical size bone defects. *Bone*. 2005;37(5): 688-698.
72. Tommasini SM, Hu B, Nadeau JH, Jepsen KJ. Phenotypic integration among trabecular and cortical bone traits establishes mechanical functionality of inbred mouse vertebrae. *J Bone Miner Res*. 2009;24(4):606-620.
73. Davey RA, MacLean HE, McManus JF, Findlay DM, Zajac JD. Genetically modified animal models as tools for studying bone and mineral metabolism. *J Bone Miner Res*. 2004; 19(6):882-892.

6 Methods in Bone Biology in Animals: Biochemical Markers

Markus Herrmann

6.1 Introduction

Osteoporosis represents a chronic disease, which is usually preceded by an extended period of time during which bone metabolism is already disturbed. In humans this period can last for more than a decade. Clinically osteoporosis is characterized by loss of bone mass and reduced biomechanical properties resulting in an increased risk of fragility fractures. However, these changes occur late and reflect the sum of a disturbed bone metabolism over an extended period of time. Biochemical bone turnover markers (BTMs) are helpful tools in closing this gap by capturing adverse changes in bone metabolism at a much earlier point in time, when structural damage has not yet occurred.[1,2] Usually BTMs react quickly to changes in bone metabolism. Therefore, a single BTM result can be considered a snapshot of current bone metabolism. In addition, repeated measurements allow real-time monitoring of bone metabolism, providing information about changes as they occur. While histology, microcomputerized tomography (μCT), bone mineral density (BMD), or x-rays are limited to specific anatomical sites, BTMs give an overall estimate of bone metabolism in the entire organism. In the light of the systemic nature of osteoporosis this is usually considered an advantage. However, it should be kept in mind that in some local forms of osteoporosis the utility of BTMs can be limited. Furthermore, in individuals with anatomically confined conditions other than osteoporosis (e.g., fractures or infections) BTM results may not reliably reflect overall bone metabolism.[3,4] While fracture healing and osteoarthritis of large joints, such as the knee, significantly affect bone turnover,[3,4] other local conditions, such as osteonecrosis or bone marrow edema, do not.[5,6]

Theoretically, BTMs are very useful tools for the assessment of bone disease. However, their use is hampered by a number of limitations.[1,2] The fact that there are more than ten different BTMs indicates that the ideal BTM does not exist as yet. Therefore, the right choice of BTMs is the first hurdle that researchers have to take before starting any experiment. Moreover, most BTMs are affected by a number of exogenous and endogenous interfering factors (e.g., gender, circadian rhythm, food intake, etc.).[1,2,7] Some interfering factors, such as food intake can induce variability of up to 100% and more. Consequently, the experimental design and standardization of blood sampling is crucial in order to obtain meaningful results. Moreover, knowledge about interfering factors is required for appropriate interpretation of BTM results. Lastly, it needs to be mentioned that the natural kinetics of BTMs differ in some animal species from humans (e.g., rats), which is mainly due to continuous growth throughout their entire life span.

This chapter intends to provide a comprehensive overview of all relevant aspects that require consideration during the planning, performance, and analysis of animal studies in the field of osteoporosis. Since the vast majority of studies have been conducted in rats, mice, and sheep this chapter focuses mainly on these species. Nevertheless, most points apply to many other species as well. In the light of the limited space and the countless studies available, this chapter does not aim to be all-encompassing. However, the author has tried to touch all relevant aspects that researchers need to take into account.

M. Herrmann
Ageing Bone Research Centre, Sydney Medical School – Nepean Campus, The University of Sydney, Penrith, NSW 2750, Australia
e-mail: markus.herrmann@sydney.edu.au

G. Duque and K. Watanabe (eds.), *Osteoporosis Research*,
DOI: 10.1007/978-0-85729-293-3_6,

6.2 Bone Turnover and Bone Remodeling

The concept of bone turnover is essential for the understanding of the utility of BTMs. Bone is a metabolically active tissue undergoing constant turnover.[8-11] The continuous replacement of old and damaged bone by new bone tissue enables the bones to adapt to various mechanical challenges. Bone remodeling involves bone resorption and formation, which under normal circumstances are tightly regulated in order to ensure that these two counteracting processes are well balanced.[8-11] Any imbalance between bone resorption and formation will result in a change of bone mass. Bone turnover occurs in four phases and requires osteoblasts, osteoclasts, and osteocytes as these are the major cells involved.[2,11] These three cell types cooperate in close spatial proximity forming a structure called bone remodeling unit (BRU; Fig. 6.1).

During the initial resorption phase CD14+ monocytes are recruited from the circulation. Once attached to the bone surface they fuse with other monocytes and differentiate into mature multinucleated osteoclasts.[2,10,11] The differentiation of monocytes into osteoclasts requires the action of macrophage colony stimulating factor (MCSF) and receptor activator of NF-κB ligand (RANKL). The newly formed osteoclasts create a sealed space underneath their basal "ruffled border" membrane into which they secrete protons (acid) and proteolytic enzymes (cathepsin K [CPK], metalloproteinases). While acids dissolve inorganic minerals (hydroxyapatite) from the bone matrix proteases digest matrix proteins, such as collagen type I. The result is a resorption lacuna, which during the subsequent formation phase is colonized by osteoblasts. This process requires the help of growth factors, such as transforming growth factor beta (TGF-β). The resorption lacuna is then filled with newly formed non-mineralized bone (osteoid). During the final mineralization phase calcium phosphate is deposited in the osteoid forming hydroxyapatite crystals. At the end of the formation phase most osteoblasts are eliminated by apoptosis. However, some cells survive and become incorporated in the bone matrix where they reside as osteocytes. Osteocytes form a three-dimensional (3D) network of cell protrusions which has important regulatory functions that are not fully understood as yet.

The activity of each BRU is regulated by complex interaction of local (paracrine/autocrine) and systemic (endocrine) factors. Osteoclasts are activated by endocrine (vitamin D, estrogens, and androgens) and paracrine (IL-1, IL-6, TGF-β, and RANKL) signals. While some of these signals act directly on osteoclasts and their precursor cells (steroid hormones, TGF-β, interleukines), others stimulate osteoclasts indirectly by modulating osteoblast function (e.g., parathyroid hormone (PTH), parathyroid-related peptide [PTHrP]) The activation of osteoblasts then induces the secretion of paracrine signal molecules, such as RANKL, which stimulate mature osteoclasts as well as the recruitment of osteoclast precursor cells. Osteoprotegerin (OPG) is another paracrine protein secreted by osteoblasts. OPG functions as a "pseudo-receptor" for RANKL that captures and thereby inactivates RANKL. RANKL bound to OPG cannot bind to its primary receptor RANK anymore and therefore is inactive. Thus, OPG acts as an inhibitor of the RANK/RANKL system and thereby reduces the formation of active osteoclasts.

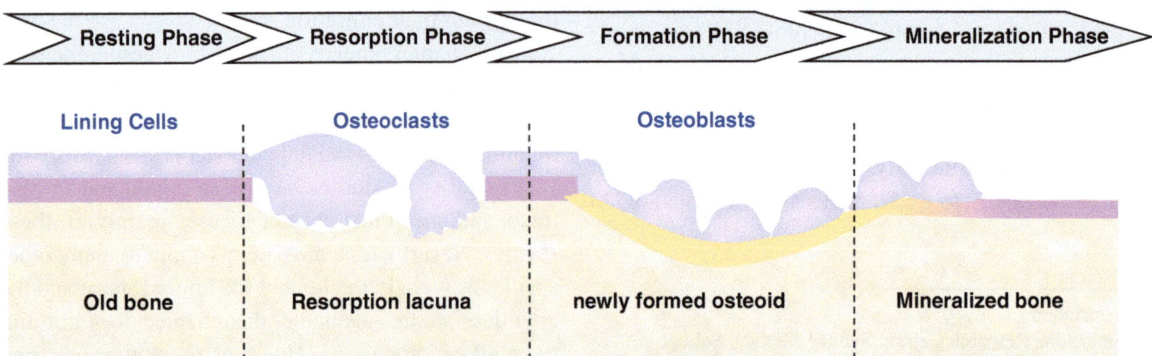

Fig. 6.1 Illustration of bone remodeling. Under normal conditions, the resorption phase (osteoclast) takes approximately 10 days, which is then followed by a formation phase (osteoblast) that can last for up to 3 months

6.3 What Bone Turnover Markers Are Available?

This section gives an overview of the most relevant BTMs. It explains their biochemical nature and what type of information can be obtained with each marker.

As mentioned above, there is a broad spectrum of BTMs available.[2,12,13] Generally, BTMs provide information about the activity of osteoblasts and osteoclasts and can be divided in bone formation and resorption markers (Table 6.1). Of note, BTMs are not specific for any disease. They just reflect changes in bone metabolism

Table 6.1 Overview of bone turnover markers (BTMs) in animals

Marker	Biochemical process	Description	Species forwhich assays are available
CTX-I	Bone resorption	C-terminal cross-linked telopeptide of type-I collagen; CTX-I is generated by cathepsin K and released during osteoclastic bone resorption; *not species-specific*	Rat, mouse, pig, dog, guinea pig, cattle, monkey, rabbit
NTX-I	Bone resorption	N-terminal cross-linked telopeptide of type-I collagen; NTX-I is generated by cathepsin K and released during osteoclastic bone resorption; *not species-specific*	Rat, mouse, pig, guinea pig, dog, cattle, rabbit, monkey
ICTP	Pathologic bone resorption (e.g., malignancies)	C-terminal telopeptide of type-I collagen; ICTP is generated by MMPs and is released during pathologic bone resorption (e.g., metastases); *not species-specific*	Rat, mouse, dog, cattle, sheep, reindeer, horse
Pyridinoline cross-links (PYD, DPD)	Bone resorption	Deoxypyridinolines (DPD) and pyridineolines (PYD) are found in mature collagen and are released during bone resorption; *not species-specific*	Rat, mouse, dog, cattle, pig, rabbit, guinea pig, sheep, horse, squirrel, monkey
Hydroxyproline	Bone resorption	Hydroxyproline is found in the triple helices of collagen and is released during bone resorption; *not species-specific*	Not species specific
TRAP/TRAP5b	Osteoclastnumber	Tartrate-resistant acid phosphatase 5b (TRAP5b) is an enzyme specifically produced by osteoclasts and involved in the intracellular processing of degraded organic bone matrix	*TRAP5b* (*ELISA*): Mouse, rat *TRAP* (*enzymatic test*): all species
Cathepsin K	Osteoclast number	Cathepsin K is the essential protease for collagen degradation and is mainly produced by osteoclasts; *high homology across species*	Rat, mouse, cattle, dog, pig, rabbit, fish, birds
Osteocalcin	Bone turnover/formation and resorption Hormone in energy metabolism	Osteoblast-specific protein which is released into the bone matrix and the circulation; during bone resorption osteocalcin is also released from the extracellular matrix	Rat, mouse guinea pig, cattle, dog, monkey, rabbit, chicken
BSAP	Osteoblast differentiation	Alkaline phosphatase is a family of enzymes, where BASP is specifically produced by osteoblasts	*Wheat-germ lectin precipitation*: dog, horse monkey *ELISA*: mouse, rat
PINP/PICP	Bone or collagen type I formation	The C- and N-terminal propeptides of type-I collagen are released from newly synthesized preprocollagen prior to incorporation of collagen molecules into the bone matrix; *not species-specific*	Mouse, rat, cattle, dog, pig, rabbit, guinea pig, monkey, chicken

Modified from Sorensen et al.[12]

independently of the underlying disease. A meaningful analysis of bone turnover should be based on the measurement of at least one bone formation and one resorption marker. It is important to consider that for some markers species-specific assays are required. Often the same protein differs slightly between species and therefore the antibody of an immunoassay may not recognize the somewhat different epitope (e.g., procollagen type I propeptide [PINP], osteocalcin [OC]). Even between closely related rodent species, such as mice and rats, assays are sometimes not interchangeable.

Besides their classification into bone formation and resorption markers BTMs can also be categorized into enzymatic, collagenous, and non-collagenous markers.[2,12,13] While enzymatic markers, such as bone-specific alkaline phosphatase (BSAP) or tartrate resistant acid phosphatase 5b (TRAP5b), measure osteoclast number and specific aspects of cellular activity, collagenous markers, such as PINP and type-I collagen breakdown (CTX), reflect the actual formation and breakdown of collagen type I, the main component of the organic extracellular bone matrix. Therefore the choice of BTMs should always be driven by the question that an experiment is designed to answer. For example, if an experiment is to analyze immediate changes in osteoblast activity after administration of a drug, BSAP would probably be the preferred marker. If information about newly formed bone matrix is required, PINP would be the first choice. Table 6.1 gives an overview of BTMs that are commercially available.

6.3.1 Bone Formation Markers

Bone formation markers are synthesized by osteoblasts and hence reflect their biologic activity. The formation of new bone matrix occurs in three phases including osteoblast proliferation and synthesis of new bone matrix, maturation of the newly formed extracellular matrix, and lastly calcification of the matrix. Bone formation markers are considered to reflect different aspects of osteoblast function and therefore the pattern of circulating bone formation marker levels varies between the different phases of bone formation.[14-17] BSAP is the characteristic marker of the proliferation phase (days 1–12), PINP and PICP characterize the phase of matrix maturation (days 12–20), and OC is mainly expressed during the matrix mineralization (starting around day 20). All markers of bone formation are measured in serum or plasma. Enzyme-linked immunosorbent assay (ELISA), radioimmunoassay (RIA), or enzymatic tests are the most commonly used techniques for the measurement of bone formation markers.

6.3.1.1 Non-collagenous Markers

Bone-specific alkaline phosphatase (*BSAP*):[2,12,13,18] BSAP is a tetrameric enzyme attached to the outer cell surface. Although it is a widely used bone formation marker its actual function is yet unknown. However, it appears to be involved in osteoid formation and mineralization. BSAP is an isoenzyme of total alkaline phosphatase (ALP). Other abundant tissue-specific ALP isoforms are liver and kidney ALP. In fully grown individuals with a normal liver function BSAP and liver ALP are the abundant isoforms and each of these isoenzymes accounts for approximately 50% of the total ALP activity in serum. In young growing animals and species that grow throughout their entire life span (e.g., rats) the bone-specific isoenzyme predominates because of skeletal growth.

In the past a variety of techniques (e.g., precipitation, electrophoresis) have been used to selectively measure individual ALP isoforms. Today, circulating BSAP is predominantly quantified by immunoassays using specific antibodies for BSAP. However, similar to most immunoassays even these assays show a certain degree of cross-reactivity with isoforms other than bone.

Osteocalcin (*OC*):[2,12,13,18] OC is the most abundant non-collagenous extracellular matrix protein in bone and is exclusively synthesized by osteoblasts. The molecule possesses three γ-carboxylation sites at position 17, 21, and 24. Carboxylation of OC is a posttranslational process that confers on the protein a high affinity for minerals, such as calcium. Therefore, carboxylated OC, which represents the predominant fraction of OC secreted by osteoblasts, is readily incorporated into the calcium-rich extracellular bone matrix where it constitutes approximately 15% of the non-collagenous protein fraction. Non- or undercarboxylated OC (depending on the degree of carboxylation) has a low affinity for minerals and is therefore released into the circulation. Circulating OC levels have been shown to correlate well with the bone formation rate as assessed by histomorphometry. Due to its exclusive expression in osteoblasts OC, for a long time, was considered the most specific marker of osteoblast function. However, since OC is an abundant component of the extracellular bone matrix it is also released during bone resorption. Consequently, OC is now considered more as a BTM rather than a bone formation marker.

Interestingly, decades of intensive research have not been able to ascribe OC a distinct function in bone. However, the undercarboxylated fraction of OC (ucOC), which after its release is not trapped in the bone matrix, has recently been found to act as a superordinate hormone in glucose and lipid metabolism.[19,20] ucOC has been shown to stimulate β-cell proliferation, insulin expression, and secretion. Moreover, high concentrations of ucOC also lower blood lipids and reduce body fat. In the light of the current paradigm shift regarding OC function, researchers should be cautious using OC as a bone formation marker.

When measuring OC it is important to consider that the protein is subject to rapid degradation resulting in very short *in vivo* and *ex vivo* half-lives. Consequently, intact protein and OC fragments of various sizes coexist in the circulation. Of note, only one-third of the total OC serum pool represents intact OC. *Ex vivo* the intact OC molecule degrades within 1–2 h while fragments, such as the mid-fragment, are much more stable. Generally it is recommended to process blood samples immediately. Blood samples should be centrifuged within 30–60 min after sampling and if required stored at −80°C until measurement. Repeated freezing and thawing causes a substantial loss of intact OC while stable OC fragments are much less affected. Four freeze and thaw cycles result in an average loss of mid-fragment immunoreactivity between 10% and 25%. In addition, mid-fragment levels are not affected by 2 years of storage at −80°C. Commercial OC assays measure either intact OC or fragments, such as the mid-fragment. Whenever samples cannot be processed in a very short period of time assays measuring stable fragments, such as the mid-fragment, are preferred.

6.3.1.2 Collagenous Markers

Telopeptides of procollagen type I (PINP and PICP):[2,12,13,18] Collagen type I is the predominant component of the organic bone matrix accounting for approximately 90%. The molecule is synthesized by osteoblasts as preprocollagen type I. After intracellular cleavage of terminal signal sequences procollagen type-I triple helices are secreted into the extracellular space. Procollagen type I is characterized by N- and C-terminal extension-peptides named amino (N-)terminal propeptide (PINP) and carboxy (C-)terminal propeptide (PICP). Once procollagen is secreted into the extracellular space procollagen peptidase cleaves PICP and PINP forming collagen type I. This cleavage permits the formation of proper collagen fibrils. PINP and PICP are eluted into the circulation where they can be measured by ELISA. Since both PICP and PINP are generated from newly synthesized collagen in a stoichiometric fashion, they are considered quantitative measures of the amount of newly formed collagen type I. Although collagen type I is the most abundant form of collagen in bone it is also present in other tissues such as skin, dentin, cornea, vessels, fibrocartilage, and tendons. However, nonskeletal tissues expressing collagen type I turn over their extracellular matrix at a much lower rate than bone, and therefore contribute very little to the circulating propeptide pool.

Compared to OC, PINP and PICP are relatively stable analyses and are not affected by extended transport and storage times.

6.3.2 Bone Resorption Markers

Bone resorption markers are either synthesized by osteoclasts (e.g., TRAP5b, CPK) or released from the extracellular bone matrix during degradation of the same by osteoclats (CTX-I, NTX-I). Similar to bone formation markers bone resorption markers can be divided into collagenous (CTX-I, NTX-I) and noncollagenous markers (TRAP5b, CPK). While noncollagenous markers, such as TRAP5b and CPK, are considered markers of osteoclast number, collagenous markers, such as CTX-I and NTX-I, reflect actual bone resorption. Although a number of techniques such as high-performance liquid chromatography (HPLC) (pyridinoline cross-links) or photometry (calcium) are used to measure bone resorption markers immunoassays are the predominant technology (CTX-I, NTX-I).

6.3.2.1 Non-collagenous Markers

Tartrate resistant phosphatase type 5b (TRAP5b):[2,12,13,18] TRAP5b belongs to a group of phosphatases that are only active under acid conditions. The group consists of five isoenzymes, which can be separated by electrophoresis. The various isoforms are expressed by different tissues and cells such as prostate, bone, spleen, platelets, erythrocytes, and macrophages. The name TRAP5 is derived from the unique characteristic of band 5 to be inhibited by tartrate. In addition, there are two subforms of TRAP5 named TRAP5a and TRAP5b. While TRAP5b is specifically expressed in osteoclasts the origin of TRAP5a is still unclear.

TRAP5b contributes to the intracellular processing of primary bone matrix degradation products and is finally released through the basolateral membrane of resorbing OCs into the circulation.[21-23] The enzyme has been used as a marker of osteoclast function for more than 20 years and has been shown to be a specific and sensitive indicator of bone resorption.[24-30] Today TRAP5b is considered more a marker of osteoclast number rather than an indicator of bone resorption activity.

Traditionally TRAP is measured by enzymatic methods using colorimetry for detection. However, these methods detect both isoforms without differentiating between TRAP5a and TRAP5b. This problem has been resolved by the recent introduction of immunoassays where TRAP5b is detected by specific antibodies. While the TRAP5b protein is stable the enzymatic activity has been shown to decline by 20% per hour. Addition of citrate to the sample can prevent the decrease in TRAP activity. Regardless of which method is used, appropriate pre-analytical sample handling is essential for the accurate measurement of TRAP5b. If measurement can't be performed immediately samples should be processed within 1 h and stored at−80°C.

Cathepsin K: (CPK):[12,31-34] Bone resorption by osteoclasts is caused mainly by acid (inorganic matrix) and lysosomal proteases (organic matrix), which are released through the ruffled border area into the space between the cell membrane and extracellular bone matrix (resorption lacuna). The most important protease involved in this process is CPK.[35,36] CPK is a cysteine protease featuring the unique ability to cleave both helical and telopeptide regions of collagen I.[2] Although CPK and its role in bone resorption have been long known it is just recently that CPK has been recognized as a bone resorption marker. As a consequence, the utility of CPK as a bone resorption marker in osteoporosis is not yet fully established. However, initial data indicate that serum concentrations of CPK reflect osteoclastic activity in patients with postmenopausal osteoporosis, Paget's disease, and rheumatoid arthritis.[31,33,34]

6.3.2.2 Collagenous Markers

N- and C-terminal telopeptides of collagen type I (CTX-I and NTX-I):[2,7,12,13,18] NTX-I and CTX-I are degradation products of type-I collagen (Fig. 6.2). Collagen type I is the major organic component of extracellular bone matrix and is present as a triple helix. Pyridinium (PYD) cross-links covalently link individual collagen molecules within the triple helix (Fig. 6.2). The main molecular sites involved in collagen cross-linking are the short non-helical peptides at both ends of the collagen molecule, termed amino (N-) and carboxy (C-) terminal telopeptides. In normal collagen, these telopeptides are each linked via PYD or pyrrole compounds to the helical portion of neighboring collagen molecules. During collagen breakdown, N- and C-terminal telopeptide fragments of various sizes, still attached to the helical portions of a nearby molecule by a PYD or pyrrole cross-link, are released into the circulation. NTX-I and CTX-I are readily cleared by the kidneys. Hence, they can be measured in both serum and urine. Since NTX-I and CTX-I are also present in tissues other than bone, non-skeletal processes may influence their circulating or urinary levels.

For both markers a large body of clinical and experimental data shows their clinical utility as integral markers of bone resorption. Similar to all other BTMs abnormal CTX-I and NTX-I levels do not provide information about the underlying cause. Hence, abnormal CTX-I and NTX-I results should always be interpreted against the background of their basic science and phenotypic picture. CTX-I and NTX-I are among the most commonly used BTMs in animal studies. However, their utility is hampered by substantial intra- and interindividual variability (see later).

No general recommendation can be given as to which material is preferred. The correlation between urinary and serum measurements of BTMs is an

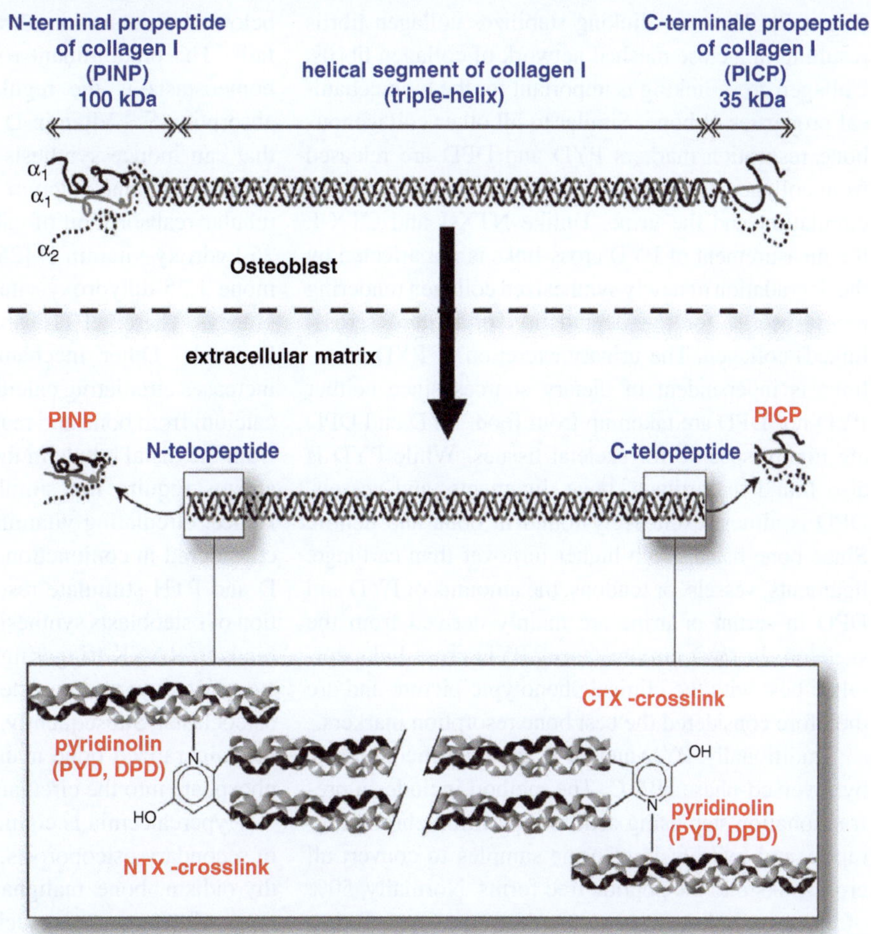

Fig. 6.2 Formation and structure of collagenous BTMs (Modified from McCudden and Kraus[37])

important and partly unresolved issue. Although urine and serum levels of CTX-I and NTX-I correlate well the correlation coefficient varies over a wide range (r=0.5–0.9). From a practical point of view, serum or plasma is preferable as it avoids problems regarding urine collection from experimental animals.

Carboxyterminal type-I collagen telopeptide (ICTP):[2,7,38-42] Although this marker is much less used than CTX-I and NTX-I it may be particularly useful or even be superior to the other two telopeptide markers of type-I collagen in some circumstances. ICTP represents exactly the same telopeptide region as CTX-I but the actual epitope detected by the antibody consists of a slightly different amino acid sequence to the alpha 1 chain of collagen type I. Similar to CTX-I the epitope of ICTP covers a cross-link-containing region and requires a trivalent cross-link for detection. Divalently and non-cross-linked peptides do not react with the antibody of the test, nor do peptides isolated from skin.

Although osteoporosis is a pathologic condition the bone resorption process involved is similar to normal bone turnover and therefore considered physiologic. ICTP appears to be a sensitive marker of pathological bone resorption as seen in multiple myeloma and metastatic bone disease. Its generation requires the action of matrix metalloproteinases (MMP).[38] While the marker is particularly useful in malignant bone disease it does not reflect the increased bone resorption seen in osteoporosis, which is probably due to the fact that MMPs do not play a major role in osteoclast-mediated resorption under osteoporotic conditions.

Pyridinium (PYD) and deoxypyridinium (DPD) cross-links:[2,12,18] PYD and DPD are small trivalent molecules linking individual collagen type I molecules within the collagen triple helix as well as different fibrils

(Fig. 6.2). The cross-linking stabilizes collagen fibrils resulting in a close meshed network of collagen fibrils. Collagen cross-linking is important for the biomechanical properties of bone. Similar to all other collagenous bone resorption markers PYD and DPD are released from collagen during bone resorption and appear in the circulation and the urine. Unlike NTX-I and CTX-I, the measurement of PYD cross-links is not affected by the degradation of newly synthesized collagen rendering them specific for the degradation of mature (cross-linked) collagen. The urinary excretion of PYD cross-links is independent of dietary sources since neither PYD nor DPD are taken up from food. PYD and DPD are highly specific for skeletal tissues. While PYD is also found in cartilage, bone, ligaments, and vessels, DPD is almost exclusively found in bone and dentin. Since bone has a much higher turnover than cartilage, ligaments, vessels, or tendons, the amounts of PYD and DPD in serum or urine are mainly derived from the skeleton. In most circumstances PYD cross-links correlate best with the clinical/phenotypic picture and are therefore considered the best bone resorption markers.

Traditionally, PYD and DPD are quantified in urine by reversed-phase HPLC. The method includes a pre-fractionation step using cellulose partition chromatography, and hydrolysis of urine samples to convert all cross-links into the peptide free forms. Normally, 50% of the cross-links are present in their free form. Today, immunoassays measuring free and peptide-bound cross-links are widely used. Most of these assays have been found to perform similarly to the traditional HPLC technique. In addition, PYD and DPD can be measured in urine and blood.

6.3.3 Other Parameters of Interest

Calcium (Ca), vitamin D [25(OH–D)], and parathyroid hormone (PTH): Homeostasis of the serum calcium concentration is critical for the maintenance of bone health.[43] Healthy bones require appropriate calcification of their extracellular matrix. Mineralization of the extracellular bone matrix depends on constant and sufficient circulating calcium levels. Calcium and phosphate homeostasis is achieved by the interaction of vitamin D and PTH, with both hormones being inversely related.[43-45] Under normal conditions, the serum calcium level is supersaturating with respect to bone mineral requirements. If plasma calcium falls below the saturation threshold bone mineralization fails. The predominant role of vitamin D in calcium homeostasis is the regulation of intestinal calcium absorption.[43-45] Vitamin D is the only known hormone that can induce synthesis of the proteins involved in active intestinal calcium absorption. PTH regulates tubular reabsorption of calcium and the conversion of 25-hydroxy-vitamin D [25(OH)D] into the active hormone 1,25-dihydroxy-vitamin D [1,25(OH)$_2$D] in the kidneys. Thereby PTH can compensate for low 25(OH) D levels. Other mechanisms by which vitamin D increases circulating calcium levels are mobilization of calcium from bone and reabsorption of filtered calcium from the distal tubule in the kidneys. Both these mechanisms require the simultaneous presence of PTH. Hence, circulating vitamin D levels should always be considered in conjunction with PTH. In bone, vitamin D and PTH stimulate resorption indirectly by activation of osteoblasts synthesizing RANKL. RANKL then binds to RANK triggering the transformation of preosteoclasts into mature osteoclasts and activates resting osteoclasts. Subsequently, active osteoclasts dissolve the mineralized bone matrix and release calcium and phosphate into the circulation.

Hypercalcemia is commonly found in certain types of secondary osteoporosis, such as primary hyperparathyroidism, bone malignancies, or metastases. Other types of osteoporosis, such as secondary osteoporosis due to vitamin D deficiency, are characterized by normal calcium levels. Therefore, the quantification of circulating calcium should be an essential component of every biochemical study in osteoporosis. Approximately 45% of total circulating calcium is bound to proteins (especially albumin) and therefore inactive. Ionized calcium represents the biologically active form of calcium and is directly regulated by PTH and 1,25(OH)$_2$D. Thus, wherever possible ionized calcium should be measured. Unlike ionized calcium, total calcium varies with varying blood protein concentrations and therefore does not reliably reflect the biologically active ionized calcium concentration. A decrease of circulating albumin by 1 mg/dl results in a reduction of total calcium by 0.25 mmol/l. Therefore, total calcium figures should always be corrected mathematically for the total protein concentration.

The reference method for the quantification of total calcium is atomic absorption spectroscopy (AAS). Alternative techniques are flame photometry or photometric tests (e.g., O-cresolphtaleine). Ionized calcium is usually measured by ion-selective electrodes.

The term vitamin D summarizes a group of fat-soluble pro-hormones, which are derived from cholesterol. The two major circulating forms of vitamin D are 25-hydroxy vitamin D_2 (synonym: ergocalciferol; abbreviation $25(OH)D_2$) and 25-hydroxy vitamin D_3 (synonym: cholecalciferol; abbreviation $25(OH)D_3$), with the latter being the predominant species under physiological circumstances.[43-45] For most purposes the 25(OH)D concentration is considered the best measure of vitamin D status. Its concentration is about three orders of magnitude higher than that of the active hormone $1,25(OH)_2D$ and it has a long half-life in the circulation of approximately 3 weeks. In addition, the conversion of 25(OH)D into $1,25(OH)_2D$ is tightly regulated, with circulating calcium being one of its main determinants. Therefore, when circulating calcium is high, such as in primary hyperparathyroidism, $1,25(OH)_2D$ levels do not longer reflect the organism's vitamin D supply.

Vitamin D is very stable and can (although it is not recommended) be stored at room temperature for several days. Repeated freezing and thawing causes a slight increase in vitamin D. Commercially available immunoassays can measure either $25(OH)D_3$ alone or $25(OH)D_3$ and $25(OH)D_2$ together. The recent introduction of liquid chromatography tandem mass spectrometry (LC-MS/MS) permits simultaneous measurement of all 25(OH)D species with reporting of separate figures for $25(OH)D_3$ and $25(OH)D_2$. However, measurement of 25(OH)D by LC-MS/MS requires sophisticated and expensive technical equipment as well as experienced staff. Quantification of $1,25(OH)_2D$ is difficult since circulating levels are very low. The most commonly used method is RIA. However, this method requires a relatively large sample volume and involves a manual extraction step. Therefore, the measurement of $1,25(OH)_2D$ is only recommended when 25(OH)D does not provide sufficient information.

PTH is a polypeptide containing 84 amino acids. It is secreted by the parathyroid glands in order to increase the circulating concentration of calcium.[43-45] *In vivo* PTH has a half-life of approximately 4 min and a molecular mass of 9.4 kDa. Secretion of PTH is regulated by a negative feedback loop where calcium-sensing receptors located on parathyroid cells constantly monitor the blood calcium level.

PTH(1–84) and a variety of peptide fragments, such as the PTH(7–84) or PTH^{1-35} fragment, are present simultaneously in peripheral blood. Indeed, the concentration of PTH fragments is severalfold greater than the concentration of the intact hormone itself. Some of these fragments arise from the metabolism of PTH(1–84) in various tissues, most notably liver, whereas others are released from the parathyroid glands directly, probably reflecting the intracellular degradation of PTH(1–84) within parathyroid cells. Of note, PTH fragments have variable biological activity. PTH(7–84), for example, decreases serum calcium concentrations in parathyroidectomized rats and antagonizes the effect of PTH(1–84) on bone.

Circulating PTH levels can be measured in several different forms: intact PTH(1–84); N-terminal PTH(1–34); mid-molecule PTH(44–68); and C-terminal PTH(39–84).[46,47] Today specific tests for most of these forms are commercially available. Immunoassay (ELISA) is the preferred detection method. Generally it is recommended to use a later-generation intact PTH assay that does not interfere with any abundant PTH fragment. Earlier assays were frequently affected by such fragments and therefore provided sometimes-unreliable results. Attention should be paid to the cross-reactivity of intact PTH(1–84) assays with PTH(7–84). There are still multiple assays available detecting both PTH(1–84) and PTH(7–84). The use of assays for specific PTH fragments should be limited to specific questions, such as bone metabolism in animal models of renal failure and chronic kidney disease.

6.4 Variability

All BTMs are subject to significant variability. Therefore, knowledge of the sources of variability and the strategies used to cope with "background noise" are essential for the meaningful interpretation of bone markers.

6.4.1 Technical Sources of Variability

In addition to parameters of assay performance, factors such as the choice of sample (i.e., serum, plasma, or urine), the mode of sample collection (e.g., pre-sampling diet/fasting/physical activity before sample collection), as well as the correct handling, processing, and storage of specimens are all important as these technical sources of variability are modifiable and hence controllable.

6.4.1.1 Thermodegradation

Some BTMs are subject to rapid thermodegradation. Intact OC is probably the most temperature-sensitive of all the BTMs with significant loss of signal within 1 h after blood sampling.[2] Therefore, samples must be centrifuged and frozen promptly. Serum and plasma samples should be stored at –80°C until measurement. Moreover, samples can only be thawed once. If these very strict pre-analytical requirements cannot be guaranteed a more stable degradation fragment, such as the mid-fragment, should be measured.[48]

Samples for *BSAP* measurement also need careful pre-analytical sample handling as the enzyme is relatively unstable. Serum and plasma samples can be kept for up to 2 h at ambient temperature and for 2 days at 4°C in the refrigerator. Thereafter freezing at –20°C to –80°C is required. Repeated freezing and thawing does not affect BSAP readings.

PINP and PICP are stable at room temperature for up to 24 h. If samples cannot be processed on the same day, they can be kept in the refrigerator for 5 days. If longer storage is required they need to be frozen preferably at –80°C.

Serum *β-CTX-I* levels have been shown to decrease by up to 30% if kept at room temperature for more than 1 day. At 4°C, serum β-CTX-I levels are stable for up to 5 days. No comparable studies are available for serum NTX-I. Both, urinary CTX-I and NTX-I are stable at room temperature for at least 3 days. At –20°C, the epitope quantified by the NTX-I assay denatures significantly within 4 months. This change is usually masked by the simultaneous decrease in creatinine. Several freeze–thaw cycles of urine samples have no effect on the concentrations of urinary CTX-I and NTX-I.

TRAP activity declines rapidly at room temperature and even at –20°C but is stable when stored at –70°C or lower.[49] Multiple freeze–thaw cycles usually have a deleterious effect on serum TRAP activity.

Pyridinoline cross-links in urine are stable for 3 days at room temperature and 1 week in the refrigerator. At –20°C they can be stored for years.

Calcium and vitamin D are very stable analytes. Although it is not recommended, serum and plasma samples can be kept for days at room temperature. Repeated freezing and thawing tends to slightly increase vitamin D levels. *PTH* shows variable stability. While some studies found intact PTH levels in ethylenediaminetetraacetic acid (EDTA) samples stable over 2 days at room temperature, others reported a 10% reduction after 48 h of storage at 4°C. In serum, PTH levels are more variable than in EDTA plasma and some manufacturers do not recommend serum as a suitable specimen any longer.

6.4.1.2 Diurnal Variation

Most BTMs are subject to significant diurnal variation with daily amplitudes between 20% and 50%.[2,7] However, the most pronounced diurnal changes (up to 90%) have been reported for CTX-I. Of note, some animal species, such as minipigs show an inverse circadian cycle when compared to humans or other animal species (Fig. 6.3). A recent study in minipigs has reported peak levels for OC and NTX-I at 18:00 h and nadirs at 6:00 h.[50] The etiology of the diurnal variation is unknown. Several hormones, such as PTH, growth hormone, or cortisol, show diurnal changes and may therefore be involved.[2] *In the light of substantial diurnal variation blood and urine sampling needs to be standardized and always performed at the same time of the day.* The preferred time depends on the animal species.[50,51] Similar to humans, where blood and urine is normally collected during the morning peak, in animals sample collection should be performed during the daily peak. Since different species have different circadian rhythms researchers need to know about the circadian pattern of the species that they intend to work with.

Measurement of DPD, PYD, CTX-I, and NTX-I is often performed in urine. Therefore, values need to be corrected for urinary creatinine, which introduces additional pre-analytical and analytical variability. Creatinine output has been reported to be fairly constant over time (variations within 10%) but correlates with lean body mass. However, other reports suggest that the correction for creatinine in a urine spot sample could be misleading because the creatinine excretion rate has been found to show a considerable diurnal variation. Serum markers usually show less pronounced changes during the day than urine-based indices and therefore can avoid most of these limitations.

6.4.1.3 Nutrition

In humans it has been shown that food ingestion has immediate effects on bone turnover. A single meal

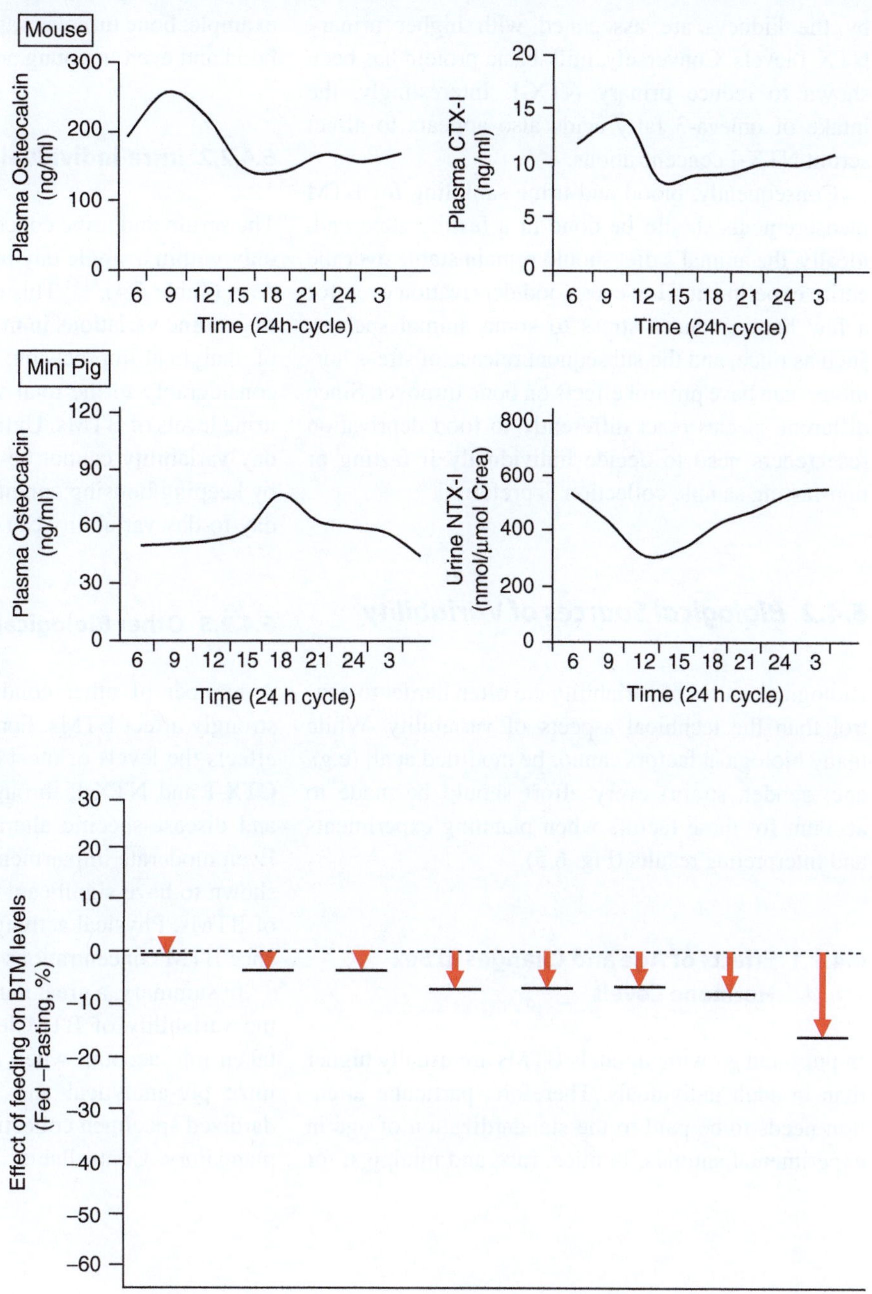

Fig. 6.3 Circadian rhythm of selected BTMs in mice and minipigs. The daily peaks differ significantly between markers and species (Modified from Tsutsumi et al.[50] and Srivastava et al.[51])

Fig. 6.4 Effect of feeding on BTMs (Modified from Clowes et al.[52])

within 60–120 min before blood collection has been shown to reduce serum CTX-I levels by up to 50%. The postprandial reduction of bone resorption is probably mediated by the intestinal release of glucagon-like peptide 2. Although CTX-I appears to be most affected other markers also show a postprandial reduction (Fig. 6.4). Animal studies showing postprandial changes in bone turnover are lacking. However, it is very likely that in many animal species similar changes occur. This assumption arises from existing data demonstrating that most animals show a postprandial release of gastrointestinal hormones, such as glucagon-like peptides, which is similar to humans.

In addition to the above, the composition of the diet over a longer period of time also affects bone resorption. Dietary changes that increase net acid excretion by the kidneys are associated with higher urinary NTX-I levels. Conversely, milk basic protein has been shown to reduce urinary NTX-I. Interestingly, the intake of omega-3 fatty acids also appears to affect serum NTX-I concentrations.

Consequently, blood and urine sampling for BTM measurements should be done in a fasting state and, ideally, the animal's diet should remain stable over the entire experiment. However, food deprivation even for a few hours induces stress to some animal species, such as mice, and the subsequent release of stress hormones can have prompt effects on bone turnover. Since different species react differently to food deprivation researchers need to decide individually if fasting or non-fasting sample collection is preferred.

6.4.2 *Biological Sources of Variability*

Biological causes of variability are often harder to control than the technical aspects of variability. While many biological factors cannot be modified at all (e.g., age, gender, strain) every effort should be made to account for these factors when planning experiments and interpreting results (Fig. 6.5).

6.4.2.1 Effects of Age and Changes in Sex Hormone Levels

In pups and growing animals BTMs are usually higher than in adult individuals. Therefore, particular attention needs to be paid to the standardization of age in experimental animals. In mice, rats, and minipigs, for example, bone turnover rapidly decreases during childhood and even in young adults (Fig. 6.6).

6.4.2.2 Intra-individual Variation

The serum and urine concentrations of BTMs vary not only within a single day but also between consecutive days (Table 6.4).[53,54] This day-to-day variability is due to genuine variations in marker levels and not because of analytical imprecision. Day-to-day variability adds considerably to the total variation of both serum and urine levels of BTMs. Unlike diurnal variation, day-to-day variability cannot be controlled easily. However, by keeping housing conditions as constant as possible day-to-day variability can be minimized.

6.4.2.3 Other Biological Sources of Variability

A number of other conditions have been shown to strongly affect BTMs. For example, renal impairment affects the levels of most collagenous BTMs, such as CTX-I and NTX-I, through both impaired clearance and disease-specific alterations in bone metabolism. Even moderate impairment of renal function has been shown to have significant effects on circulating levels of BTMs. Physical activity and immobility also influence BTM concentrations in an independent fashion.

In summary, a great number of factors contribute to the variability of BTM levels and hence need to be taken into account when measuring BTMs. To minimize pre-analytical and analytical variability, standardized specimen collection and sample handling are mandatory. Controllable factors such as the mode of

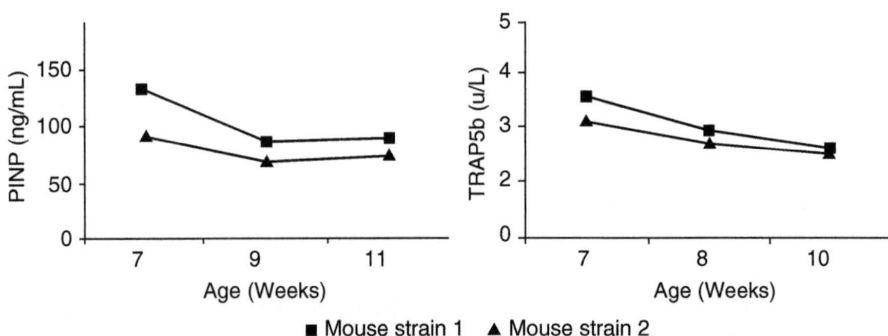

Fig. 6.5 Age-related decrease of PINP and TRAP5b in mice

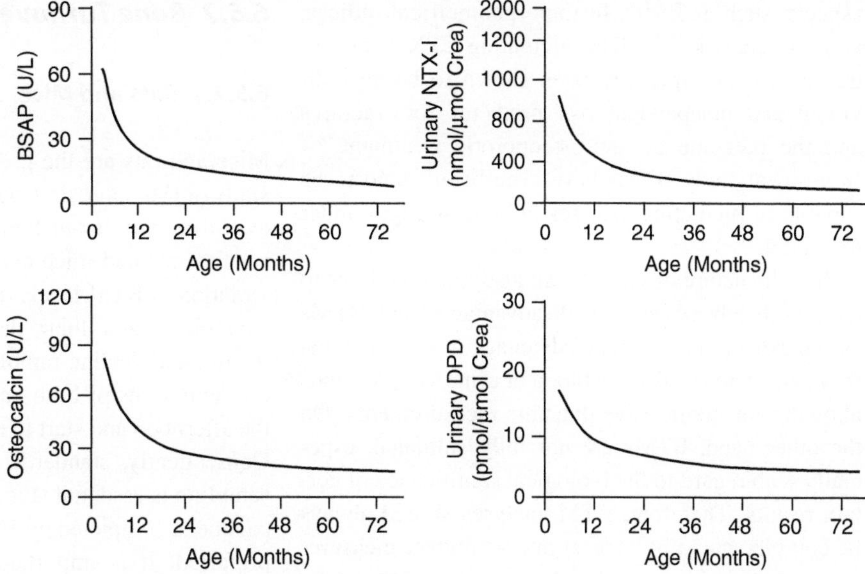

Fig. 6.6 Age-related decrease of various BTMs in minipigs (Modified from Tsutsumi et al.[50])

sample collection, sample handling, storage, diurnal rhythm, and food intake should be standardized whenever possible.

6.5 Animal Specific Considerations

While the use of BTMs in experimental animals is often similar to that in humans there are significant differences and pitfalls requiring consideration. The selection of BTMs should be tailored to the animal model and experimental design employed. In the existing literature numerous models have been described and used in order to investigate a great variety of aspects of osteoporosis. Since mice, rats, sheep, cats, and dogs are the prevailing species in the scientific literature this section will mainly focus on these.

6.5.1 General Aspects

Before measuring any BTM it is essential to bear in mind that BTMs are not disease-specific. However, they are most useful in assessing a variety of physiologic and pathologic conditions in a dynamic fashion. Furthermore, BTMs are very helpful for the monitoring of new treatment strategies since they allow noninvasive serial measurements.[12] Although BTMs closely correlate with most key clinical characteristics of bone quality, such as histomorphometrical and biomechanical indices, the partly unresolved problem of variability requires results to be validated against other relevant methods, such as histomorphometry, dual energy X-ray absorption (DEXA), μCT scans, or biomechanical testing.[12] Most of these methods provide unique and direct information about various important aspects of bone biology, such as bone structure and mass, as well as biomechanical aspects that BTMs cannot supply. On the down side, most of these methods are laborious, require expensive equipment, and can only be done once since animals need to be sacrificed before the analysis can be performed. Furthermore, some methods, such as histomorphometry, are often overestimated by researchers. Histomorphometry, for example, has substantial variability mainly due to technical factors. Although variability can be reduced by the use of experienced staff the degree of standardization remains significantly lower than for most BTMs. One of the main problems is that histomorphometrical indices represent a snapshot of the very specific regions from which sections have been obtained. Even more importantly, structural data as obtained from histomorphometry or μCT do not always correlate with the biomechanical properties of bone. On the other hand, BTM results have been shown to correlate well with many relevant aspects, such as BMD, histomorphometrical indices, and fracture risk.[28,55-57] The circulating CTX-I concentration, for example, has been shown to be an individual and independent risk predictor for fractures and the outcome of anti-osteoporotic treatment.[58,59] In a recent study BTMs have even been found to be capable of predicting changes in bone strength under treatment.[56]

It is the nature of virtually all analytical methods to have both advantages and disadvantages and BTMs are no exception. The main advantage of BTMs is that they can be done easily on blood or urine samples, thus allowing for noninvasive dynamic measurements. On the other hand, BTMs are not fully validated, especially with regard to the biological significance of certain results. Therefore, BTM analyses should always be complemented by at least one secondary measurement such as histomorphometry or μCT. While the results from alternative measures, such as μCT or dynamic histomorphometry, are validated and provide detailed information they are labor-intensive and require sacrifice of the animals. However, in most cases BTMs correlate well with histomorphometrical and μCT data.

6.5.2 Bone Turnover in Selected Species

6.5.2.1 Rats and Mice

Mice and rats are the preferred animal species in the study of osteoporosis. Therefore a large body of data is available. Similar to humans and most other animal species rats and mice exhibit a pronounced circadian variation of BTM levels (Fig. 6.7). CTX-I and OC, for example, reach their daily peak at approximately 9 a.m., and decline rapidly thereafter. The circulating concentrations of both parameters remain low during the afternoon and start to rise again in the late evening. Consequently, standardization of the time of blood sampling is essential (Fig. 6.8). If morning collections cannot be completed by 10 a.m., afternoon samples are preferred. It is important to avoid blood collection between 10 a.m. and 3 p.m., the period when BTM levels change most rapidly. Between-subject variation ranges between 10% and 20% for OC, BSAP, and CTX-I. BSAP has been shown to have very little circadian variation. It is important to bear in mind that other species may have a different circadian cycle. Minipigs,

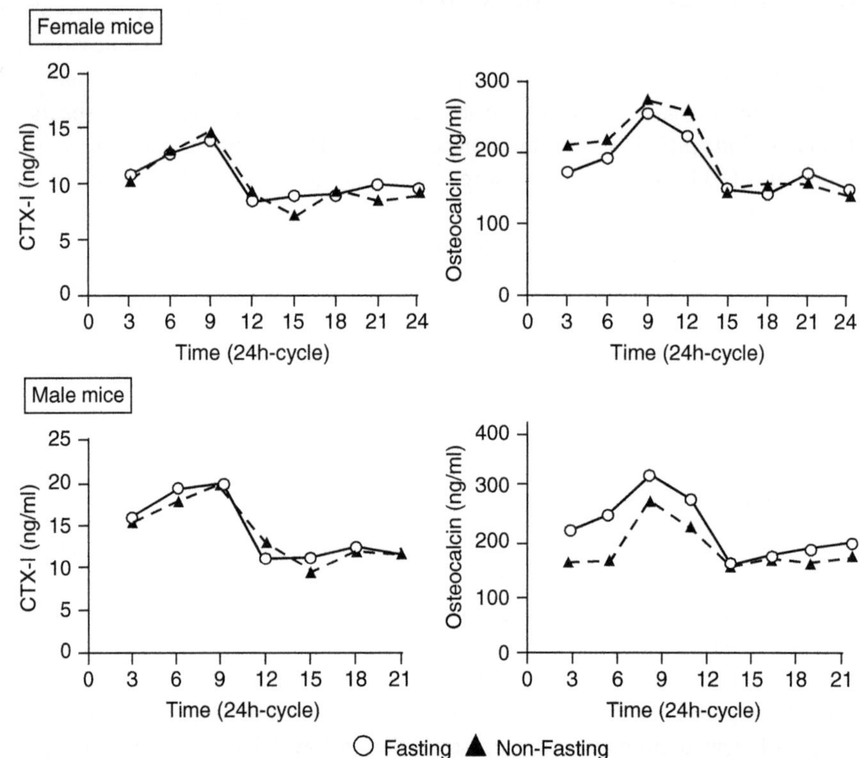

Fig. 6.7 Circadian rhythm of circulating CTX-I and OC levels in fasting and non-fasting mice (Modified from Srivastava et al.[51])

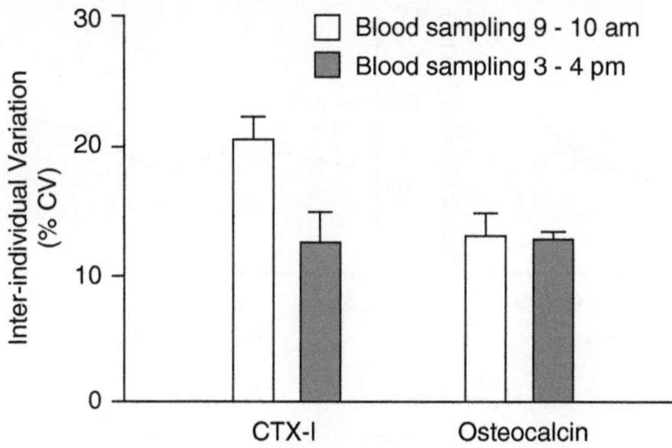

Fig. 6.8 The time of blood collection affects between-subject variability. Afternoon collection is preferred (Modified from Srivastava et al.[51])

for example, exhibit peak levels of OC, NTX-I, and PYD/DPD in the early evening (Fig. 6.3).

A critical point during the planning phase of every study is the calculation of sample size. Considering the substantial natural variation of most BTMs a minimum of seven to ten animals are required when morning blood samples are used (Table 6.2). Due to the lower variability during the afternoon it can be expected that when samples are collected at this time of the day five animals are sufficient to give significant results.

Mice and rats go into menopause very late (15–18 months), thus preventing studies of naturally occurring menopause and postmenopausal osteoporosis. To overcome this obstacle the ovariectomized (OVX) model has been established. Removal of the estrogen-secreting ovaries has been found to be an appropriate model to mimic menopause and postmenopausal bone loss. Male rats are not suitable to study age-related osteoporosis because growth plates do not close before 30 months.

When studying bone turnover in rats and mice it should be considered that both species are very susceptible to mental stress. The stress experienced during blood collection can be sufficient to alter circulating concentrations of BTMs, such as OC. However, an experienced person is normally able to achieve blood collection with minimal mental stress to the animal.

Another factor hampering the measurement of BTMs in mice and rats is a continuous decline of some markers, such as OC, until the age of 12 months (Fig. 6.9). Thus, it is essential to always match experimental animals by age. In young mice a difference in age of just 1 week can result in a significant decline of OC. However, not all markers show the same kinetics. Urinary PYD cross-link levels, for example, are very stable throughout the first 12 months of life.

6.5.2.2 Sheep

Since 1994, the United States Food and Drug Administration (FDA) require data from both the rat and a well-validated large animal model for preclinical evaluation of new experimental drug therapies. When it comes to bone turnover in large animal species, most work has been done in sheep. The circadian pattern of BTMs in sheep closely resembles that in humans with peak levels late at night or early morning.[61] Similar to most other species, plasma levels of markers, such as OC, are high in neonates and continuously decline during childhood and adolescence.[61] Lowest levels are reached at 2–3 years of age (Fig. 6.10). Thereafter, BTMs slightly increase with age. In 7-year-old animals serum OC levels are similar to those of postmenopausal women of approximately 65 years of age. The physiologic response

Table 6.2 Power calculations for selected BTMs in OVX mice accounting for naturally occurring biological variance (Modified from Srivastava et al.[51])

Parameter	Percentage (%) change after OVX	Interindividual CV (%)	Required sample size	Signal to noise ratio
CTX-I	47.8	20.6 (9–10 a.m. sample)	10	2.3
		12.9 (3–4 p.m. sample)	5	3.7
Osteocalcin	47.1	16.4 (9–10 a.m. sample)	7	2.9
		13.3 (3–4 p.m. sample)	5	3.5
BSAP	31.5	12.9 (9–10 a.m. sample)	10	2.4
		12.6 (3–4 p.m. sample)	10	2.5

Sample size for means of two groups to be statistically different ($p<0.01$, two-tailed)

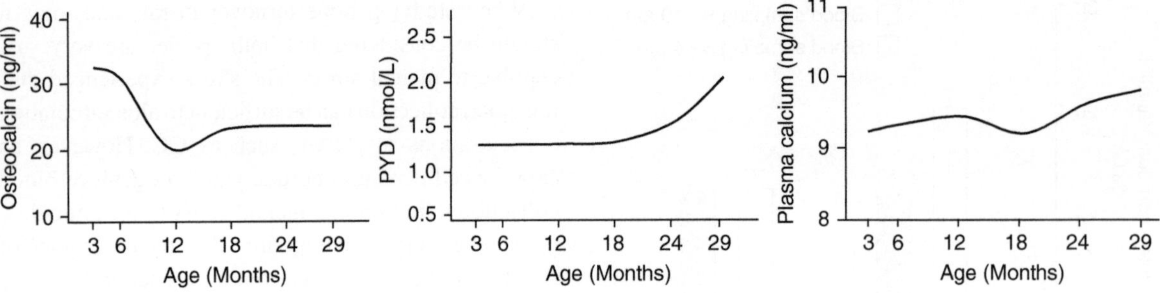

Fig. 6.9 Kinetics of serum OC, PYD, and calcium levels in mice (Modified from Hamrick et al.[60])

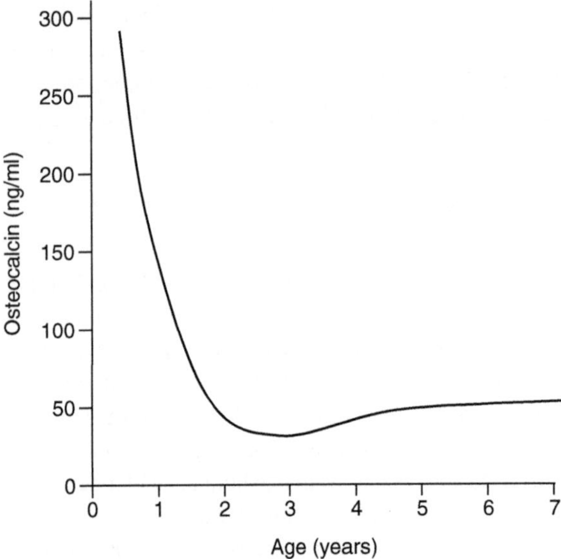

Fig. 6.10 Age-related changes of serum OC in sheep (Modified from Corlett et al.[61])

to a variety of endocrine stimuli is also comparable to those of humans. For example, sheep show reduced OC levels during phosphate depletion and systemic glucocorticoid treatment. Also during pregnancy, delivery, and the postpartum period circulating OC levels show dramatic changes.[62] In pregnancy, ovine plasma OC is lower than in nonpregnant animals of the same age. Within 5–10 days after delivery OC starts to increase, reaching peak levels at 20–24 days. During the subsequent plateau phase (3–6 weeks after delivery) plasma OC levels are three to four times higher than during pregnancy and return to nonpregnant levels thereafter.[62] Ovine OC shares a high degree of homology with the human peptide and closely correlates with histomorphometric indices of bone biopsies from the iliac crest.

Besides OC other BTMs, such as PYD and DPD, have been measured in the urine of sheep.[63] It appears that these markers are also able to demonstrate changes in bone turnover during lactation, glucocorticoid treatment, and OVX.

6.5.2.3 Cats and Dogs

Many of the commercial BTM assays initially developed for humans show substantial cross reactivity with dogs and cats. Therefore, these assays have been widely used in these animals. In domestic cats bone formation can be assessed by measuring BSAP activity in serum by ELISA or by wheat-germ lectin precipitation.[64] The latter method is also able to precipitate BSAP in dogs, horses, monkeys, and humans. For the assessment of bone resorption urinary levels of total (by HPLC) and free (by ELISA) DPD as well as serum and urine levels of CTX-I (ELISA) have been measured.[65]

Longitudinal analyses have shown that similar to most other mammalians bone turnover decreases within the first 1–2 years of life and ceases when skeletal maturity is attained (Fig. 6.11). In cats growth plates close at approximately 9 months. At the same time most BTMs (e.g., DPD, CTX-I) reach a nadir. Unlike most of the other BTMs the growth related decrease of BSAP may take up to 2 years before a plateau is reached.[64] It has been speculated that the delayed decline in BSAP may reflect ongoing mineralization. If correct this would indicate that complete skeletal maturity does not occur until the second year of life, even though longitudinal long bone growth ceases at 9 months of age.

The bone turnover of cats and dogs also shows a circadian rhythm. Except for BSAP, all BTMs attain peak levels in the morning between 4 and 8 a.m. (Table 6.3). Trough levels are usually observed in the afternoon. For BSAP the daily peak is delayed, reaching maximum concentrations between 11 a.m. and 3 p.m.

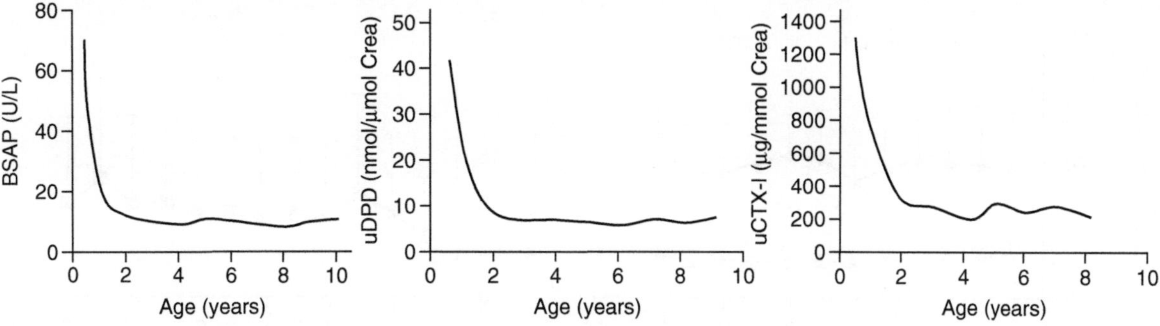

Fig. 6.11 Kinetics of serum OC, urinary DPD, and CTX-I in dogs (Modified from Ladlow et al.[65])

Table 6.3 Circadian pattern of selected BTMs in skeletally mature dogs (Modified from Ladlow et al.[65])

	Time						
	7 a.m.	11 a.m.	3 p.m.	7 p.m.	11 p.m.	3 a.m.	7 a.m.
BSAP(U/L)	14.13±1.71	15.43±4.25	15.45±4.95	14.13±3.77	12.70±2.42	13.10±2.36	13.46±3.58
OC(ng/ml)	18.80±7.10	15.33±5.42	15.60±4.37	16.01±6.09	17.30±6.05	18.48±6.96	19.77±7.62
ICTP(ng/ml)	8.46±2.99	5.51±2.00	5.78±2.56	6.91±2.88	7.28±3.03	7.59±3.55	7.62±3.10
uDPD(nmol/ mmol Crea/L)	0.44±0.15	0.58±0.03	0.40±0.09	0.32±0.12	0.34±0.02	0.50±0.11	0.40±0.07
NTX-I(nmol BCE/ mmol Crea/l)	10.95±4.65	10.11±2.57	11.70±4.36	12.12±3.83	12.86±4.55	13.41±3.43	12.44±2.80

Weekly measurements over a period of 3 months have shown that serum levels of OC, ICTP, and BSAP are very stable over time with an intra-individual coefficient of variation of 14–15% (Fig. 6.12).[65] Urinary markers, such as DPD and NTX-I, appear to be more variable with an intra-individual coefficient of variation of approximately 26%. The correlation between most BTMs is rather poor with correlation coefficients ranging between 0.07 and 0.47. This is a good example for the partly unresolved biological validation of BTM results.

6.5.3 BTMs in Selected Animal Models of Osteoporosis

The most commonly used animal models of osteoporosis would be glucocorticoid-induced osteoporosis and sex hormone deprivation by ovariectomy (OVX, for females) or orchidectomy (ORX, for males). Other relevant models are retinoic acid–induced hypercalcemia, thyroparathyroidectomy (rats), and genetically modified mouse models which mimic osteoporosis, such as OPG knockout mice. OVX of female rats and mice is used to mimic postmenopausal osteoporosis in women while ORX in male animals is used to study age-related osteoporosis in men.

The deprivation of sex hormones accelerates bone turnover substantially (Table 6.2). Although bone formation and resorption are both increased, formation appears to be less affected, resulting in an imbalance in favor of bone resorption. Both OVX and ORX models provide useful tools to assess the pathological mechanism of age-related osteoporosis and to explore potential treatment options.

6.5.3.1 BTMs in OVX/ORX Models

Sex hormone deprivation results in a substantial acceleration of bone turnover across species. Shortly after OVX bone resorption markers increase by up to 150% (Fig. 6.13). With ongoing time bone metabolism attains a steady state at significantly lower BTM levels. In OVX mice, for example, the steady-state levels of OC, CTX-I, and BSAP were 47%, 48%, and 32% higher than before the procedure (Table 6.2). The increase

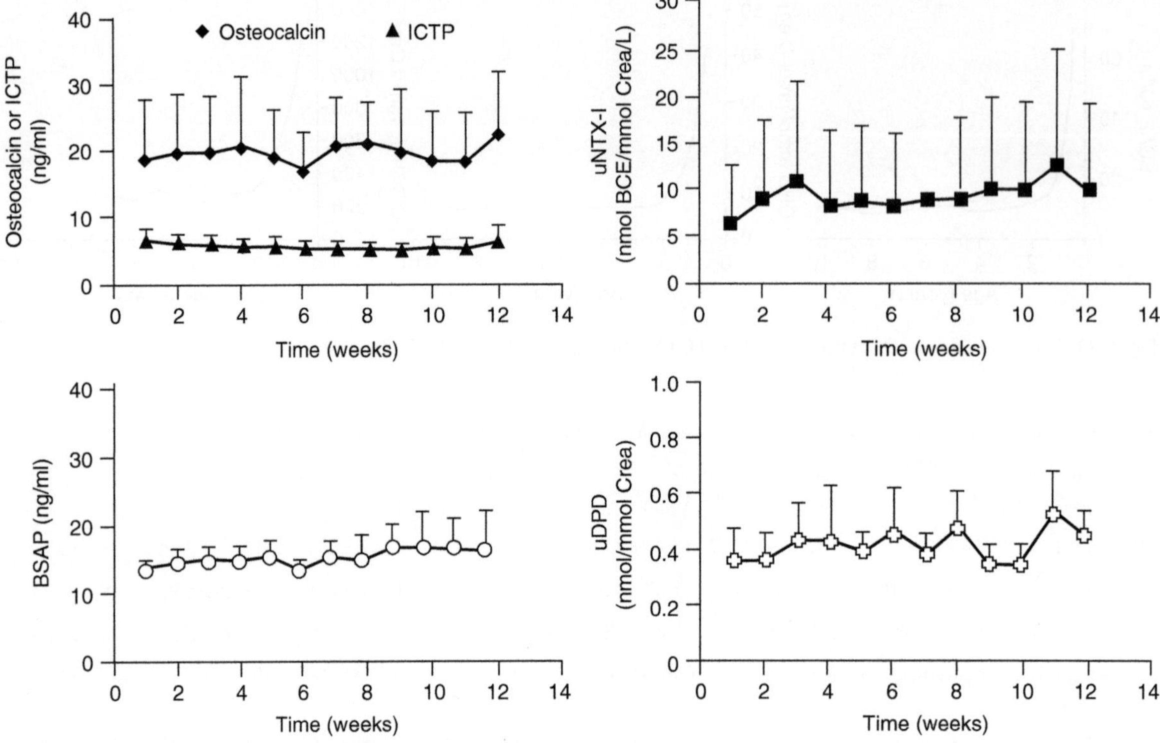

Fig. 6.12 Week-to-week variability of selected BTMs in skeletally mature dogs. Data represent means ± standard deviation from eight animals (Modified from Ladlow et al.[65]). Serial blood sampling in skeletally mature dogs over an extended period of several months

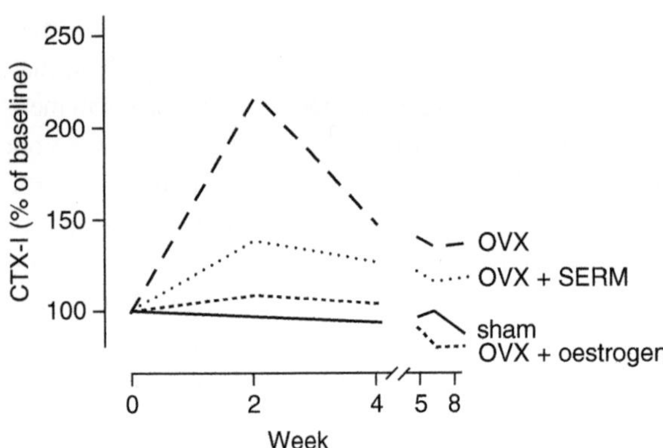

Fig. 6.13 Kinetic of CTX-I in 5-month-old OVX and sham-operated rats. Treatment with estrogen or a SERM ameliorates the increase in bone resorption (Modified from Hoegh-Andersen et al.[66])

in bone turnover is usually accompanied by substantial bone loss, which can be prevented by hormone replacement therapy. In sheep and rats, for example, the OVX-induced rise in bone turnover could be ameliorated by estrogen replacement or selective estrogen receptor modulator (SERM) treatment (Fig. 6.13).[66]]

Although OVX is a well-established model of osteoporosis the age of animals at the time of surgery has a significant impact on changes in bone turnover. In 7-month-old Sprague-Dawley rats, for example, circulating CTX-I levels have been found to increase by 150% within 2 weeks.[66] In contrast, 5-month-old animals of the same strain showed an acceleration of bone turnover not before 5 weeks after surgery and in 50% the degree of this increase was less pronounced (Fig. 6.14).

Sheep show similar kinetics with greater changes of BTM levels in older animals.[63,67] The early peaks of OC and urinary CTX-I in 8-year-old animals exceed 100–150% with a rapid decline thereafter (Fig. 6.15). In younger animals (3 years of age) BSAP and urinary DPD rise by only 25–50%. Most BTMs reach peak concentrations within 2–3 months and return to baseline within 4–5 months.

In OVX sheep changes of BTM levels start to occur within 4 weeks after surgery. The acceleration of BTM levels in sheep and rats is similar in magnitude when compared to human menopause. In sheep the initial rise in BTM levels is reversible within 4–5 months,

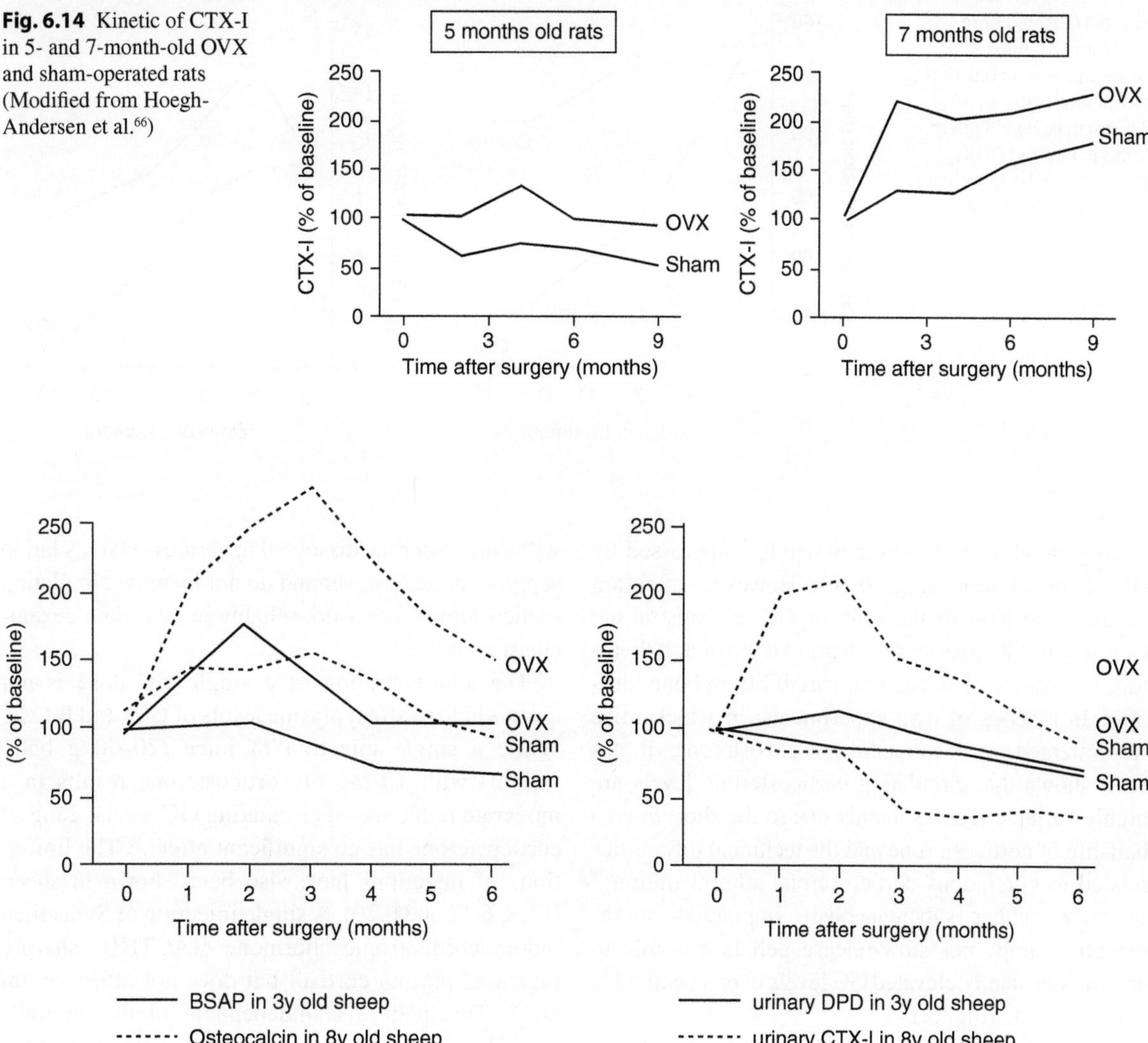

Fig. 6.14 Kinetic of CTX-I in 5- and 7-month-old OVX and sham-operated rats (Modified from Hoegh-Andersen et al.[66])

Fig. 6.15 Kinetics of selected bone formation and resorption markers in 3- and 8-year-old sheep after OVX or sham operation (Modified from Sigrist et al.[63] and Chavassieux et al.[67])

indicating that bone turnover reaches a steady state. In 7-month-old rats BTM levels remain elevated over at least 9 weeks while 5-month-old animals show a return to baseline within 6 weeks.

6.5.3.2 BTMs in Glucocorticoid-Induced Osteoporosis

Systemic glucocorticoid (GC) treatment has been long known to induce bone loss and osteoporosis. Human and animal studies have consistently shown that GCs reduce BMD and trabecular bone mass in a dose-dependent manner. Loss of trabecular bone is considered to be the main cause of increased bone fragility in GC-treated individuals. However, more recent data indicate that cortical bone loss is also involved.[68-73] Numerous studies in animals and humans suggest that the most relevant catabolic skeletal actions of GC target the osteoblast via accelerated apoptosis and decreased expression of Runx-2 and collagen I.[74,75] This results in an impaired osteoblastic lineage commitment, osteoblast differentiation, and function. GCs also favor osteoclastogenesis and increase the life span of mature OC, thereby increasing bone resorption.[76] In the light of the frequent therapeutic use of GCs in humans, animal models of GC-induced osteoporosis have received great attention.

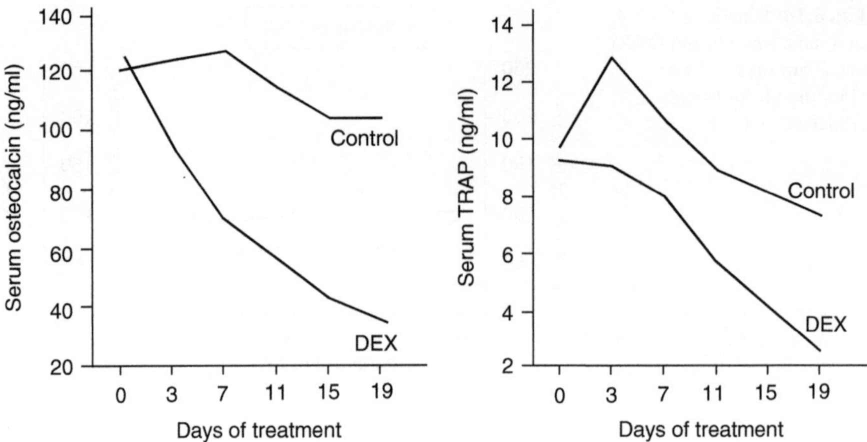

Fig. 6.16 Rapid drop of serum OC and TRAP concentrations in rats during continuous infusion of dexamethasone via micro-osmotic pumps (DEX, 1.2 μg/100 g body weight) (Modified from King et al.[77])

In general, bone turnover is rapidly suppressed by GC administration (Fig. 6.16). However, attention needs to be paid to the type of GC administration. Continuous GC treatment is hard to control and therefore is a source of substantial variability in bone turnover. In a series of own experiments, in which mice were treated with exogenous corticosterone, it has been shown that circulating corticosterone levels are highly variable. This is mainly due to the short *in vivo* half-life of corticosterone and the technical difficulties related to continuous corticosterone administration.[78] In mice neither subcutaneously implanted micro-osmotic pumps nor slow-release pellets are able to achieve constantly elevated GC levels over an extended period of time (Fig. 6.17).

The implantation of a single slow-release pellet containing 10 mg of corticosterone induces a strong elevation of circulating corticosterone levels within 1 day. According to the manufacturer these pellets provide a constant corticosterone release over 21 days. However, by day 7 the increase in plasma corticosterone is fully reversible. Nonetheless, between 1 and7 days after pellet implantation the plasma OC level remains suppressed but returns to baseline concentration by day 14. Only the once-weekly implantation of a slow-release pellet is reliably able to suppress plasma OC levels in mice over an extended period of time. Low-dose treatment with weekly implanted 1.5 mg corticosterone pellets has also been found to reduce bone turnover (Fig. 6.18). With such a treatment regime other BTMs, such as TRAP5b and PINP, are also significantly lowered (Fig. 6.16). While micro-osmotic pumps loaded with corticosterone dissolved in various solvents fail to suppress bone turnover and do not increase circulating corticosterone they work reliably in rats when dexamethasone is used.

The administration of a single GC dose is not always able to affect plasma levels of GCs and BTMs. While a single injection of mice (20–30 g body weight) with 10 mg of corticosterone results in a moderate reduction of circulating OC levels, 2 mg of corticosterone has no significant effect.[78] The limitations of injections have also been shown in sheep (Figs. 6.19 and 6.20). A single injection of Synacthen (adrenocorticotropic hormone [ACTH]) sharply increases plasma cortisol but does not affect serum OC.[61] This pattern is independent of the animal's age. However, daily injections of depot Synacthen into sheep results in a continuous elevation of plasma cortisol and a prompt and sustained suppression of OC within 3–4 days.[61] It has also been shown that a daily injection of 16 mg of methylprednisone for 3 months reduces histomorphometric parameters of bone formation but has no effect on serum levels of BSAP and OC.[79]

On the other hand, five prednisone injections per week over a 7-month period (calculated dose 0.60 mg/kg/day) into skeletally mature sheep causes a substantial drop in serum OC and ALP (Fig. 6.20).[82] Continuous infusion of prednisone (0.7–1 mg/h) into sheep over 6 days has also been shown to lower plasma OC significantly.[80]

In summary, a single dose of GCs is not able to reliably change BTM levels. Only very high doses of

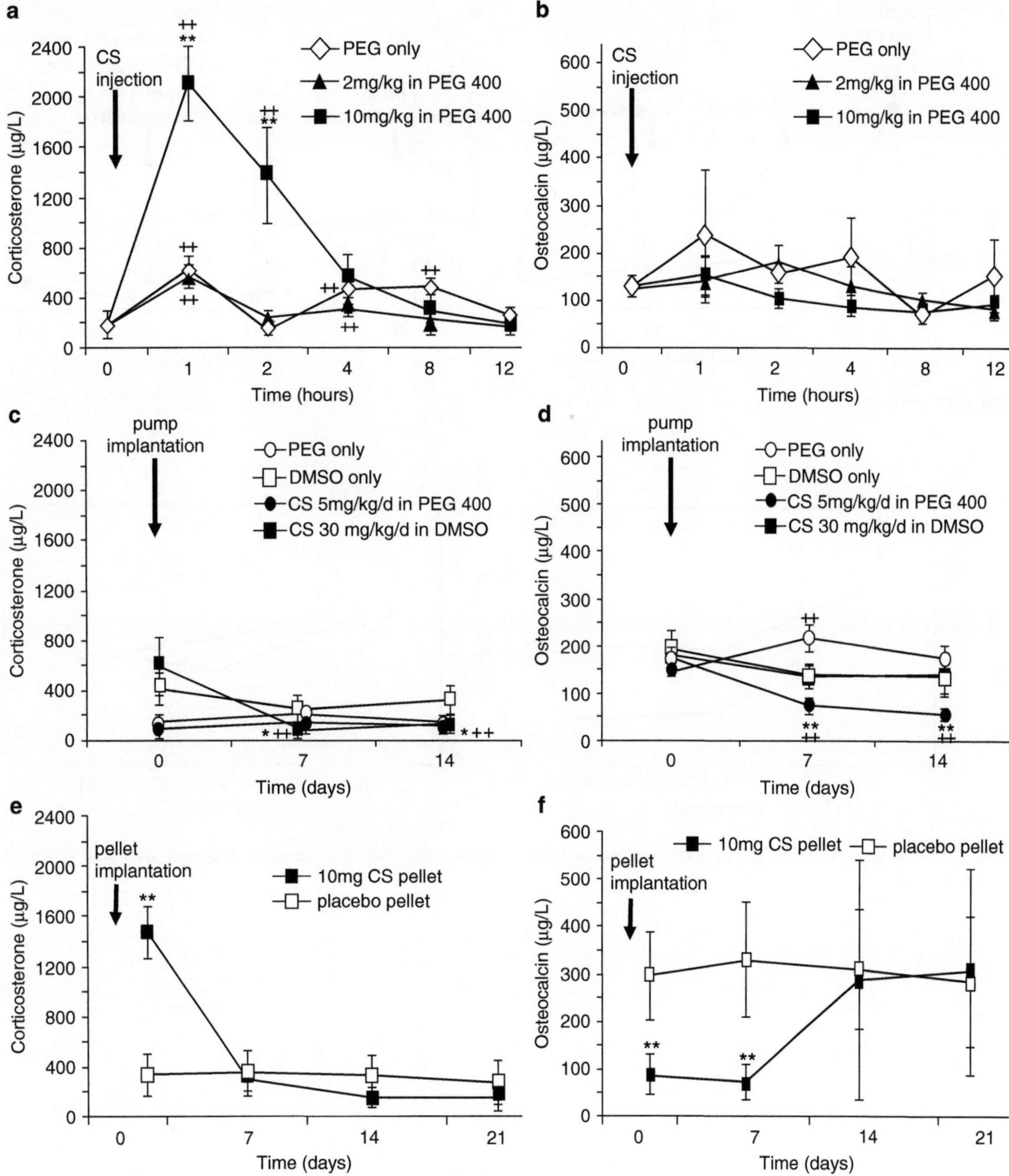

Fig. 6.17 Changes in corticosterone and OC plasma levels over time. (**a, b**): Single subcutaneous injections of 2 or 10 mg/kg body weight corticosterone. (**c,d**): Subcutaneous implantation of micro-osmotic pumps loaded with different concentrations of corticosterone. (**e,f**): Subcutaneous implantation of one slow-release pellet containing 10 mg of corticosterone. (**g,h**): Weekly implantation of one slow-release pellet containing 10 mg of corticosterone[78]

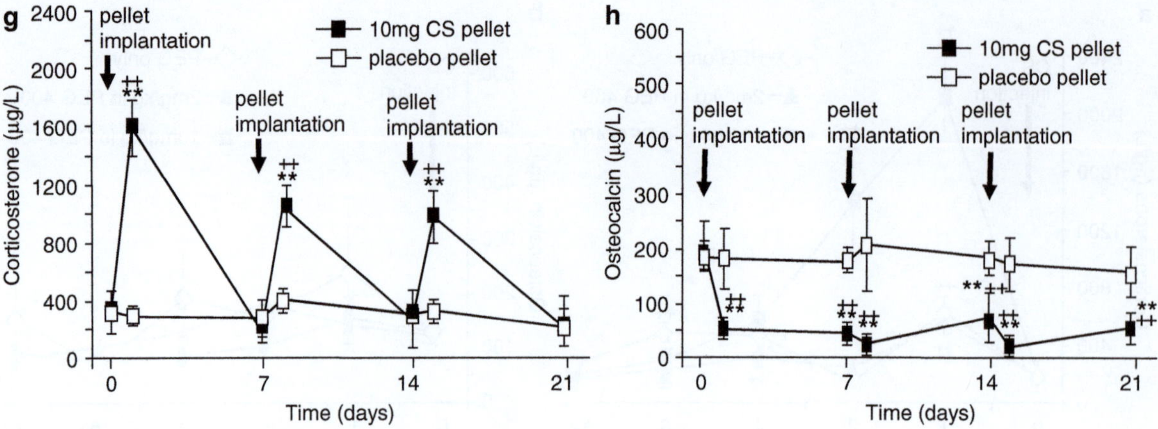

Fig. 6.17 (continued)

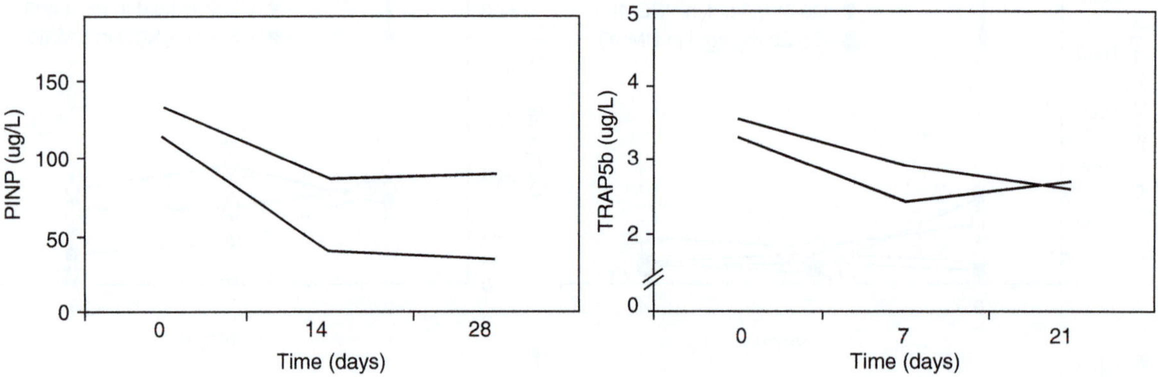

Fig. 6.18 Characteristic changes in corticosterone and OC plasma levels during continuous treatment with low doses of corticosterone

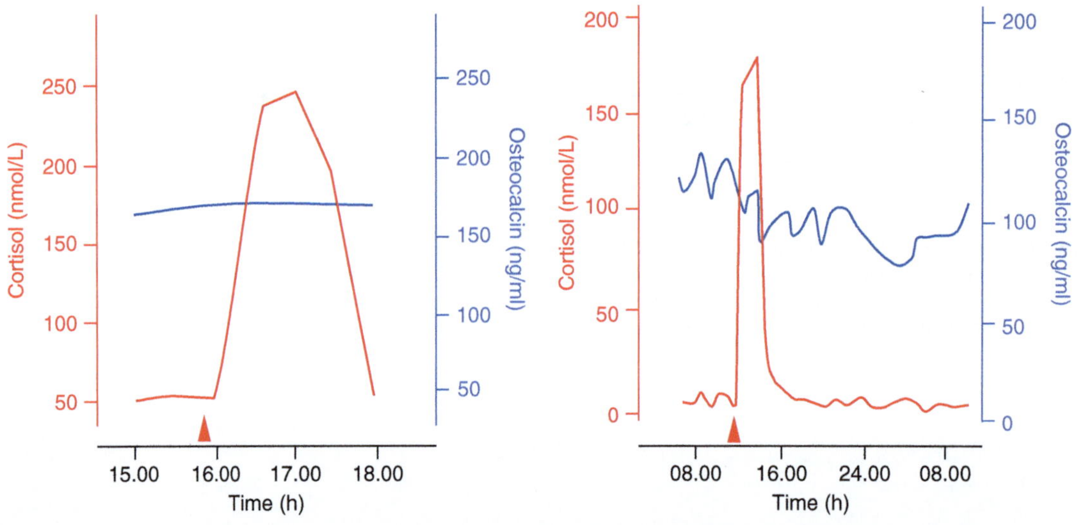

Fig. 6.19 The effect of a single GC injection on serum OC levels in sheep (Modified from Corlett et al.[61])

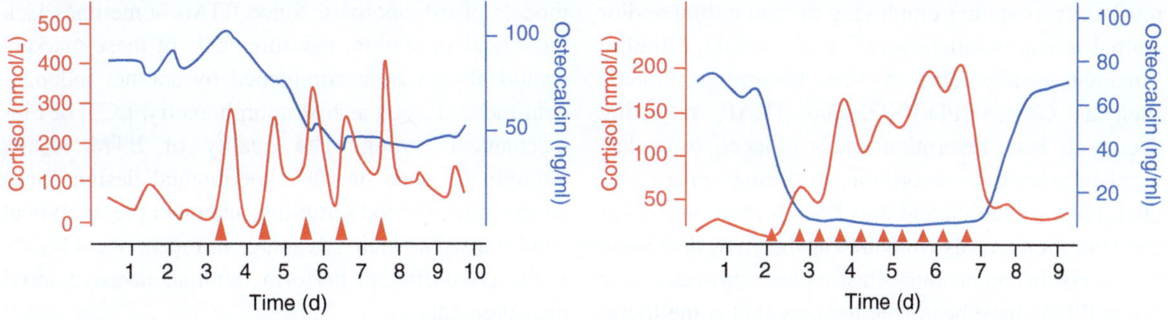

Fig. 6.20 *Left*: Kinetics of serum OC in 3-year-old sheep after daily injection of 1 mg depot ACTH (*Synacthen*). *Right*: Kinetics of serum OC in 2-year-old sheep after twice-daily injection of 1 mg depot ACTH (*Synacthen*) (Modified from Corlett et al.[61])

exogenous GCs have shown some effect. Continuous administration of GCs usually lowers both bone formation and resorption markers. However, continuous administration of exogenous GCs is not a trivial exercise. Only continuous infusion is able to provide constantly elevated circulating GC levels. Injections, micro-osmotic pumps, and subcutaneously implanted slow-release pellets result in highly variable GC levels in blood and are sometimes ineffective.

6.5.4 Additional Aspects

BTMs have been successfully used to monitor a variety of therapeutic approaches, such as hormone replacement, bisphosphonate, or calcitonin treatment in different models of osteoporosis.[12,56,57] These markers were also found to be responsive when novel drugs, such as CPK inhibitors or RANKL neutralizing antibodies, are used (Table 6.4). Consistency of BTM

Table 6.4 Bone markers used in preclinical osteoporosis models[12]

Target	Class of drug	Name of drug	Marker
Estrogen receptors	Estrogen agonists	Estradiol	TRAP
Estrogen receptors	Estrogen agonists	Estradiol	Osteocalcin CTX-I
Estrogen receptors	Estrogen agonists	Estradiol	Osteocalcin Pyridinolines
Osteoclasts	Bisphosphonates	Zoledronate	Osteocalcin Pyridinolines
Osteoclasts	Bisphosphonates	Incadronate	Osteocalcin Pyridinolines
Osteoclasts	Bisphosphonates	Alendronate	TRAP
Osteoclasts	Bisphosphonates	Clodronate	Osteocalcin Alkaline phosphatase Pyridinolines
Calcitonin receptor	Calcitonin	Calcitonin	Hydroxyprolines
RANKL	Anti-RANKL	Osteoprotegerin	BSAP TRAP
V-ATPase	V-ATPase inhibitor	FR167356	Pyridinolines
V-ATPase	V-ATPase inhibitor	SB242784	Pyridinolines
CIC-7	CIC-7 inhibitor	NS3736	Osteocalcin CTX-I
CIC-7	CIC-7 inhibitor	NS3696	TRAP Pyridinolines
Cathepsin K	Cathepsin K inhibitor	SB331750	Pyridinolines

results across studies employing the same drug and/or animal model is satisfactory.[12] For example, estradiol treatment usually decreases bone resorption markers, such as CTX, DPD/PYD, and TRAP, reflecting decreased bone resorption and a reduced osteoclast number. Since bone resorption and formation are coupled, bone formation and thus bone formation marker concentrations are also impaired as shown by decreased OC levels. In recent studies testing new anti-resorptive drugs BTMs have been able to show that some therapeutic drugs are able to uncouple bone resorption and formation. In OVX rats treated with different chloride channel 7 (ClC-7) inhibitors, bone resorption markers, such as CTX-I and DPD, were consistently reduced while bone formation, as assessed by OC, was preserved.[56,81] Since TRAP5b levels mainly reflect osteoclast numbers and collagen breakdown products, such as CTX-I, assess the actual degradation rate of bone matrix, the ratio between the two can be utilized as a resorption index for the individual osteoclast.[12] This index can provide new insights into bone metabolism and the effectiveness of therapeutic drugs. Bone formation markers, on the other hand, have been found particularly useful in animal studies testing anabolic agents, such as PTH or strontium ranelate.

Whenever unexpected differences in BTM results occur it is important to look for differences in the individual experiment, such as treatment regimen, dosage, gender, and age of experimental animals. Other potential causes for discrepancies are of pre-analytical nature, such as sample storage and time of blood/urine collection.

Since it is recommended to use BTMs in conjunction with other methods, together they often provide a more powerful tool for aspects such as the prediction of fracture risk. In human and animal studies BTMs are often measured in combination with BMD. Each of these types of analysis can independently predict future fracture risk, but when combined their predictive value is much higher than for each of the methods alone.

6.6 Conclusion

In summary, biochemical markers of bone turnover are very useful for assessing onset and progression of metabolic bone diseases, the activity of specific cell types, and the response to treatment in numerous animal models of osteoporosis. Since BTMs sometimes lack biological validation, measurements of these markers should always be accompanied by another independent method, such as histomorphometry, μCT, or biomechanical testing. The quality of BTM results strongly depends on the experimental design, standardization of blood sampling, and other pre-analytical conditions. The main advantage of biochemical BTMs is the possibility to perform minimal invasive serial measurements.

References

1. Seibel MJ. Biochemical markers of bone remodeling. *Endocrinol Metab Clin North Am*. 2003;32:83-113.
2. Seibel MJ. Biochemical markers of bone turnover: Part I: Biochemistry and variability. *Clin Biochem Rev*. 2005;26: 97-122.
3. Herrmann M, Klitscher D, Georg T, Frank J, Marzi I, Herrmann W. Different kinetics of bone markers in normal and delayed fracture healing of long bones. *Clin Chem*. 2002;48:2263-2266.
4. Garnero P, Piperno M, Gineyts E, Christgau S, Delmas PD, Vignon E. Cross sectional evaluation of biochemical markers of bone, cartilage, and synovial tissue metabolism in patients with knee osteoarthritis: relations with disease activity and joint damage. *Ann Rheum Dis*. 2001;60: 619-626.
5. Berger CE, Kroner A, Kristen KH, Minai-Pour M, Leitha T, Engel A. Spontaneous osteonecrosis of the knee: biochemical markers of bone turnover and pathohistology. *Osteoarthritis Cartilage*. 2005;13:716-721.
6. Berger CE, Kroner AH, Minai-Pour MB, Ogris E, Engel A. Biochemical markers of bone metabolism in bone marrow edema syndrome of the hip. *Bone*. 2003;33:346-351.
7. Herrmann M, Seibel M. The amino- and carboxyterminal cross-linked telopeptides of collagen type I, NTX-I and CTX-I: a comparative review. *Clin Chim Acta*. 2008;393: 57-75.
8. Ott SM. Histomorphometric measurements of bone turnover, mineralization, and volume. *Clin J Am Soc Nephrol*. 2008;3(Suppl 3):S151-S156.
9. Pogoda P, Priemel M, Rueger JM, Amling M. Bone remodeling: new aspects of a key process that controls skeletal maintenance and repair. *Osteoporos Int*. 2005;16(Suppl 2): S18-S24 (Epub November 16, 2004; S18–S24).
10. Seeman E. Bone modeling and remodeling. *Crit Rev Eukaryot Gene Expr*. 2009;19:219-233.
11. Raisz LG. Physiology and pathophysiology of bone remodeling. *Clin Chem*. 1999;45:1353-1358.
12. Sorensen MG, Henriksen K, Schaller S, Karsdal MA. Biochemical markers in preclinical models of osteoporosis. *Biomarkers*. 2007;12:266-286.
13. Garnero P. Biomarkers for osteoporosis management: utility in diagnosis, fracture risk prediction and therapy monitoring. *Mol Diagn Ther*. 2008;12:157-170.

14. Stein GS, Lian JB. Molecular mechanisms mediating proliferation/differentiation interrelationships during progressive development of the osteoblast phenotype. *Endocr Rev.* 1993;14:424-442.
15. Owen TA, Aronow M, Shalhoub V, et al. Progressive development of the rat osteoblast phenotype *in vitro*: reciprocal relationships in expression of genes associated with osteoblast proliferation and differentiation during formation of the bone extracellular matrix. *J Cell Physiol.* 1990;143: 420-430.
16. Lian JB, Stein GS. Concepts of osteoblast growth and differentiation: basis for modulation of bone cell development and tissue formation. *Crit Rev Oral Biol Med.* 1992;3: 269-305.
17. Siggelkow H, Rebenstorff K, Kurre W, et al. Development of the osteoblast phenotype in primary human osteoblasts in culture: comparison with rat calvarial cells in osteoblast differentiation. *J Cell Biochem.* 1999;75:22-35.
18. Leeming DJ, Alexandersen P, Karsdal MA, Qvist P, Schaller S, Tanko LB. An update on biomarkers of bone turnover and their utility in biomedical research and clinical practice. *Eur J Clin Pharmacol.* 2006;62:781-792.
19. Ferron M, Hinoi E, Karsenty G, Ducy P. Osteocalcin differentially regulates beta cell and adipocyte gene expression and affects the development of metabolic diseases in wild-type mice. *Proc Natl Acad Sci USA.* 2008;105:5266-5270.
20. Lee NK, Sowa H, Hinoi E, et al. Endocrine regulation of energy metabolism by the skeleton. *Cell.* 2007;130: 456-469.
21. Nesbitt SA, Horton MA. Trafficking of matrix collagens through bone-resorbing osteoclasts. *Science.* 1997;276: 266-269.
22. Vaananen HK, Zhao H, Mulari M, Halleen JM. The cell biology of osteoclast function. *J Cell Sci.* 2000;113: 377-381.
23. Vaaraniemi J, Halleen JM, Kaarlonen K, et al. Intracellular machinery for matrix degradation in bone-resorbing osteoclasts. *J Bone Miner Res.* 2004;19:1432-1440.
24. Halleen JM, Alatalo SL, Janckila AJ, Woitge HW, Seibel MJ, Vaananen HK. Serum tartrate-resistant acid phosphatase 5b is a specific and sensitive marker of bone resorption. *Clin Chem.* 2001;47:597-600.
25. Halleen JM, Ranta R. Tartrate-resistant acid phosphatase as a serum marker of bone resorption. *Am Clin Lab.* 2001;20: 29-30.
26. Halleen JM. Tartrate-resistant acid phosphatase 5B is a specific and sensitive marker of bone resorption. *Anticancer Res.* 2003;23:1027-1029.
27. Minkin C. Bone acid phosphatase: tartrate-resistant acid phosphatase as a marker of osteoclast function. *Calcif Tissue Int.* 1982;34:285-290.
28. Chu P, Chao TY, Lin YF, Janckila AJ, Yam LT. Correlation between histomorphometric parameters of bone resorption and serum type 5b tartrate-resistant acid phosphatase in uremic patients on maintenance hemodialysis. *Am J Kidney Dis.* 2003;41:1052-1059.
29. Janckila AJ, Nakasato YR, Neustadt DH, Yam LT. Disease-specific expression of tartrate-resistant acid phosphatase isoforms. *J Bone Miner Res.* 2003;18:1916-1919.
30. Janckila AJ, Takahashi K, Sun SZ, Yam LT. Tartrate-resistant acid phosphatase isoform 5b as serum marker for osteoclastic activity. *Clin Chem.* 2001;47:74-80.
31. Meier C, Meinhardt U, Greenfield JR, et al. Serum cathepsin K concentrations reflect osteoclastic activity in women with postmenopausal osteoporosis and patients with Paget's disease. *Clin Lab.* 2006;52:1-10.
32. Fuller K, Lawrence KM, Ross JL, et al. Cathepsin K inhibitors prevent matrix-derived growth factor degradation by human osteoclasts. *Bone.* 2008;42:200-211.
33. Skoumal M, Haberhauer G, Kolarz G, Hawa G, Woloszczuk W, Klingler A. Serum cathepsin K levels of patients with long-standing rheumatoid arthritis: correlation with radiological destruction. *Arthritis Res Ther.* 2005;7:R65-R70.
34. Munoz-Torres M, Reyes-Garcia R, Mezquita-Raya P, et al. Serum cathepsin K as a marker of bone metabolism in postmenopausal women treated with alendronate. *Maturitas.* 2009;64:188-192.
35. Saftig P, Hunziker E, Everts V, et al. Functions of cathepsin K in bone resorption: lessons from cathepsin K deficient mice. *Adv Exp Med Biol.* 2000;477:293-303.
36. Gowen M, Lazner F, Dodds R, et al. Cathepsin K knockout mice develop osteopetrosis due to a deficit in matrix degradation but not demineralization. *J Bone Miner Res.* 1999; 14:1654-1663.
37. McCudden CR, Kraus VB. Biochemistry of amino acid racemization and clinical application to musculoskeletal disease. *Clin Biochem.* 2006;39:1112-1130.
38. Garnero P, Ferreras M, Karsdal MA, et al. The type I collagen fragments ICTP and CTX reveal distinct enzymatic pathways of bone collagen degradation. *J Bone Miner Res.* 2003;18:859-867.
39. Kong QQ, Sun TW, Dou QY, et al. Beta-CTX and ICTP act as indicators of skeletal metastasis status in male patients with non-small cell lung cancer. *Int J Biol Markers.* 2007;22:214-220.
40. Risteli J, Elomaa I, Niemi S, Novamo A, Risteli L. Radioimmunoassay for the pyridinoline cross-linked carboxy-terminal telopeptide of type I collagen: a new serum marker of bone collagen degradation. *Clin Chem.* 1993; 39:635-640.
41. Risteli J, Risteli L. Analysing connective tissue metabolites in human serum. Biochemical, physiological and methodological aspects. *J Hepatol.* 1995;22:77-81.
42. Risteli L, Risteli J. Biochemical markers of bone metabolism. *Ann Med.* 1993;25:385-393.
43. DeLuca HF. Overview of general physiologic features and functions of vitamin D. *Am J Clin Nutr.* 2004;80: 1689S-1696S.
44. Lips P. Vitamin D deficiency and secondary hyperparathyroidism in the elderly: consequences for bone loss and fractures and therapeutic implications. *Endocr Rev.* 2001;22: 477-501.
45. Holick MF. Vitamin D deficiency. *N Engl J Med.* 2007;357: 266-281.
46. Lepage R, Roy L, Brossard JH, et al. A non-(1-84) circulating parathyroid hormone (PTH) fragment interferes significantly with intact PTH commercial assay measurements in uremic samples. *Clin Chem.* 1998;44:805-809.
47. Solal ME, Sebert JL, Boudailliez B, et al. Comparison of intact, midregion, and carboxy terminal assays of parathyroid hormone for the diagnosis of bone disease in hemodialyzed patients. *J Clin Endocrinol Metab.* 1991;73:516-524.
48. Stability of N-MID osteocalcin in serum, heparin- and EDTA-plasma over a 24 month period at −70°C.

www.radmed.com.tr/usr_img/nonizotopik/n_mid_osteo/eng_nmid_osteocalcin_elisa_1006a.pdf.pdf. 2010. 18-3-2010. Ref Type: Internet Communication.

49. Bais R, Edwards JB. An optimized continuous-monitoring procedure for semiautomated determination of serum acid phosphatase activity. *Clin Chem*. 1976;22:2025-2028.
50. Tsutsumi H, Katagiri K, Morimoto M, Nasu T, Tanigawa M, Mamba K. Diurnal variation and age-related changes of bone turnover markers in female Gottingen minipigs. *Lab Anim*. 2004;38:439-446.
51. Srivastava AK, Bhattacharyya S, Li X, Mohan S, Baylink DJ. Circadian and longitudinal variation of serum C-telopeptide, osteocalcin, and skeletal alkaline phosphatase in C3H/HeJ mice. *Bone*. 2001;29:361-367.
52. Clowes JA, Hannon RA, Yap TS, Hoyle NR, Blumsohn A, Eastell R. Effect of feeding on bone turnover markers and its impact on biological variability of measurements. *Bone*. 2002;30:886-890.
53. Hannon R, Eastell R. Preanalytical variability of biochemical markers of bone turnover. *Osteoporos Int*. 2000;11: S30-S44.
54. Bernardi D, Zaninotto M, Plebani M. Requirements for improving quality in the measurement of bone markers. *Clin Chim Acta*. 2004;346:79-86.
55. Eriksen EF, Charles P, Melsen F, Mosekilde L, Risteli L, Risteli J. Serum markers of type I collagen formation and degradation in metabolic bone disease: correlation with bone histomorphometry. *J Bone Miner Res*. 1993;8:127-132.
56. Schaller S, Henriksen K, Sveigaard C, et al. The chloride channel inhibitor NS3736 [corrected] prevents bone resorption in ovariectomized rats without changing bone formation. *J Bone Miner Res*. 2004;19:1144-1153.
57. Visentin L, Dodds RA, Valente M, et al. A selective inhibitor of the osteoclastic V-H(+)-ATPase prevents bone loss in both thyroparathyroidectomized and ovariectomized rats. *J Clin Invest*. 2000;106:309-318.
58. Garnero P, Gineyts E, Schaffer AV, Seaman J, Delmas PD. Measurement of urinary excretion of nonisomerized and beta-isomerized forms of type I collagen breakdown products to monitor the effects of the bisphosphonate zoledronate in Paget's disease. *Arthritis Rheum*. 1998;41:354-360.
59. Chapurlat RD, Garnero P, Breart G, Meunier PJ, Delmas PD. Serum type I collagen breakdown product (serum CTX) predicts hip fracture risk in elderly women: the EPIDOS study. *Bone*. 2000;27:283-286.
60. Hamrick MW, Ding KH, Pennington C, et al. Age-related loss of muscle mass and bone strength in mice is associated with a decline in physical activity and serum leptin. *Bone*. 2006;39:845-853.
61. Corlett SC, Couch M, Care AD, Sykes AR. Measurement of plasma osteocalcin in sheep: assessment of circadian variation, the effects of age and nutritional status and the response to perturbation of the adrenocortical axis. *Exp Physiol*. 1990;75:515-527.
62. Farrugia W, Fortune CL, Heath J, Caple IW, Wark JD. Osteocalcin as an index of osteoblast function during and after ovine pregnancy. *Endocrinology*. 1989;125:1705-1710.
63. Sigrist IM, Gerhardt C, Alini M, Schneider E, Egermann M. The long-term effects of ovariectomy on bone metabolism in sheep. *J Bone Miner Metab*. 2007;25:28-35.
64. DeLaurier A, Jackson B, Pfeiffer D, Ingham K, Horton MA, Price JS. A comparison of methods for measuring serum and urinary markers of bone metabolism in cats. *Res Vet Sci*. 2004;77:29-39.
65. Ladlow JF, Hoffmann WE, Breur GJ, Richardson DC, Allen MJ. Biological variability in serum and urinary indices of bone formation and resorption in dogs. *Calcif Tissue Int*. 2002;70: 186-193.
66. Hoegh-Andersen P, Tanko LB, Andersen TL, et al. Ovariectomized rats as a model of postmenopausal osteoarthritis: validation and application. *Arthritis Res Ther*. 2004; 6:R169-R180.
67. Chavassieux P, Garnero P, Duboeuf F, et al. Effects of a new selective estrogen receptor modulator (MDL 103, 323) on cancellous and cortical bone in ovariectomized ewes: a biochemical, histomorphometric, and densitometric study. *J Bone Miner Res*. 2001;16:89-96.
68. Lane NE. An update on glucocorticoid-induced osteoporosis. *Rheum Dis Clin North Am*. 2001;27:235-253.
69. Tsugeno H, Goto B, Fujita T, et al. Oral glucocorticoid-induced fall in cortical bone volume and density in postmenopausal asthmatic patients. *Osteoporos Int*. 2001;12:266-270.
70. Canalis E. Mechanisms of glucocorticoid-induced osteoporosis. *Curr Opin Rheumatol*. 2003;15:454-457.
71. Schorlemmer S, Gohl C, Iwabu S, Ignatius A, Claes L, Augat P. Glucocorticoid treatment of ovariectomized sheep affects mineral density, structure, and mechanical properties of cancellous bone. *J Bone Miner Res*. 2003;18:2010-2015.
72. Iwamoto J, Seki A, Takeda T, Yamada H, Sato Y, Yeh JK. Effects of alfacalcidol on cancellous and cortical bone mass in rats treated with glucocorticoid: a bone histomorphometry study. *J Nutr Sci Vitaminol (Tokyo)*. 2007;53:191-197.
73. Kaji H, Yamauchi M, Chihara K, Sugimoto T. Glucocorticoid excess affects cortical bone geometry in premenopausal, but not postmenopausal, women. *Calcif Tissue Int*. 2008;82:182-190.
74. Weinstein RS, Jilka RL, Parfitt AM, Manolagas SC. Inhibition of osteoblastogenesis and promotion of apoptosis of osteoblasts and osteocytes by glucocorticoids. Potential mechanisms of their deleterious effects on bone. *J Clin Invest*. 1998;102: 274-282.
75. O'Brien CA, Jia D, Plotkin LI, et al. Glucocorticoids act directly on osteoblasts and osteocytes to induce their apoptosis and reduce bone formation and strength. *Endocrinology*. 2004;145:1835-1841.
76. Weinstein RS, Chen JR, Powers CC, et al. Promotion of osteoclast survival and antagonism of bisphosphonate-induced osteoclast apoptosis by glucocorticoids. *J Clin Invest*. 2002;109:1041-1048.
77. King CS, Weir EC, Gundberg CW, Fox J, Insogna KL. Effects of continuous glucocorticoid infusion on bone metabolism in the rat. *Calcif Tissue Int*. 1996;59:184-191.
78. Herrmann M, Henneicke H, Street J, et al. The challenge of continuous exogenous glucocorticoid administration in mice. *Steroids*. 2009;74:245-249.
79. Chavassieux P, Buffet A, Vergnaud P, Garnero P, Meunier PJ. Short-term effects of corticosteroids on trabecular bone remodeling in old ewes. *Bone*. 1997;20:451-455.
80. O'Connell SL, Tresham J, Fortune CL, et al. Effects of prednisolone and deflazacort on osteocalcin metabolism in sheep. *Calcif Tissue Int*. 1993;53:117-121.
81. Karsdal MA, Henriksen K, Sorensen MG, et al. Acidification of the osteoclastic resorption compartment provides insight into the coupling of bone formation to bone resorption. *Am J Pathol*. 2005;166:467-476.
82. Ding M, Cheng L, Bollen P, Schwarz P, Overgaard S. Glucocorticoid induced osteopenia in cancellous bone of sheep: validation of large animal model for spine fusion and biomaterial research. *Spine (Phila Pa 1976)*. 2010;35:363-370.

7 Methods in Bone Biology: Cancer and Bone

Yu Zheng, Markus J. Seibel, and Hong Zhou

7.1 Introduction

Metastasis of cancer to bone is one of the most significant causes of morbidity and often indicates poor prognosis particularly for breast cancer, prostate cancer, and lung cancer patients. Animal models are important tools to investigate the pathogenesis of, and develop novel treatment strategies for, bone metastases in humans. The ideal animal model of bone metastatic human cancer would reproduce the genetic and phenotypic changes that occur with human cancers. These include invasion of cancer cells into circulation, vascular spread to bone, and proliferation and survival in the bone marrow microenvironment with subsequent modifications to bone architecture. However, most naturally occurring spontaneous mammary carcinomas in mice and rats do not metastasize.[1] Therefore, experimental models of "bone metastasis" require xenografts of human tumors or cell lines derived from human cancers into immunodeficient rodents (e.g., nude mice and rats, or severely compromised immunodeficient [SCID] mice). To produce malignant bone lesions that can serve to study biologically or clinically relevant aspects of bone metastases, xenografted cells can be injected orthotopically (e.g., into the bone marrow of long bones such as the tibia), intravascularly into the femoral or other arteries, or transcutaneously into the left ventricle of the heart. Furthermore, breast cancer models may involve injection of malignant cells or cell lines into the mammary fat pad.

H. Zhou (✉)
Bone Research Program, ANZAC Research Institute,
University of Sydney, Hospital Road, Concord,
NSW 2139, Australia
e-mail: hzhou@anzac.edu.au

In this chapter, we describe the correct preparation of cancer cells and the most efficient injection procedures for intratibial, intravascular, intracardiac, and mammary fat pad models.

7.2 Intratibial Model

This model has the advantage that a tumor is generated in a predetermined site with a known number of cells, and the contralateral tibia can be used for control. This model is very useful for evaluating the effects of modification of the bone microenvironment after establishment of a tumor as the steps of extravasation and growth to micrometastases are bypassed.[2-5] Disadvantages of this approach are that the piercing of the cortex and displacement of bone marrow in themselves produce a marked reparative response changing local bone metabolism and hence the bone microenvironment. This model should therefore not be considered for investigation of early metastatic process. In addition, since the cells were injected directly into marrow cavity this model is not an invasion model.

7.2.1 Preparation of Cells for Injection

Cell preparation is an important step to ensure consistent and reproducible results. Cells are routinely passaged once or twice after revival from frozen stocks before preparation for injection into mice. When the cells reach ~80% confluence:

1. Remove culture media. Following a phosphate buffered saline (PBS) wash, the cell layers are rinsed briefly with Versene (0.02% EDTA, GIBCO

G. Duque and K. Watanabe (eds.), *Osteoporosis Research*,
DOI: 10.1007/978-0-85729-293-3_7, © Springer-Verlag London Limited 2011

#15040-66 for 100 ml) prior to detachment in 2 ml (75 cm^2 flask) or 4 ml (175 cm^2 flask) Versene at 37°C for 30 min. Versene rather than trypsin is selected to detach cells for *in vivo* injection, since trypsin contains proteases which may damage the cells.

2. Following detachment from the flask, the Versene suspension is transferred to a 15 ml Falcon tube. The cells are then washed twice by centrifugation at 250 g for 5 min in 10 ml PBS before an aliquot is removed for assessment of viability by Trypan blue exclusion. Only suspensions with >97% viability are used for mouse injections.
3. After a final PBS wash and centrifugation, cells are resuspended in PBS at the concentration needed (e.g., 50,000 cells/10 μl for MDA-MB-231 cells) for intratibial injection.

7.2.2 Preparation of Mice

Immunocompromised mice (congenitally athymic nude), 4–5 weeks of age, will be anesthetized with an intraperitoneal (IP) mixture of ketamine and xylazine (100 μl xylazine + 750 μL ketamine using 0.9% saline dilute to 10 ml, freshly made before IP injection). The analgesic carprofen (Rimadyl) (5 mg/kg subcutaneously) will be administered prior to the inoculation (as part of the anesthetic delivery) to ensure the animals do not feel any pain. All procedures should be performed in a sterile biohazard hood.

7.2.3 Injection

The animals are anesthetized and the left and right legs are cleaned with 70% ethanol. One tibia is inoculated with tumor cells, while the contralateral tibia will be injected with PBS to serve as a control. The intratibial injection is performed using 25 μl Hamilton syringes (Hamilton Syringe Co., Reno, NV). Syringes should be kept sterile before use. After each use, they should be immersed in 100% ethanol for at least 2 h or overnight and dried completely before using again. Cells should be kept on ice until inoculation has been completed in all mice.

1. The cancer cells are aspirated into a 25 μl syringe fitted with a 26 gauge needle. The aspirated volume depends on the age of the mouse and is usually 10–15 μl, maximum 20 μl.
2. The anesthetized mouse is placed on its back and the knee is flexed to expose access to the proximal end of the tibia (Fig. 7.1a). The needle is inserted through the skin (Fig. 7.1b) and passed through the tibia plateau, articular cartilage, and growth plate until it reaches the bone marrow approximately 3–5 mm below the diaphysis of the tibia (Fig. 7.1b). Once this point has been reached, 10 μl of cell suspension (or for control purposes, 10 μl of medium) is injected. The needle should be advanced using a drilling motion toward the marrow cavity so as not to break through the cortical bone. Once the needle is in the marrow cavity, the hand initially used to hold the leg in place can be freed to execute the injection (Fig. 7.1c). To prevent leakage of cell

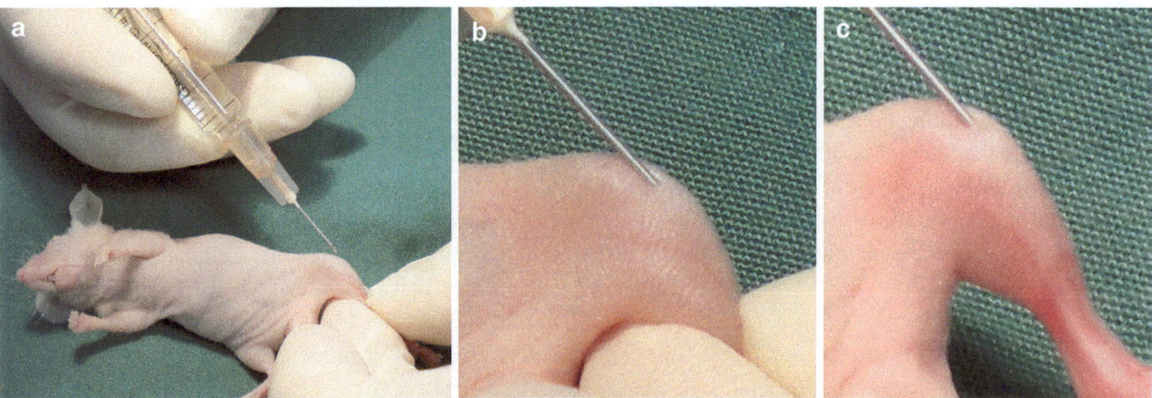

Fig. 7.1 Intratibial injection procedure. (**a**) Bend the knee of the nude mouse to expose access to the proximal end of the tibia. (**b**, **c**) The needle is inserted through the skin into the tibial plateau

suspension, injection speed should be slow (20–30 s for 10 μl of suspension). If the needle becomes blocked it is best to change the needle and try to reenter the same site. Use new needles for each mouse and injection.

3. After injection mice should be kept warm until they fully recover from anesthesia. Nude mice should be closely monitored daily for potential infection and cancer cachexia, and body weight should be checked twice a week. If mice lose more than 15% of body weight they should be euthanized.

7.2.4 Outcome Analysis by X-Ray

The development of osteolytic lesions can be monitored by digital radiography after 7 days and checked every 3–7 days from then on. For breast cancer cell lines, such as MDA-MB-231 cells, visible lytic lesions should normally develop within 7–10 days post injection of 50,000 cells.[4] By 2 weeks post inoculation, lytic lesions should be clearly visible on x-ray and by 3 weeks the defect should reach a size of approximately 2.5 mm^2 (Fig. 7.2).

7.3 Intra-arterial Model

In this model, which has been developed for rats but in principle can also be used for mice, tumor cells are directly inoculated into the femoral artery. This model reliably generates vital osteolytic lesions, has high site specificity, allows for serial assessments of bone and tumor-related parameters, and does not cause artificial bone damage as the intratibial injection model.[6] Compared with the intracardiac model (see later), the intra-arterial method (Fig. 7.3) has several advantages: (1) malignant dissemination into visceral peripheries does not occur; (2) animals usually show no significant morbidity, as reflected by normal mobility and axial bone mineral density (BMD), and the absence of cachexia; (3) a success rate of 95–100% can be obtained in properly trained hands; and (4) the use of larger-size rodents offers an alternative to mice, and permits serial assessment of parameters that are hard to measure in mice, such as bone turnover markers. The disadvantages of this model are similar to other models of metastatic disease, i.e., the need for immunocompromised rats, which are expensive and require special housing conditions. Also, the canulation of the femoral artery requires minor surgery and can be time-consuming, particularly in untrained hands or in mice.

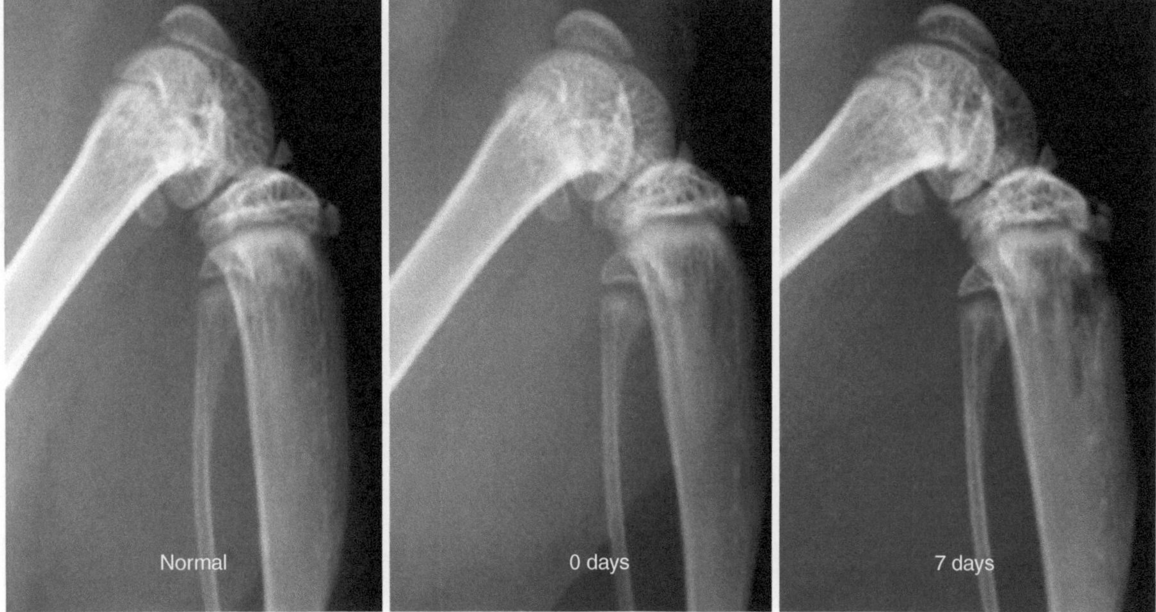

Fig. 7.2 Bone erosions increase after intratibial implantation of breast cancer cells. After 7–10 days post inoculation of MDA-MB-231 cells, small lytic lesions become visible on x-ray. By 2 weeks, the lesions should be clearly lytic and by 3 weeks, the defect should reach a size of approximately 2.0–2.5 mm^2

Fig. 7.2 (continued)

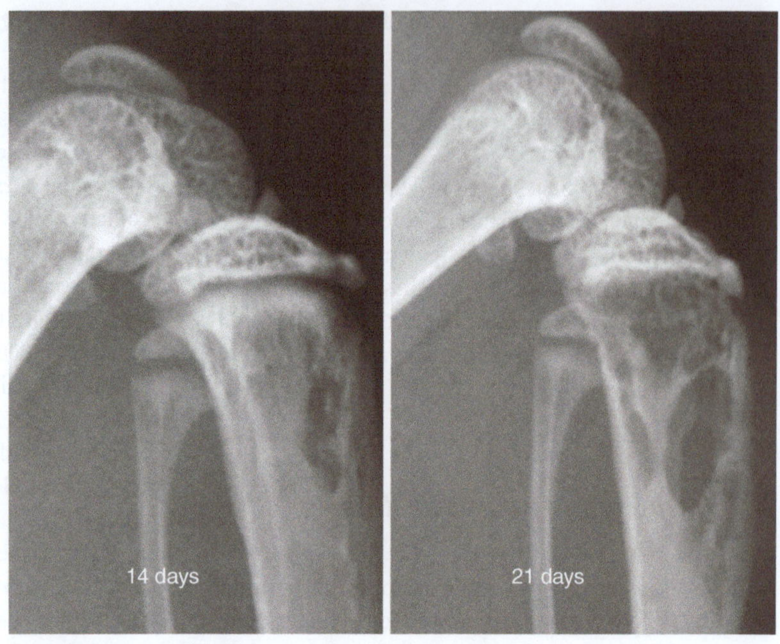

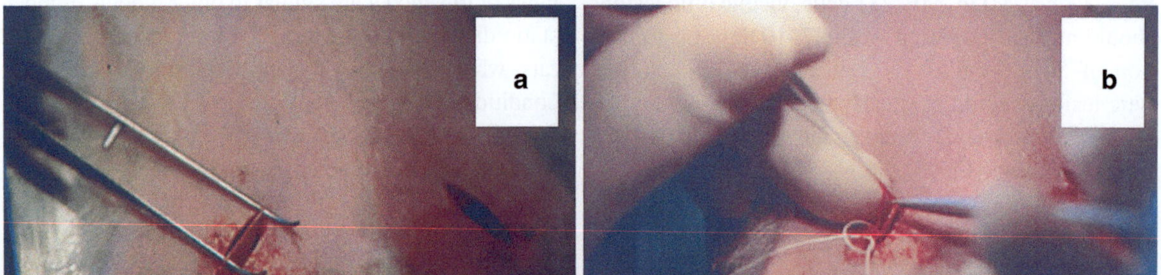

Fig. 7.3 Intra-arterial injection procedure. (**a**) Separate the femoral artery from the accompanying femoral vein and nerve by blunt dissection. (**b**) Place a thread underneath each artery as proximal as possible, and completely ligate the vessel. (**c**) Make a perpendicular incision into the femoral artery distal of the ligation site and insert a small polyethylene catheter (approx. 0.1 mm diameter) pointing distally. (**d**) After injection of the tumor cells and rinse by injection of 0.2 ml of PBS, swiftly remove the catheter and pull the previously loaded knot tight, thus completely ligating the femoral artery

7.3.1 Preparation of Rats

Immunocompromised (congenitally athymic nude) rats, 7–8 weeks of age, are anesthetized with an IP injection of a mixture of ketamine (50 mg/kg) and xylazine (15 mg/kg), or other anesthetics as appropriate. An analgesic (e.g., carprofen 5 mg/kg subcutaneously) should be administered prior to the inoculation as part of the anesthetic delivery. All procedures should be performed in a sterile biohazard hood.

7.3.2 Preparation of Cells for Injection

The cells are usually prepared in the same way as the cells used for intratibial injections. The concentration of the cancer cell suspension depends on the cell type applied; for MDA-MB-231 cells, we use ~1×10^5 cells per injection.

7.3.3 Procedure

1. Anesthetize animal as described above.
2. Place the rat in a ventral position; scrub both groins with 70% alcohol.
3. Open up the skin and separate the femoral artery from the accompanying femoral vein and nerve by blunt dissection. Avoid damage to the femoral nerve since hind leg paralysis will severely affect the animal's mobility and the validity of the experimental outcome.
4. Place a thread underneath each artery as proximal as possible, and completely ligate the vessel.
5. Make a perpendicular incision into the femoral artery distal of the ligation site.
6. Insert a small polyethylene catheter (~0.1 mm Ø) pointing distally.
7. Aspirate 0.5 ml of the cancer cell suspension into a 1.0 ml syringe fitted with a needle or connector that snugly fits the polyethylene catheter without leak.
8. Use a second thread and place it ~2 mm distal of the insertion site of the catheter and tie a snug knot to prevent retrograde leakage of the injected material.
9. Gently inject the cell suspension. The contralateral leg may be used as PBS control.
10. Following injection of the tumor cells, the catheter's dead volume should be rinsed by injection of 0.2 ml PBS. Then swiftly remove the catheter and pull the knot tight, thus completely ligating the femoral artery. Do not worry, this will not cause any measureable damage to the leg or pain to the animals. Unlike humans, rats will maintain arterial flow through collateral arteries.
11. Make sure there is no residual leak (bleeding). Close the skin with a few stitches.
12. After surgery, rats should be kept warm until they fully recover from anesthesia. Nude rats should be closely monitored (daily) for bleeding, infection, or any other complication. Body weight should be checked twice weekly. Animals losing more than 15% of body weight should be euthanized.

7.3.4 Outcome Analysis

Body weight, 24 h urine samples, blood specimens, and x-rays can be taken at appropriate time intervals. With 1×10^5 MDA-MB-231 cells injected, lytic lesions become visible by day 18, and by day 30, lesions are extensive (Fig. 7.4).[6] Urine and serum samples can be collected for specific purposes, such as bone marker analyses. Tibial BMD should be monitored by dual energy x-ray absorptiometry (DEXA). Animals should be euthanized at end point and the femora and tibiae collected for further analyses.[6]

7.4 Intracardiac Model

This is an invasion model. Inoculation of tumor cells into the left ventricle of the heart causes the cells to be disseminated throughout the body along with the general blood flow. As regards bone metastases, the intracardiac model allows to investigate the cell invasion by genetic modification of certain genes and early establishment of tumor foci in the bone, and/ or the effects of a change in the bone microenvironment on cancer cell distribution and survival in the bone.[5] Advantages of this technique are the reproduction of vascular delivery of tumor cells to tissues and the opportunity to study the growth of tumors from small numbers of cells originally invading the bone. As in other models, the development of lytic bone lesions can be monitored radiographically, but the time for visible lesions could vary according to the type of cancer cells. With MDA-MB-231 cells,

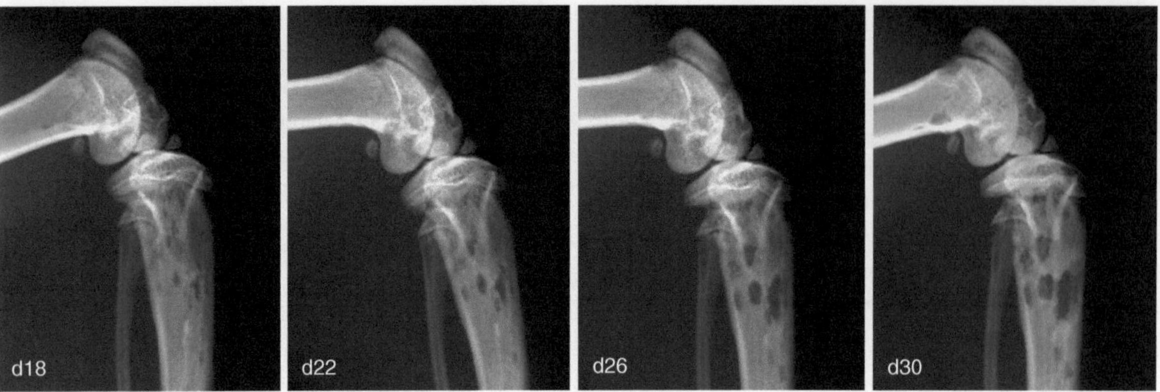

Fig. 7.4 Bone erosions increase after intra-arterial injection of breast cancer cells. MDA-MB-231 cells (1×10^5) were injected into the femoral artery, and multiple visible bone lytic lesions on x-ray become clear by day 18, and extensively large

visible lesions occur within 3–4 weeks post inoculation. Disadvantages of this technique mainly lie in its technical challenges and the relatively long duration of the experiment. Mortality will be relatively high, especially in untrained hands, and successful establishment of tumor in bone could be compromised by techniques, which may make it hard to differentiate the actual metastatic potential with people's skills for certain cell lines.

7.4.1 Preparation of Cells for Injection

The cells are usually prepared in the same way as in intratibial injection. The concentration of the cancer cell suspension depends on the type of cells. For the MDA-MB-231 cell line, we usually apply ~2×10^5 cells intracardially.

7.4.2 Procedure

1. Anesthetizing procedure is the same as that described earlier in the Intratibial Injection section.
2. Place the mouse in a ventral position, parallel to the side of the operating pad, and fix with sticking tape as shown in Fig. 7.5a. Scrub the anterior chest wall with 70% alcohol.
3. Up to 100 μl of the cancer cell suspension is aspirated into a 1.0 ml syringe fitted with a 26 gauge needle.
4. Aiming centrally, insert the needle left of the xyphoid process and through the diaphragm into the heart, either parallel to the operating bench (Fig. 7.5b) or at 15–20° angle. The spontaneous, pulsatile entrance of bright red oxygenated blood into the transparent needle hub indicates correct needle position into the left ventricle (Fig. 7.5c, d). Once this happens, immediately stop advancing the needle and hold steadily.
5. Slowly inject the cell suspension over a period 20–30 s.
6. Withdraw the needle, position the mouse laterally, and keep the mouse warm to wake it up.
7. After injection mice should be monitored as described in the intratibial model.

Intracardiac cell inoculations are technically demanding and cannot be easily mastered from a textbook. For the sake of the welfare of the animals, the authors strongly recommend that beginners seek hands-on technical help before attempting an injection for the fist time.

7.5 Subcutaneous or Mammary Fat Pad Model

Inoculation of tumor cells subcutaneously or into mammary fat pad is used to test for cancer cell tumorigenesis, aggressiveness (including metastasis), and response to treatment. Successful establishment of tumors requires that cells be suspended in matrigel, which increases the uptake of the tumor cells as well as enhances tumor growth.[4,7,8]

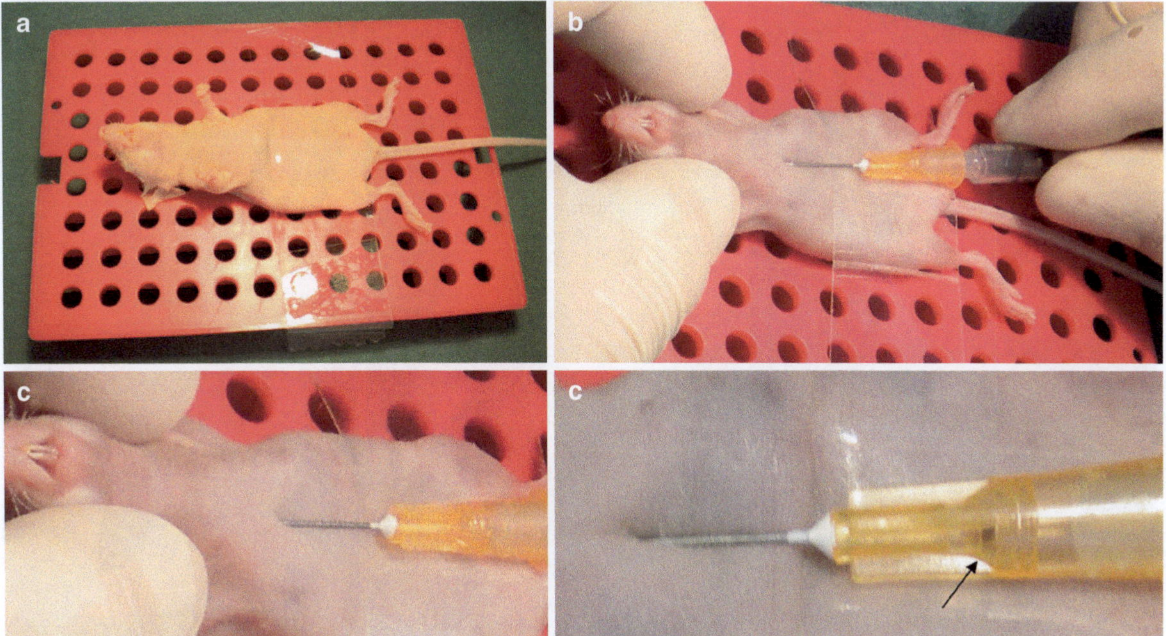

Fig. 7.5 Intracardiac injection procedure. (**a**) Position the mouse parallel to the side of the operating pad, and fix with sticking tape. (**b**) Insert the needle into the left of the xyphoid process, parallel to the operating bench. (**c, d**) Pulsatile retrograde entrance of bright red oxygenated blood (*arrow*) into the syringe indicates correct needle placement

7.5.1 Preparation of Cells for Injection

The cells are usually prepared in the same way as that in intratibial injection. For subcutaneous or mammary fat pad injections, resuspend cells in Matrigel mix (Matrigel to PBS = 1:1) at the concentration needed. For the MDA-MB-231 cell line, we usually apply ~2×10^5 cells in Thaw Matrigel matrix (from −20 freezers, BD #354234 for 10 ml) on ice for 2–3 h before use.

7.5.2 Procedure

1. Place 1 ml syringes on ice to keep cold.
2. Anesthetize the mice and give analgesic as described for the intratibial injection model.
3. Place the mouse in a lateral position as shown in Fig. 7.6a. Scrub the skin with 70% alcohol.
4. Load cell suspension into a cold syringe and fit the syringe with a 25 gauge needle.
5. With the mouse on its side, lift the skin at the flank in front of the hind limb as shown in Fig. 7.6a. This corresponds to the fourth mammary fat pad of the mouse. The fat pad should be visible under the skin (Fig. 7.6b, c).
6. Slowly inject 100 μl of cell suspension within 30 s.
7. Allow the mouse to rest in the same position to allow solidification of Matrigel before recovery.
8. After injection mice should be monitored as described for the intratibial model.

The length, width, and height of the resulting mammary tumors are measured every 3 days with a pair of callipers to determine tumor progression. Tumor volumes are calculated using the formula detailed below. The experimental end point is usually reached when tumors grow to a size of 1,500–2,000 mm^3, at which point mice should be euthanized.

7.5.3 Outcome Analysis by Tumor Measurements

1. Measure length, width, and height of the tumor as shown in Fig. 7.7a–c, using digital callipers. To monitor tumor growth, we recommend measuring

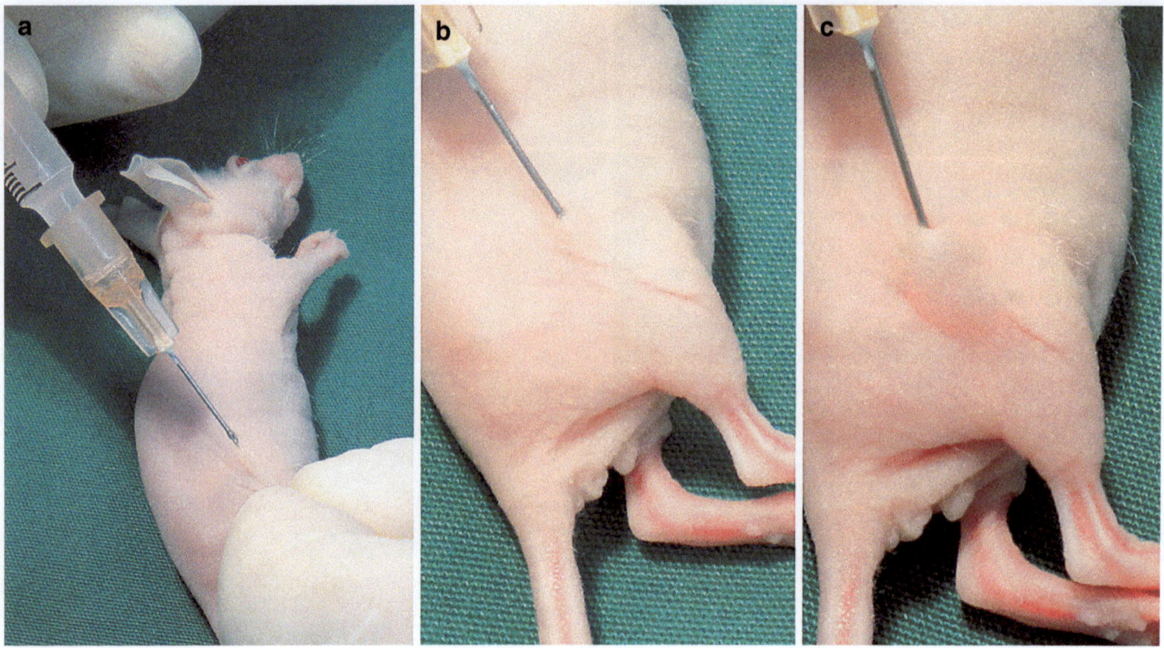

Fig. 7.6 Intra-mammary fat pad injection. (**a**) Lift skin at the flank around the site of the fourth mammary fat pad with the right hand. (**b, c**) Injection of cell suspension

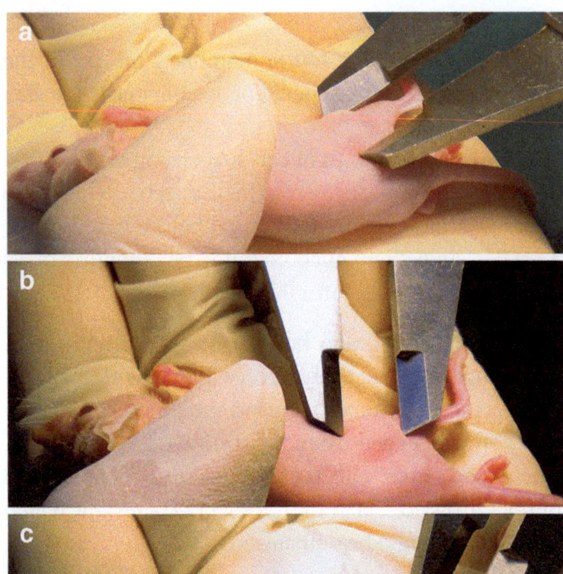

Fig. 7.7 Measurement of tumor growth. (**a–c**) Using a digital caliper, measure the length, width, and height of the developing mass

every third day post injection. Assuming an ellipsoid shape of the developing mass, the following formula can be used to calculate tumor volume:

$$\frac{4}{3}\pi \times \text{length} \times \text{width} \times \text{height}$$

2. At end point, weigh the tumor after dissecting it from the adjacent skin and tissues.

7.6 General Comments

Generally, in procedures mentioned above, if cell lines have the ability to grow in bone they could be implanted in these models. For intravascular[6] and intracardiac[5] models, MDA-MB-231 cells have been used extensively. For intratibial and mammary fat pad models, MDA-MB-231,[2,4,8] MCF-7,[3,9] and prostate cancer cell line PC-3[10] cells were shown to induce lesions successfully.

As for assessment of the effect of antimetastasis treatments in these animal models, treatment regimes would depend on the agents tested. For antiresorptive treatment using either osteoprotegerin or bisphosphonates, these agents could be given to animals before tumor implantation as a preventive measure,[4,6] or administered when tumor is established at an early or late stage.[2,6] Serial x-ray imaging and the end point histology can help monitor and evaluate the treatment effect.

Acknowledgments The authors would like to thank Dr Marcus Neudert and Professor Frieder Bauss, Germany, for their assistance with the description of the intra-arterial rat model. This work has been supported by the following research grants: Prostate Cancer Foundation of Australia (PCFA) (M.J.S, Y.Z, H.Z), University of Sydney Cancer Research Fund (M.J.S), and National Health and Medical Research Council, Australia (NHMRC) (M.J.S, H.Z.). Y.Z receives support from the National Health & Medical Research Council Australia, Training Fellowship.

References

1. Rosol TJ, Tannehill-Gregg SH, Corn S, Schneider A, McCauley LK. Animal models of bone metastasis. *Cancer Treat Res*. 2004;118:47-81.
2. Zheng Y, Zhou H, Brennan K, et al. Inhibition of bone resorption, rather than direct cytotoxicity, mediates the anti-tumour actions of ibandronate and osteoprotegerin in a murine model of breast cancer bone metastasis. *Bone*. 2007;40:471-478.
3. Zheng Y, Zhou H, Fong-Yee C, Modzelewski JR, Seibel MJ, Dunstan CR. Bone resorption increases tumour growth in a mouse model of osteosclerotic breast cancer metastasis. *Clin Exp Metastasis*. 2008;25:559-567.
4. Zheng Y, Zhou H, Modzelewski JR, et al. Accelerated bone resorption, due to dietary calcium deficiency, promotes breast cancer tumor growth in bone. *Cancer Res*. 2007; 67:9542-9548.
5. Yoneda T, Williams PJ, Hiraga T, Niewolna M, Nishimura R. A bone-seeking clone exhibits different biological properties from the MDA-MB-231 parental human breast cancer cells and a brain-seeking clone *in vivo* and *in vitro*. *J Bone Miner Res*. 2001;16:1486-1495.
6. Neudert M, Fischer C, Krempien B, Bauss F, Seibel MJ. Site-specific human breast cancer (MDA-MB-231) metastases in nude rats: model characterisation and *in vivo* effects of ibandronate on tumour growth. *Int J Cancer*. 2003;107:468-477.
7. Mehta RR, Graves JM, Hart GD, Shilkaitis A, Das Gupta TK. Growth and metastasis of human breast carcinomas with Matrigel in athymic mice. *Breast Cancer Res Treat*. 1993;25:65-71.
8. Ooi LL, Zhou H, Kalak R, et al. Vitamin D deficiency promotes human breast cancer growth in a murine model of bone metastasis. *Cancer Res*. 2010;70:1835-1844.
9. Ooi LL, Zheng Y, Zhou H, et al. Vitamin D deficiency promotes growth of MCF-7 human breast cancer in a rodent model of osteosclerotic bone metastasis. *Bone*. 2010;47:795-803.
10. Zheng Y, Zhou H, Ooi LL, et al. Vitamin D deficiency promotes prostate cancer growth in bone. *Prostate*. 2011 Jun 15;71(9):1012-21..

8 How to Test Osteoporosis Treatments in Experimental Animals

Robert J. van 't Hof

8.1 Introduction

Osteoporosis is characterized by an imbalance between bone formation and bone resorption, leading to a decrease in bone volume, and increased fracture risk. The ultimate goal of treatment for osteoporosis is the prevention of fractures. The two major approaches of treating osteoporosis are inhibition of resorption and stimulation of bone formation.[1] Any new treatments are normally first tested in appropriate *in vitro* models before further testing in animal models.

There are many animal models for osteoporosis, such as age-related osteoporosis, disuse osteoporosis,[2] inflammation-induced osteoporosis,[3] and steroid-induced osteoporosis.[4] The most common animal model for testing novel treatments for osteoporosis, however, is the ovariectomized[5] (OVX) model (see Chap. 9). The most commonly used species are the mouse and rat, although primates are also used for testing compounds in an advanced stage of development. Ovariectomy leads to a very rapid loss of bone that is comparable to the bone loss observed in postmenopausal osteoporosis. However, the timescale depends very much on the species used. Mice lose a substantial amount of bone within 3–4 weeks, rats in 2–3 months, and primates such as Cynomolgus monkeys in 1–2 years.[6,7] One major difference with human postmenopausal osteoporosis is, though, that none of the animal models leads to fracture. Therefore the major criterion for efficacy in these models is not the prevention of fracture but the prevention of bone loss. However, some studies have used mechanical testing of bone samples to assess effects on bone strength, and this may be an acceptable surrogate for fracture risk.

8.2 Species Considerations

Mouse models are especially suited to early-stage research, as the bone loss after OVX is very rapid and housing costs are relatively low. This results in a fairly rapid and relatively cheap model system. Furthermore, because of the small size of the animal, relatively small amounts of compounds are required, and this can be beneficial in early-stage research, especially in an academic setting where large-scale compound synthesis is usually not available. An important consideration in mouse models is the strain of mice to be used. There are large differences between strains in bone architecture with some strains reported to show little or no OVX-induced bone loss.[8]

The OVX rat has been a very successful model for testing new anti-osteoporotic drugs. Although bone loss in this model takes longer and housing costs are higher than for the mouse, imaging and analyzing bone tissue is generally easier than in mice due to the larger size of bones and trabecular structures. Furthermore, blood and urine sampling are also easier to perform in rats than in mice, and blood sample volumes are less limited than in mice, allowing some degree of repeated sampling. Rats attain their peak bone mass at about 7–8 months of age, and to avoid difficulties with interpretation of changes in bone mass, it is advisable to use rats around this age and not much younger.

R.J. van 't Hof
Department of Rheumatology, Molecular Medicine Centre, Institute of Genetics and Molecular Medicine, University of Edinburgh, Western General Hospital, Edinburgh, Midlothian, UK
e-mail: rvanthof@staffmail.ed.ac.uk

G. Duque and K. Watanabe (eds.), *Osteoporosis Research*,
DOI: 10.1007/978-0-85729-293-3_8, © Springer-Verlag London Limited 2011

Although rodent models have been successfully used in osteoporosis research, there are some problems with the extrapolation of the results to human disease treatment. One of the problems with rodent models is that bone metabolism in the species used can be different from that in humans. Rats and mice have relatively little trabecular bone, and there is virtually no intracortical bone remodeling in small rodents. Primates such as monkeys are much more closely related to humans than rodents, and their bone architecture and metabolism very closely resemble that of humans. Primate studies are, however, considerably more expensive than rodent studies, and are rarely used in early-phase drug development. Ethical concerns further limit the use of primate models.

8.3 Assessing Bone Loss in the Ovariectomized Model

In this part several methods and readouts will be described that can be used to investigate the efficacy of novel treatments for osteoporosis focusing on the rodent OVX model as a test system, although very similar approaches and techniques can be used in other osteoporosis models as well. The OVX model will be described in detail in Chap. 9. After bilateral ovariectomy, young adult mice (10–16 weeks of age) and rats rapidly (within 3 weeks and 2 months respectively) lose a considerable amount of trabecular bone. Some cortical bone loss can be observed as well, although this usually takes considerably longer. The amount of bone lost depends on the site studied (femur, tibia, spine) as well as the method used to determine bone density or volume.

8.3.1 Assessing Bone Loss Using DEXA

The most widely accepted method for assessing bone density in the clinic is the dual energy x-ray absorptiometry (DEXA) scan. DEXA scanners for patient use, however, are not suitable for measuring bone density in small animals such as mice because of resolution restrictions. Specialized small animal DEXA scanners do exist, and the most commonly used system is the GE Healthcare Piximus system.[9] The Piximus scanner allows rapid (less than 5 min/animal) assessment of bone mineral density (BMD) and bone mineral content (BMC). These measurements can be obtained both as whole-body measurement and for specific areas such as the lumbar spine, the tibia, or the femur. The whole-body measurements are usually not as sensitive to OVX and tend to give smaller differences. A recent study by Yao et al., for instance, describes a 10% BMD loss at the spine and 5% loss at the femur compared to approximately 2–3% at the whole-body level.[10] As the coefficient of variation for measurement of whole-body BMD was reported to be 4.9% compared to 2.7% at the spine,[11] DEXA scanning appears not to be sensitive enough to establish OVX-induced BMD loss at the whole-body level, but only at specific sites such as the spine. The sensitivity at the spine is most probably due to the fact that the vertebrae consist mostly of trabecular bone, where changes in bone volume are more rapid than in cortical bone. Although the Piximus was designed for use with mice, it has also been used for rats, even though the imaging area is not large enough for whole-body measurements in these animals.[12]

Although DEXA scanning is a rapid technique, the resolution is not sufficient to distinguish between cortical and trabecular bone, or to study bone architecture.[13] Another disadvantage of DEXA scanning is that is uses a two-dimensional (2D) projection of the three-dimensional (3D) structure of the skeleton.[13] Partially because of these deficiencies, more advanced techniques such as peripheral quantitative computed tomography (pQCT) and microcomputerized tomography (μCT) are becoming the methods of choice for determining bone density and architecture in small animals.

8.3.2 pQCT and μCT

pQCT[14] and μCT[15] are both based on similar principles. Objects are imaged by x-rays from a range of angles, and a 3D image is reconstructed by the use of a computer algorithm (usually filtered back projection). Both techniques are normally used to image small parts of the skeleton, such as the proximal tibia or the distal femur. pQCT requires relatively low doses of x-rays, but has lower resolution (up to 70 μm) than μCT and only images a single slice, usually 0.5–1 mm thick. This resolution is sufficient to separate trabecular and cortical bone, but not sufficient to visualize individual trabeculae in mouse or rat bone. pQCT has been successfully used in both mouse and rat ovariectomy studies. In a comparison study of DEXA and pQCT in OVX mice, DEXA showed only small OVX-induced decreases of BMD (2.6% compared to sham-operated animals), while pQCT detected a 52% decrease in BMD of the trabecular bone at the proximal tibia.[16] In the same study, DEXA only measured a 7.6% increase in BMD after parathyroid hormone (PTH) treatment, while pQCT detected a 94% increase in BMD at the trabecular bone of the tibia.[16] The changes in cortical BMC as detected by pQCT were not significant. These results show that the capability of the pQCT system to separate trabecular from cortical bone substantially increases the power to detect changes in bone density over DEXA. The main reason for this is that the majority of mineral is present in the cortical bone, whereas the bone loss is predominant in the trabecular compartment. The DEXA scan using the 2D projection cannot distinguish between the two bone compartments, and the unchanged, large amount of mineral in the cortex masks the changes in the trabecular bone. One problem of pQCT is that exact positioning of the volume to be assessed is crucial, and small inaccuracies of positioning may lead to differences greater than those due to the treatments. This is especially true for scans of the small bones of mice.

μCT is a high-resolution technique (maximum resolution typically in the range of <1–5 μm) that is sufficiently powerful to image individual trabeculae even in small rodents such as mice. μCT produces a 3D stack of images which allows the 3D visualization and analysis of bone architecture. Using μCT analysis at the proximal tibia, OVX mice lose around 30% of the trabecular bone (BV/TV) in 3 weeks, and this is accompanied by a loss of trabecular thickness and connectivity, and a change of shape of the trabeculae from platelike to rodlike.[17] Similar changes are seen in the rat OVX model after 8 weeks.[13] In comparison to DEXA measurements, the relative bone loss measured by μCT is usually much higher. We have previously observed an OVX-induced bone loss of 11% at the proximal tibia by DEXA, while μCT analysis measured a 40% decrease of trabecular bone at the same site in the same animals.[18]

Although μCT is mostly used as an *ex vivo* technique in bone research, it can also be used *in vivo* using specialized *in vivo* scanners. This allows for the analysis of bone volume and architecture before and after treatment. However, the maximum resolution for *in vivo* systems is restricted to around 10 μm. This resolution is sufficient for imaging rat trabeculae, but only just sufficient for mouse trabeculae. In rat studies, *in vivo* μCT has been used to identify changes to individual trabeculae as a result of OVX.[19-21] One possible caveat for using μCT in longitudinal studies is that compared to DEXA and pQCT the radiation doses are substantially higher and may affect bone metabolism.[22]

8.3.3 Bone Histomorphometry

Although the x-ray–based analysis methods such as DEXA, pQCT, and μCT can measure the end results of the effects of OVX and treatments on bone mass, these methods do not provide information on changes in osteoblast and osteoclast numbers and activity. A powerful technique for measuring these parameters is bone histomorphometry, the quantitative microscopical analysis of bone and bone cells. The parameters used in bone histomorphometry have been standardized and a useful guide to these has been published by Parfitt et al.[23] Bone histomorphometry requires embedding and sectioning of undecalcified bone specimens in hard plastics such as methylmethacrylates. Care needs to be taken with the embedding to preserve activity of marker enzymes such as tartrate resistant acid phosphatase (TRAP) for osteoclasts and alkaline phosphatase (ALP) for osteoblasts,[24] and sectioning requires tungsten steel knives. Several software packages are nowadays available to assist with histomorphometry. Although histomorphometry can be used to measure architectural parameters such as trabecular bone volume and thickness, this does suffer from sampling errors as only a few sections per sample are analyzed, and these parameters are more reliably assessed by μCT.

The main strength of bone histomorphometry is analyzing changes in bone cells and resorption and formation rates. The analysis of bone formation requires the use of *in vivo* labeling with fluorochromes that bind to newly forming bone surfaces, such as calcein and tetracycline.[25] Fluorescence microscopy is then used to assess parameters such as mineral apposition rate and bone formation rate.

Especially in the mouse, osteoclasts may be hard to recognize by morphology alone as in this species the osteoclasts are much smaller than those in human or rat bone and quite often only one nucleus per osteoclast is seen in sections. This may lead to a substantial underestimate of the number of osteoclasts present, in our own experience by up to 50%. To avoid this it is recommended to use TRAP staining of the sections to assist identification of osteoclasts. Another problem can be that it is often difficult to assess which areas of TRAP-stained cell in a section belong to one osteoclast, as osteoclasts can be very large and complex-shaped cells. It is therefore often better to measure the bone surface covered with TRAP-positive cells.

Ovariectomy usually leads to a significant increase in osteoclast number and resorption surfaces in rats,[17,26-28] but this increase may not always be observed in mouse studies.[8,17] Whether increased resorption is observed is also determined by the timing of the sampling, as the increase in resorption is most pronounced during the early stages after OVX. The osteoporosis in OVX rodents is characterized by increased bone turnover, and indices for bone formation are therefore usually increased as well.[17,26,27]

8.3.4 Serum Markers of Bone Turnover

Although bone histomorphometry is a powerful technique for assessing rates of bone formation and bone resorption, it is a relatively difficult and time-consuming procedure. Furthermore, it only provides information on the levels of bone turnover in a small part of the skeleton. An alternative technique for determining rates of bone formation and resorption is the use of serum markers for these bone turnover parameters. Several markers are available for urine analysis as well; however, reliable sampling can be difficult, especially in mice. Kits for measuring several markers are commercially available, and an advantage of many is that equivalent kits are used in human studies. The most common markers for bone resorption are NTx[29] and CTx,[30] which measure cross-linked collagen fragments that are the result of osteoclastic degradation of bone, and TRAP,[30] a marker enzyme for osteoclasts that reflects osteoclast number. Bone formation can be assessed by serum markers such as ALP, osteocalcin,[31] and P1NP,[32] a pro-collagen fragment that is produced during bone formation. One advantage of using serum markers is that effects of treatments on bone turnover can be assessed relatively early, often before any changes in bone volume are observed. Furthermore, it allows for repeat sampling during the study without the possible problems of repeated exposure of the test animals to x-rays. Repeat sampling can be problematic in mouse studies, though, because of regulatory limitations on the sample volume. Another confounder can be circadian changes in the levels of bone turnover markers (BTMs),[33,34] and sampling strategies should therefore be carefully designed. The BTMs give a snapshot readout of the levels of resorption and formation. However, they do not provide evidence of changes in bone volume or strength, and are therefore usually used in combination with other methods such as histomorphometry or μCT. Also, because the serum markers reflect total body bone turnover levels, they may not detect changes in small parts of the skeleton.

8.4 Assessing the Effectiveness of Bone Anabolic and Anti-resorptive Treatments

8.4.1 Anti-resorptive Treatment

Currently, the most common approach in the treatment of osteoporosis is the use of anti-resorptive drugs, mainly bisphosphonates.[1] The most common experimental design for testing the efficacy of novel anti-resorptive drugs is a preventive ovariectomy study. In this type of study, the start of administration of compounds is very soon after the ovariectomy, usually around 2 days to allow for recovery of the animals. The main criteria for efficacy in these studies are prevention of bone loss and reduction of resorption parameters. Maximum bone loss at the distal femur and proximal tibia is observed after at about 3 weeks in mice[35] and 3–4 months in rats,[21,26] and bone volume does not change significantly after this time interval.

Upregulation of osteoclast numbers and resorption surfaces is most prominent in the early phases of the experiment, up to 2–3 weeks after ovariectomy in mice and around 2–3 months in rats, before returning to normal levels.[26] This is the best time frame for histomorphometric analysis and obtaining serum and urine samples for analysis of resorption markers. A time interval after ovariectomy of 2–3 weeks for mice and

2–3 months for rats is therefore recommended for obtaining both significant changes in bone volume and resorption markers in control animals.

An experimental setup in rodents as described here has been widely used in studying the effects of bisphosphonates,[36,37] and a wide range of other resorption inhibitors.[38-40] Some resorption inhibitors have been designed to be very specific to human targets, and therefore can only be tested in (*in vitro*) human test systems or in closely related species. An example of this is the development of cathepsin K (CPK) inhibitors. CPK inhibitors designed for maximum potency in human cells are not very effective in rodent models as rodent and human CPK do not show sufficient homology.[41] Monkey and human CPK, however, are identical, and therefore most *in vivo* tests on these inhibitors have been performed in OVX monkeys.[42,43] Interestingly, one of these studies used a pharmacological approach to induce estrogen deficiency by treatment with a gonadotropin-releasing hormone agonist.[43] Both studies assessed the efficacy of treatment solely by measuring serum levels of markers for osteoclast activity, rather than prevention of bone loss. This approach results in relatively short experiments compared to measuring bone density (weeks rather than >1 year), but does not provide direct evidence for prevention of bone loss or maintenance of bone strength.

8.4.2 Bone Anabolic Treatment

Although the most common osteoporosis treatment is still inhibition of resorption, this approach does not normally restore bone density to normal values in cases of severe osteoporosis. There is therefore a requirement for bone anabolic treatments to help restore lost bone volume. In contrast to studies testing anti-resorptive treatment, studies testing novel bone anabolic treatments generally do not study prevention of bone loss, but rather recovery of bone after bone loss. The general design for ovariectomy studies therefore usually incorporates a first phase after the ovariectomy without treatment (to obtain osteopenic animals) followed by a second treatment phase to restore the lost bone volume. However, the prevention strategy described in the previous paragraph has been used as well. Most studies in the literature used the rat OVX model, although other species have been used. Animal studies like these have been instrumental in establishing the bone anabolic effects of PTH[44-47] and are now being used to study novel anabolic drugs such as strontium ranelate[48-50] and calcium sensor agonists.[51] The recovery design is not only useful in testing new compounds, but can also be used to test treatments based on mechanical stimulation.[52,53]

8.5 Concluding Remarks

Advances in bone imaging and measurement of BTMs over the last 10 years have greatly benefited the analysis of the effects of new treatments for osteoporosis. Especially in rat models, high-quality imaging is now available to visualize changes in bone architecture *in vivo*. The technical advances allow more extensive and rapid analysis of the effects of new treatments. Although the basic experimental design of studies described in the last two paragraphs has barely changed over the last 30 years, variations have been used to study combinations of anabolic and anti-resorptive treatment,[47,54] and to investigate maintenance of bone volume and bone strength after withdrawing treatment.[55] These types of studies could be of great importance in developing treatment strategies where restoration of bone volume by anabolic treatment is followed by maintenance of bone volume using anti-resorptive treatment.

References

1. Rodan GA, Martin TJ. Therapeutic approaches to bone diseases. *Science*. 2000;289(5484):1508-1514.
2. Turner RT, Bell NH. The effects of immobilization on bone histomorphometry in rats. *J Bone Miner Res*. 1986;1(5):399-407.
3. Minne HW, Pfeilschifter J, Scharla S, et al. Inflammation-mediated osteopenia in the rat: a new animal model for pathological loss of bone mass. *Endocrinology*. 1984; 115(1):50-54.
4. McLaughlin F, Mackintosh J, Hayes BP, et al. Glucocorticoid-induced osteopenia in the mouse as assessed by histomorphometry, microcomputed tomography, and biochemical markers. *Bone*. 2002;30(6):924-930.
5. Wronski TJ, Lowry PL, Walsh CC, Ignaszewski LA. Skeletal alterations in ovariectomized rats. *Calcif Tissue Int*. 1985; 37(3):324-328.
6. Miller LC, Weaver DS, McAlister JA, Koritnik DR. Effects of ovariectomy on vertebral trabecular bone in the cynomolgus

monkey (*Macaca fascicularis*). *Calcif Tissue Int.* 1986; 38(1):62-65.
7. Lees CJ, Register TC, Turner CH, Wang T, Stancill M, Jerome CP. Effects of raloxifene on bone density, biomarkers, and histomorphometric and biomechanical measures in ovariectomized cynomolgus monkeys. *Menopause.* 2002; 9(5):320-328.
8. Iwaniec UT, Yuan D, Power RA, Wronski TJ. Strain-dependent variations in the response of cancellous bone to ovariectomy in mice. *J Bone Miner Res.* 2006;21(7):1068-1074.
9. Kolta S, De Vernejoul MC, Meneton P, Fechtenbaum J, Roux C. Bone mineral measurements in mice: comparison of two devices. *J Clin Densitom.* 2003;6(3):251-258.
10. Yao GQ, Wu JJ, Ovadia S, Troiano N, Sun BH, Insogna K. Targeted overexpression of the two colony-stimulating factor-1 isoforms in osteoblasts differentially affects bone loss in ovariectomized mice. *Am J Physiol Endocrinol Metab.* 2009;296(4):E714-E720.
11. Modder UI, Riggs BL, Spelsberg TC, et al. Dose-response of estrogen on bone versus the uterus in ovariectomized mice. *Eur J Endocrinol.* 2004;151(4):503-510.
12. Binkley N, Dahl DB, Engelke J, Kawahara-Baccus T, Krueger D, Colman RJ. Bone loss detection in rats using a mouse densitometer. *J Bone Miner Res.* 2003;18(2): 370-375.
13. Nazarian A, Cory E, Muller R, Snyder BD. Shortcomings of DXA to assess changes in bone tissue density and microstructure induced by metabolic bone diseases in rat models. *Osteoporos Int.* 2009;20(1):123-132.
14. Gasser JA. Bone measurements by peripheral quantitative computed tomography in rodents. *Methods Mol Med.* 2003; 80:323-341.
15. Stauber M, Muller R. Micro-computed tomography: a method for the non-destructive evaluation of the three-dimensional structure of biological specimens. *Methods Mol Biol.* 2008;455:273-292.
16. Andersson N, Lindberg MK, Ohlsson C, Andersson K, Ryberg B. Repeated *in vivo* determinations of bone mineral density during parathyroid hormone treatment in ovariectomized mice. *J Endocrinol.* 2001;170(3):529-537.
17. Idris AI, Greig IR, Bassonga-Landao E, Ralston SH, van 't Hof RJ. Identification of novel biphenyl carboxylic acid derivatives as novel antiresorptive agents that do not impair parathyroid hormone-induced bone formation. *Endocrinology.* 2009;150(1):5-13.
18. Idris AI, van 't Hof RJ, Greig IR, et al. Regulation of bone mass, bone loss and osteoclast activity by cannabinoid receptors. *Nat Med.* 2005;11(7):774-779.
19. Waarsing JH, Day JS, Weinans H. Longitudinal micro-CT scans to evaluate bone architecture. *J Musculoskelet Neuronal Interact.* 2005;5(4):310-312.
20. Boyd SK, Moser S, Kuhn M, et al. Evaluation of three-dimensional image registration methodologies for *in vivo* micro-computed tomography. *Ann Biomed Eng.* 2006; 34(10):1587-1599.
21. Boyd SK, Davison P, Muller R, Gasser JA. Monitoring individual morphological changes over time in ovariectomized rats by *in vivo* micro-computed tomography. *Bone.* 2006; 39(4):854-862.
22. Klinck RJ, Campbell GM, Boyd SK. Radiation effects on bone architecture in mice and rats resulting from *in vivo* micro-computed tomography scanning. *Med Eng Phys.* 2008;30(7):888-895.
23. Parfitt AM, Drezner MK, Glorieux FH, et al. Bone histomorphometry: standardization of nomenclature, symbols, and units. Report of the ASBMR Histomorphometry Nomenclature Committee. *J Bone Miner Res.* 1987;2(6):595-610.
24. Erben RG. Embedding of bone samples in methylmethacrylate: an improved method suitable for bone histomorphometry, histochemistry, and immunohistochemistry. *J Histochem Cytochem.* 1997;45(2):307-313.
25. Erben RG. Bone-labeling techniques. In: An YH, Martin KL, eds. *Handbook of Histology Methods for Bone and Cartilage.* Totowa: Humana Press; 2003:99-117.
26. Wronski TJ, Cintron M, Dann LM. Temporal relationship between bone loss and increased bone turnover in ovariectomized rats. *Calcif Tissue Int.* 1988;43(3):179-183.
27. Power RA, Iwaniec UT, Magee KA, Mitova-Caneva NG, Wronski TJ. Basic fibroblast growth factor has rapid bone anabolic effects in ovariectomized rats. *Osteoporos Int.* 2004;15(9):716-723.
28. Lesclous P, Guez D, Saffar JL. Short-term prevention of osteoclastic resorption and osteopenia in ovariectomized rats treated with the H(2) receptor antagonist cimetidine. *Bone.* 2002;30(1):131-136.
29. Clemens JD, Herrick MV, Singer FR, Eyre DR. Evidence that serum NTx (collagen-type I N-telopeptides) can act as an immunochemical marker of bone resorption. *Clin Chem.* 1997;43(11):2058-2063.
30. Rissanen JP, Suominen MI, Peng Z, Halleen JM. Secreted tartrate-resistant acid phosphatase 5b is a marker of osteoclast number in human osteoclast cultures and the rat ovariectomy model. *Calcif Tissue Int.* 2008;82(2):108-115.
31. Gaumet N, Seibel MJ, Coxam V, Davicco MJ, Lebecque P, Barlet JP. Influence of ovariectomy and estradiol treatment on calcium homeostasis during aging in rats. *Arch Physiol Biochem.* 1997;105(5):435-444.
32. Rissanen JP, Suominen MI, Peng Z, et al. Short-term changes in serum PINP predict long-term changes in trabecular bone in the rat ovariectomy model. *Calcif Tissue Int.* 2008; 82(2):155-161.
33. Hassager C, Risteli J, Risteli L, Jensen SB, Christiansen C. Diurnal variation in serum markers of type I collagen synthesis and degradation in healthy premenopausal women. *J Bone Miner Res.* 1992;7(11):1307-1311.
34. Shao P, Ohtsuka-Isoya M, Shinoda H. Circadian rhythms in serum bone markers and their relation to the effect of etidronate in rats. *Chronobiol Int.* 2003;20(2):325-336.
35. Klinck J, Boyd SK. The magnitude and rate of bone loss in ovariectomized mice differs among inbred strains as determined by longitudinal *in vivo* micro-computed tomography. *Calcif Tissue Int.* 2008;83(1):70-79.
36. Seedor JG, Quartuccio HA, Thompson DD. The bisphosphonate alendronate (MK-217) inhibits bone loss due to ovariectomy in rats. *J Bone Miner Res.* 1991;6(4):339-346.
37. Brouwers JE, Lambers FM, Gasser JA, van Rietbergen B, Huiskes R. Bone degeneration and recovery after early and late bisphosphonate treatment of ovariectomized wistar rats

assessed by *in vivo* micro-computed tomography. *Calcif Tissue Int*. 2008;82(3):202-211.

38. Kim MK, Kim HD, Park JH, et al. An orally active cathepsin K inhibitor, furan-2-carboxylic acid, 1-{1-[4-fluoro-2-(2-oxo-pyrrolidin-1-yl)-phenyl]-3-oxo-piperidin-4-ylcarba moyl}-cyclohexyl)-amide (OST-4077), inhibits osteoclast activity *in vitro* and bone loss in ovariectomized rats. *J Pharmacol Exp Ther*. 2006;318(2):555-562.
39. van 't Hof RJ, Idris AI, Ridge SA, Dunford J, Greig IR, Ralston SH. Identification of biphenylcarboxylic acid derivatives as a novel class of bone resorption inhibitors. *J Bone Miner Res*. 2004;19(10):1651-1660.
40. Schaller S, Henriksen K, Sveigaard C, et al. The chloride channel inhibitor NS3736 [corrected] prevents bone resorption in ovariectomized rats without changing bone formation. *J Bone Miner Res*. 2004;19(7):1144-1153.
41. Marquis RW, Ru Y, LoCastro SM, et al. Azepanone-based inhibitors of human and rat cathepsin K. *J Med Chem*. 2001;44(9):1380-1395.
42. Palmer JT, Bryant C, Wang DX, et al. Design and synthesis of tri-ring P3 benzamide-containing aminonitriles as potent, selective, orally effective inhibitors of cathepsin K. *J Med Chem*. 2005;48(24):7520-7534.
43. Stroup GB, Lark MW, Veber DF, et al. Potent and selective inhibition of human cathepsin K leads to inhibition of bone resorption *in vivo* in a nonhuman primate. *J Bone Miner Res*. 2001;16(10):1739-1746.
44. Brouwers JE, van Rietbergen B, Huiskes R, Ito K. Effects of PTH treatment on tibial bone of ovariectomized rats assessed by *in vivo* micro-CT. *Osteoporos Int*. 2009;20(11):1823-1835.
45. Liu CC, Kalu DN. Human parathyroid hormone-(1–34) prevents bone loss and augments bone formation in sexually mature ovariectomized rats. *J Bone Miner Res*. 1990;5(9): 973-982.
46. Wronski TJ, Yen CF, Qi H, Dann LM. Parathyroid hormone is more effective than estrogen or bisphosphonates for restoration of lost bone mass in ovariectomized rats. *Endocrinology*. 1993;132(2):823-831.
47. Mosekilde L, Danielsen CC, Gasser J. The effect on vertebral bone mass and strength of long term treatment with antiresorptive agents (estrogen and calcitonin), human parathyroid hormone-(1–38), and combination therapy, assessed in aged ovariectomized rats. *Endocrinology*. 1994;134(5): 2126-2134.
48. Fuchs RK, Allen MR, Condon KW, et al. Strontium ranelate does not stimulate bone formation in ovariectomized rats. *Osteoporos Int*. 2008;19(9):1331-1341.
49. Bain SD, Jerome C, Shen V, Dupin-Roger I, Ammann P. Strontium ranelate improves bone strength in ovariectomized rat by positively influencing bone resistance determinants. *Osteoporos Int*. 2009;20(8):1417-1428.
50. Marie PJ, Hott M, Modrowski D, et al. An uncoupling agent containing strontium prevents bone loss by depressing bone resorption and maintaining bone formation in estrogen-deficient rats. *J Bone Miner Res*. 1993;8(5):607-615.
51. Kumar S, Matheny CJ, Hoffman SJ, et al. An orally active calcium-sensing receptor antagonist that transiently increases plasma concentrations of PTH and stimulates bone formation. *Bone*. 2010;46:534-542.
52. Judex S, Lei X, Han D, Rubin C. Low-magnitude mechanical signals that stimulate bone formation in the ovariectomized rat are dependent on the applied frequency but not on the strain magnitude. *J Biomech*. 2007;40(6):1333-1339.
53. Brouwers JE, van Rietbergen B, Ito K, Huiskes R. Effects of vibration treatment on tibial bone of ovariectomized rats analyzed by *in vivo* micro-CT. *J Orthop Res*. 2010;28(1): 62-69.
54. Gasser JA, Kneissel M, Thomsen JS, Mosekilde L. PTH and interactions with bisphosphonates. *J Musculoskelet Neuronal Interact*. 2000;1(1):53-56.
55. Fuchs RK, Phipps RJ, Burr DB. Recovery of trabecular and cortical bone turnover after discontinuation of risedronate and alendronate therapy in ovariectomized rats. *J Bone Miner Res*. 2008;23(10):1689-1697.

9 The Ovariectomized Mice and Rats

Jameela Banu

The most common animals that are used for experimental studies are rodents, mainly rats and mice. Osteoporosis-related research is no exception. As early as 1985, ovariectomized (OVX) rats were used to study postmenopausal osteoporosis.[1] In 1991, Kalu[2] reported the OVX rat as a model for studying postmenopausal bone loss. There are many similarities between bone loss in rats after ovariectomy and postmenopausal bone loss in women, like bone resorption exceeding bone formation, increased bone loss virtually followed by slower bone formation, higher loss of cancellous bone than cortical bone, and lower absorption of calcium in the intestine.[2] The major factors resulting from ovarian hormone deficiency, induced surgically or by menopause, are decreased bone density and increased fragility due to decreased cancellous bone volume[2,3] in the secondary spongiosa and lumbar vertebrae. This is characterized by increased trabecular separation, reduced trabecular thickness, trabecular connectivity, and trabecular number.[4] This is a result of estrogen deficiency, which increases bone turnover and bone resorption rates resulting in net loss of bone mass mainly in the cancellous bone compartment. Biochemical markers for bone formation and resorption markers, especially bone resorption, are higher as a result of high bone turnover after ovariectomy. Genes related to immune response, bone resorption, growth cell cycle regulation, and apoptosis were upregulated while those related to carbohydrate metabolism, mitosis, extracellular matrix surface, and angiogenesis were downregulated.[5]

For the last two decades, OVX rats have been used to understand the mechanism of bone loss as well as to test therapeutic agents including hormones, selective estrogen receptor modulators, bisphosphonates, nutritional supplements, alternative medicine, and other treatment parameters like physical activity and mechanical stress on bone. In 1994, the United States Food and Drug Administration (FDA) mandated the use of OVX rat models to test any preventive or treatment strategy for osteoporosis.[6]

In the OVX rat model, the rate of bone loss is different in different bones and at different bone sites. Proximal tibial metaphysis (PTM) loses significant amounts of bone 14 days after surgery and a steady state is reached after 90 days.[7,8] Significant bone loss occurs in the neck of the femur 30 days after surgery[9] and at the lumbar vertebra 60 days after surgery.[10] Both these sites do not reach a steady state till 270 days after surgery. All these three sites are very rich in trabecular bone. Cortical bone often shows enlargement of endocortical surface/marrow cavity between 90 and 120 days after ovariectomy[11-13] and takes more than 180 days to reach a steady state.[14] Figure 9.1 shows the different bone sites that are normally analyzed in OVX rodent models of postmenopausal bone loss.

Ovarian hormone deficiency promotes marrow-derived progenitor cells that differentiate into osteoclasts mainly by influencing the bone marrow stroma[15]; therefore, many soluble proteins like cytokines and growth factors are necessary for osteoclast development[16-18] (Fig. 9.2). Within 7 days after ovariectomy there is increase in granulocyte macrophage colony-forming unit and in osteoclast-like cells.[19] The close proximity to bone marrow cells explains the effects of estrogen to regulate cytokine expression from the cells.

J. Banu
Department of Medicine, Physiology and Medical Research Division, Edinburg Regional Academic Center,
University of Texas Health Science Center at San Antonio, 1214, W Schunior, Edinburg, TX 78541, USA
e-mail: banu@uthscsa.edu

G. Duque and K. Watanabe (eds.), *Osteoporosis Research*,
DOI: 10.1007/978-0-85729-293-3_9,

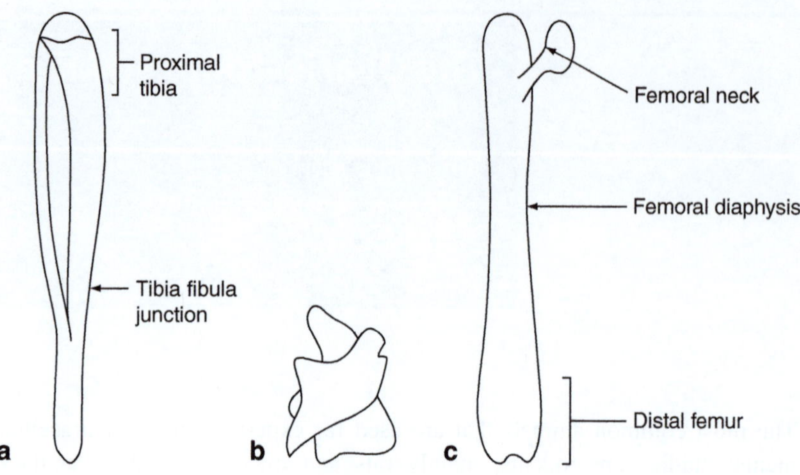

Fig. 9.1 Diagrammatic representation of the different bone sites that are analyzed in OVX rodent models. (**a**) Tibia; (**b**) lumbar vertebrae; (**c**) femur

Proximal tibia
Tibia fibula junction
a
b
c
Femoral neck
Femoral diaphysis
Distal femur

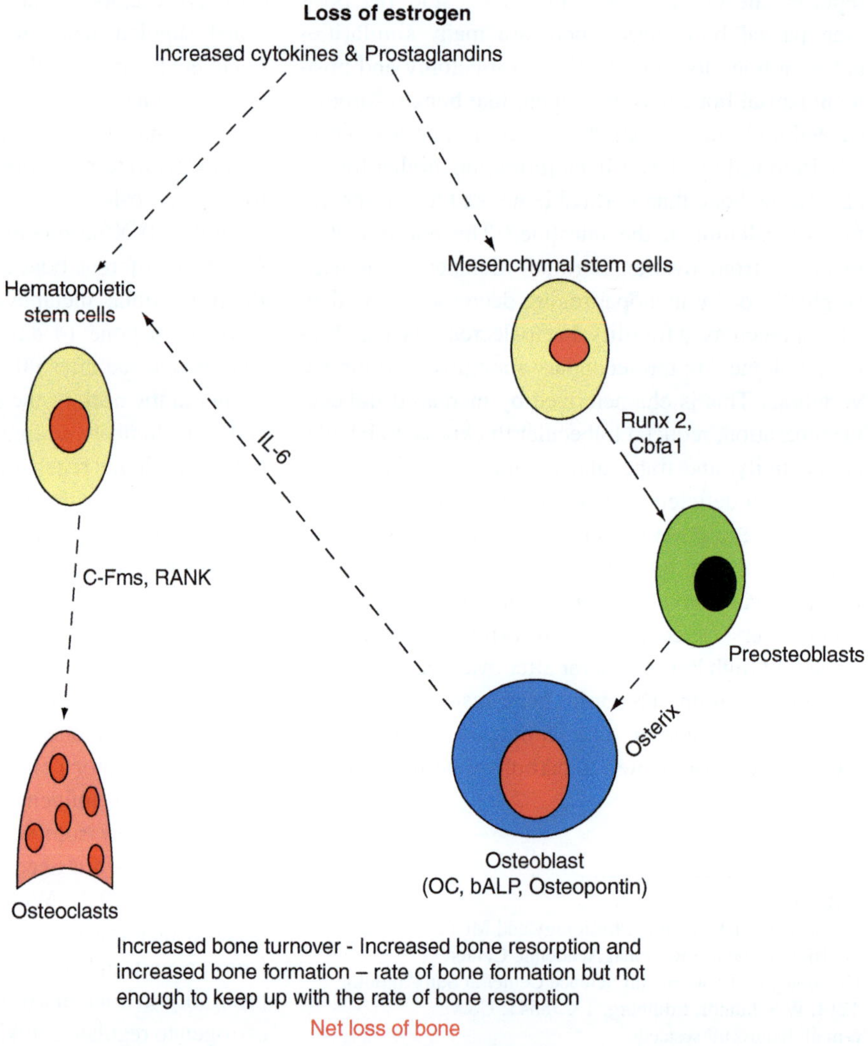

Loss of estrogen
Increased cytokines & Prostaglandins
Hematopoietic stem cells
Mesenchymal stem cells
IL-6
Runx 2, Cbfa1
C-Fms, RANK
Preosteoblasts
Osterix
Osteoclasts
Osteoblast
(OC, bALP, Osteopontin)
Increased bone turnover - Increased bone resorption and increased bone formation – rate of bone formation but not enough to keep up with the rate of bone resorption
Net loss of bone

Fig. 9.2 Diagrammatic representation of the effects of ovariectomy on osteoblastogenesis and osteoclastogenesis

Modulatory properties of estrogen in bone marrow cells show that estrogen receptors (ERs) α and β are affected in OVX mice.[20] Estrogen acts through ER α activation in the mesenchymal stem cells.

Also, after ovariectomy there is increased production of pro-inflammatory cytokines, specifically interleukin (IL)-1 and tumor necrosis factor-alpha (TNF-α), in mice.[21-25] IL-6 mediates osteoclast development in OVX mice.[26] Estrogen suppresses IL-6 expression.[27] Neutralization of IL-11 decreases cancellous bone loss in OVX mice by decreasing osteoclast formation.[28] Apart from pro-inflammatory cytokines, intracellular adhesion molecule 1 (ICAM 1) expression in OVX mice is important for osteoclastogenesis.[29]

Macrophage migration inhibitory factor–deficient mice are protected from ovariectomy-induced bone loss.[30] Prostaglandins increased nuclear factor κB (NF-κB) in bone marrow cells of OVX mice.[31] Estrogen deficiency increased Macrophage colony stimulating factor (M-CSF) production via early growth response (Egr)-1 and Egr-null mice increased bone resorption and decreased bone mass.[32]

Among the different strains of rats commonly used in the laboratory, Sprague-Dawley (SD) rats are used widely. Other strains of rats that have been commonly used include Wistar and Fisher 344. Young adult OVX rats show significant bone loss, while middle-aged and older rats show more similarities to postmenopausal bone loss, because bone formation is less and bone resorption is higher in these rats.

Bones from different strains of mice show different levels of bone mass and lose bone at different levels after ovariectomy, in both trabecular and cortical compartments. Mice with higher trabecular bone at baseline seem to lose more trabecular bone 1 month after ovariectomy, while mice with higher cortical bone at baseline lose less cortical bone 1 month after surgery.[33] It is interesting that the amount of trabecular bone at the proximal tibia and distal femur is less in C57Bl/6 (B6) mice, the most commonly used mice for studies related to bone, when compared to that in other strains.[33,34] B6 mice also have thinner cortical bone when compared to C3H/HeJ and Balb-C.[35] Young adult mice as well as middle-aged and old mice have been used to study bone loss after ovariectomy.

OVX mice have also been used to develop assay techniques for biochemical markers of bone turnover like osteocalcin assay[36] and C telopepetide enzyme-linked immunosorbent assay (ELISA).[37] Scanning techniques like peripheral quantitative computed tomography (pQCT), microcomputerized tomography (μCT), and three-dimensional (3D) structural assessment to understand the pathophysiology of osteoporosis[38] have also been developed using OVX mice.[39] Three-dimensional–reconstructed images of the distal femoral metaphysis and PTM are shown in Fig. 9.3 from sham and OVX mice.

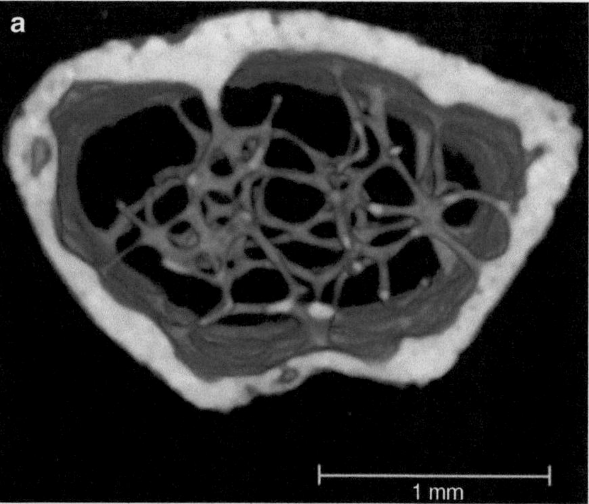

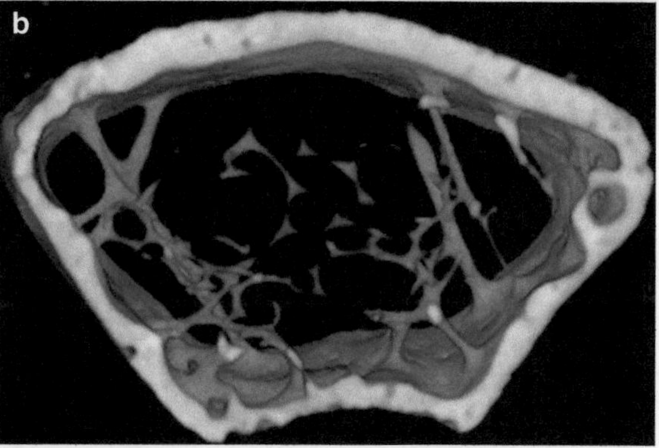

Fig. 9.3 Three-dimensional μCT images of tibia and femur from sham and OVX 4.5-month-old C57BL/6 mice. (**a**) Sham distal femoral metaphysis; (**b**) OVX distal femoral metaphysis; (**c**) sham PTM; (**d**) OVX PTM

9.1 Ovariectomized Rats and Mice as Models for Testing Therapeutic Agents

OVX rats are used as animal models to determine the therapeutic effects for the prevention and treatment of osteoporosis. Several compounds including hormones

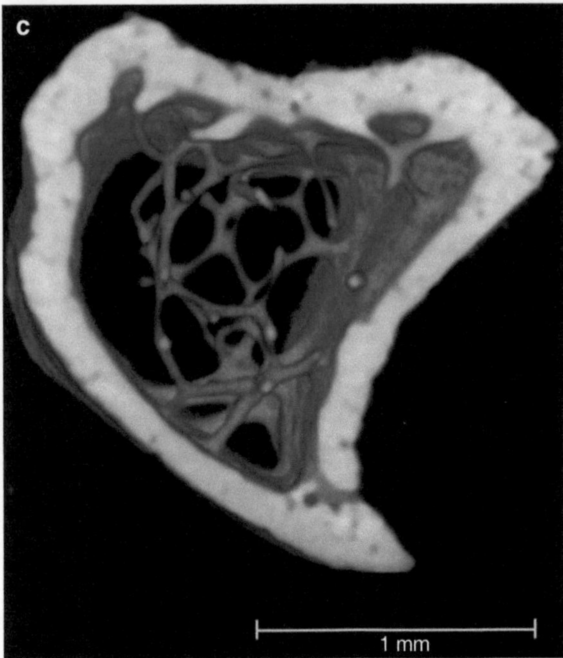

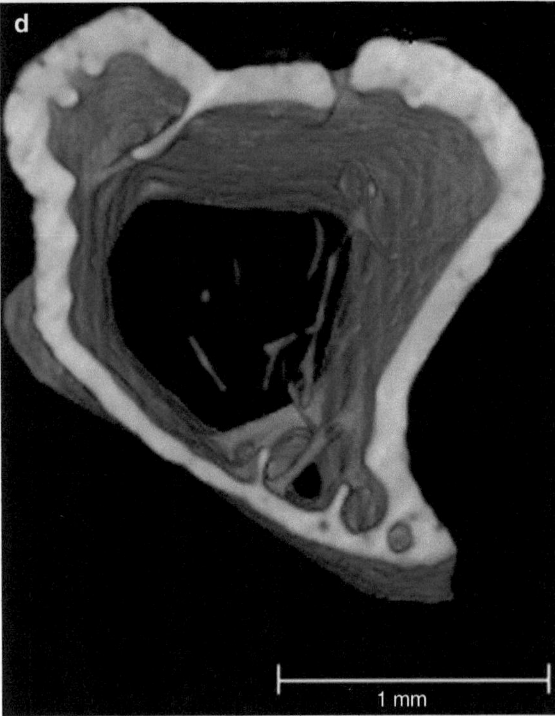

Fig. 9.3 (continued)

and combinations of hormones with other compounds have also been studied in the OVX rats and mice models for osteoporosis.

9.1.1 Hormones

9.1.1.1 Estrogen

As estrogen deficiency leads to rapid bone loss during menopause, estrogen supplementation has been widely studied. Estrogen supplementation to OVX rats showed complete protection of bone mass.[4,40-42] Infusion of 17β-estradiol into the distal femur of young SD rats, for a short period (8 days), locally inhibited bone resorption and stimulated bone formation by increasing osteoblast number and osteoid surface.[3] Estrogen prevented ovariectomy-induced bone loss by decreasing bone turnover.[2] Estrogen supplementation prevented loss of cancellous bone in the lumbar and proximal tibial metaphyses in middle-aged mice but not in younger mice.[43] 17β-estradiol stimulated endocortical bone formation[44] in young mice.

9.1.1.2 Parathyroid Hormone (PTH)

Another hormone that is widely studied for its therapeutic effects on osteoporosis is PTH. As PTH regulates calcium homeostasis in the body, any decrease in calcium levels triggers the reabsorption of calcium from the kidney and/or bone. The absorption is initiated by vitamin D and PTH stimulates osteoblasts to produce NF-κB and receptor activator of NF-κB ligand (RANKL) to stimulate osteoclastogenesis and initiate bone resorption.[45,46] Although PTH can initiate bone resorption, it is also a potent bone anabolic agent. Female SD rats, treated with PTH, have shown increased calcium content[47] and bone mass.[48] PTH enhances osteoblast insulin-like growth factor (IGF) expression in young adult OVX rats.[49] PTH-treated OVX rats had decreased tartrate resistant acid phosphatase (TRAP)$^+$ multinuclear cells suggesting that PTH also reduced osteoclastogenesis, thereby decreasing bone resorption.[50] PTH also restored bone after established bone loss.[51] PTH treatment (short-term study 28 days) increased trabecular bone mass mainly by increasing trabecular thickness and also activated osteogenic precursor cells to stimulate bone formation.[52-56] Vertebral bone mass, bone quality, and cancellous bone connectivity are increased in OVX rats after PTH treatment.[57,58] In the femur of aged OVX rats,

PTH treatment significantly increased trabecular bone mass and strength of the femoral neck.[59-61] Total recovery of bone at the tibial metaphysis was reported after PTH treatment in OVX mice.[62,63] As mentioned earlier, PTH also showed site-specific effects on different skeletal sites in OVX mice.[64]

Administration of PTH mainly stimulated endocortical bone formation and trabecular thickness, indicating the possibility of marrow occlusion in long bones. Therefore, an alternative approach to continuous administration is intermittent administration of PTH to OVX rodents. Intermittent treatment with PTH inhibited osteoclast proliferation and stimulated proliferation and differentiation of osteoblast progenitors.[65] Intermittent therapy with PTH increased bone formation in OVX rats[66] in the mandibles.[67] Intermittent treatment with hPTH on mandibular condyle of OVX rats increased bone formation.[68,69] PTH also increased alveolar bone in OVX rats.[70] PTH has the capacity to restore bone mass in the long bones and lumbar vertebrae even after withdrawal and readministration in OVX Wistar rats.[71]

PTH treatment has been tried in combination with several other compounds like hormones, bisphosphonates, and exercise in OVX rats and/or mice models. Combination of PTH with estrogen has been studied in OVX rats and the combination therapy reversed bone-forming rate in cancellous bone mass and trabecular connectivity in these rats.[72-74] PTH treatment in OVX rats also increased cortical bone area.[75-77]

Combination treatment of growth hormone (GH) and PTH on the reversal of osteopenia in middle-aged OVX rats on vertebra and tibio–fibular junction showed significant increase in the periosteal surface after GH treatment, significant decrease in the endocortical surface after PTH treatment, and in combination GH and PTH showed additive effects.[78,79] Co-treatment increased the strength of the femur and increased bone mass in the femoral neck.[80,81]

PTH and Icadronates (BP) restored cancellous bone and cortical bone in OVX rats as well as bone strength.[82] Osteoprotegerin (OPG) and PTH have additive effects on bone density and mechanical strength in OVX rats.[83] PTH restored lost cancellous bone in the proximal tibial metaphysis (PTM) of OVX rats after 8 weeks of treatment.[84] Sequential treatment with fibroblast growth factor and PTH is more efficacious than PTH alone. PTH and zolendronate increased cancellous and cortical bone mass in the vertebrae and femur.[85] Long-term pretreatment with alendronate, estrogen, or raloxifene does not decrease the effect of PTH treatment on cancellous bone of vertebrae and PTM of OVX rats.[86]

9.1.1.3 Other Hormones

GH is also a potent bone anabolic agent. GH increased the bone mass as well as strength in appendicular skeleton and lumbar vertebra.[87-89] OVX rats have been used to study the bone anabolic properties of GH which restored vertebral strength in middle-aged OVX rats.[87] Although the influence of GH on bone is partly mediated by IGF-1, there is evidence that GH can act independent of circulating IGF-1 to protect ovariectomy-induced bone loss.[90]

Thyroid-stimulating hormone prevented and restored bone mass in (aged) OVX rats by antiresorption and anabolic properties.[91]

9.1.1.4 Selective Estrogen Receptor Modulators (SERMs) and Bisphosphonates

Several SERMs like raloxifene,[92,93] ormeloxifene,[94] HMR-3339,[95] SCH 57068,[96] and OS-0544[97] have been tested in OVX rodents before they were introduced to humans.

Bisphosphonates like alendronate had restorative effects on cancellous and cortical bone mass of tibia in middle-aged rats.[98,99] Other bisphosphonates like tiludronate also increased bone mass in OVX rats.[100] Continuous and intermittent administration of Ibandronate maintained bone mass, architecture, and strength in OVX rats.[101] Zoledronic acid prevented ovariectomy-induced trabecular bone loss and micro-architectural deterioration in middle-aged Wistar rats.[102]

9.1.1.5 Other Therapies Currently Available for Treating Bone Loss

Apart from the known therapies for postmenopausal osteoporosis, several other compounds have been tested for their therapeutic properties in OVX rats and mice.

These compounds protect ovariectomy-induced bone loss by several mechanisms. Some of these compounds mainly decrease bone resorption: triphenylethylene (Fc 1271 a) reduced ovariectomy-induced bone loss and increases bone strength in rats[103]; triazolotriazepine JTT-606 prevented bone resorption by decreasing bone resorption factors in OVX rats[104]; polyethylene particles protected ovariectomy-induced bone resorption by decreasing the number of osteoclasts, thereby showing less mean bone loss in OVX animals implanted with polyethylene particles[105]; selective p38α-inhibitor SD 282 prevented trabecular bone loss after ovariectomy in rats[106]; suppression of NF-κB in OVX mice (NF-κB inhibitor pyrrolidine dithiocarbamate) prevented ovariectomy-induced bone loss[107]; cyclooxygenase-2 (COX-2) inhibitor decreased bone resorption in OVX mice[108]; tyrosine inhibitor decreased TRAP-positive osteoclast cells in bone from OVX rats[109]; trehalose decreased osteoclastogenesis in OVX mice[110]; aspirin inhibited osteoclast activity in OVX mice.[111]

Using OVX rats and mice, some compounds that can increase bone formation and decrease bone resorption are also reported: the antibiotic tetracycline analog CMT 8 reduced bone resorption and increased bone formation in OVX rats[112]; cathepsin K (CPK) inhibitor SB-553484 inhibited bone resorption by reducing trabecular separation, increasing trabecular number and connectivity, and stimulating cortical bone formation[113]; bone morphometric protein-6 decreased bone resorption, increasing bone formation in OVX mice[114]; OVX mice when transduced with RANK-Fc prevented ovariectomy-induced bone loss and increased bone mineral density (BMD)[115]; fibroblast growth factor (FGF-1) prevented and restored ovariectomy-induced bone loss[116]; bone FGF and risendronate restored trabecular mineralization and micro-architecture in OVX mice[117]; β blocker – propranolol –and PTH increased both trabecular and cortical bone in young OVX mice.[118]

In other studies, OVX rats and mice are used to show how certain compounds have protective effects against ovariectomy-induced bone loss: a phosphodiesterase 4 inhibitor, XT-44, increased BMD of OVX rats.[119] Transplantation of mesenchymal stem cells over expressing RANK-Fc and CXC chemokine receptor-4 protected against ovariectomy-induced bone loss in mice.[120] 3-hydroxybutyrate containing polyhydroxyalkanoids stimulated bone growth.[121] Human OPG gene therapy reversed ovariectomy-induced bone loss in OVX mice[122] and when administered reduced trabecular bone loss.[123] Biglycan can modulate bone turnover in OVX mice.[124]

9.2 Ovariectomized Rats and Mice as Models for Studying the Effects of Nutritional Supplements to Treat and Prevent Osteoporosis

Recently, there has been increased awareness of the benefits of taking nutritional supplements and compounds from organic sources for the prevention and treatment of bone loss. This approach has been sought mainly because of the high risks involved in the consumption of existing drugs when used for long periods of time. Many compounds that are active ingredients of food components and are normally consumed are now becoming popular for preventing and treating bone loss.

9.2.1 Vitamins and Calcium

As calcium is the major mineral that is lost from the bone after ovarian hormone deficiency, supplementation with calcium in the diet has been widely studied in OVX rodent models for bone loss. Dietary calcium in the form of calcium carbonate is the best source of calcium and the amount of calcium consumed influenced skeletal strength in OVX rats.[125] Other sources are egg shell calcium[126] and lobster shell calcium,[127] and supplementation from antlers has increased bone mass and strength in OVX rats and SAMP8 mice.[128] Calcium-rich compound, Praval bhasma, also increased strength and decreased trabecular separation in OVX rats.[129] When calcium was administered in combination with oligofructose, bone was protected from ovariectomy-induced bone loss.[130] OVX rats on a low calcium diet and treated with 1,25(OH)2D$_3$ showed increased bone mineral content and maintained positive mineral balance.

Calcitonin, a hormone that can reduce serum calcium levels, has been studied widely in OVX rodents. Calcitonin protected bone from ovariectomy-induced bone loss[131] in a site-specific manner and withdrawal of calcitonin rapidly increased bone loss[132] in rats as well as nasal salmon calcitonin.[133]

Vitamins like vitamin D and vitamin K have been reported to protect bones after ovariectomy: 1 alpha hydroxyl vitamin D3 reduced ovariectomy-induced bone loss in young mice[134]; vitamin D increased bone formation and decreased bone resorption in OVX mice[135]; vitamin K2 acted on osteoblasts and prevented ovariectomy-induced bone loss in OVX Fisher rats[136]; vitamin K and risendronate increased the strength of the femur in OVX ICR mice[137]; an analog of 1,25 (OH)(2)D(3), 2-methylene-19-nor-1-alpha, 25(OH)(2)D(3) increased bone formation in OVX rats.[138]

9.2.2 Phytoestrogens

Phytoestrogens like soy proteins have shown bone-protective properties in OVX rodent models of bone loss. Soybean protein protected bone from ovariectomy-induced bone loss in rats.[139] Soybean milk and milk peptide increased BMD and bone strength in OVX rats.[140] Soy isoflavones reduced ovariectomy-induced osteoporosis in middle-aged mice in the femur and vertebrae.[141] Soy in combination with other compounds has also been reported to benefit bone both in middle-aged and young rats and mice. Soy and fructo-oligosaccharides, in middle-aged OVX SD rats, increased BMD of tibia and lumbar vertebrae, and reversed micro-architecture like tibial trabecular number, trabecular separation, and trabecular thickness.[142] Soy by itself or soy along with plum and fructo-oligosaccharides increased BMD and alkaline phosphatase activity, and decreased urinary Dpd in young adult SD rats.[143]

9.2.3 Isoflavones

Two isoflavones have been widely studied with respect to bone. One of them is genestein. This isoflavone is reported to completely prevent ovariectomy-induced bone loss.[144] It acts as an estrogen agonist only in bone by increasing BMD in OVX mice.[145] It can also inhibit bone resorption and stimulate bone formation in young OVX rats and mice.[146-148]

The other isoflavone commonly tested for its bone-protective properties is diadzein; diadzein metabolites – equol and o-desmethylangolensin – in OVX mice showed inhibition of osteoclast formation with equol.[149] Diadzein has been tested in combination with calcium and shown to prevent cortical and trabecular bone loss and preserve mechanical strength in OVX mice, in femur and lumbar vertebrae.[150]

A herb that contains isoflavones, *Puerariae redix*, restored trabecular bone loss in OVX mice.[151] Combination of isoflavone conjugates and fructo-oligosaccharides increased femoral BMD in OVX mice.[152]

9.2.4 Flavanoids

A flavanoid found in onions and vegetables, Qvercetin, inhibited ovariectomy-induced bone loss in mice.[153] Other flavanoids from Herperidin, a citrus flavanoid, and from *Epiedium brevicornum maxim* prevented ovariectomy-induced bone loss.[154,155]

9.2.5 Fatty Acids

OVX mice have been used to study the effects of certain fatty acids (FA) on bone. n-3 FA inhibited osteoclastogenesis and activation, and reduced bone loss in OVX mice.[156,157] Endogenously produced n-3 FA reduced ovariectomy-induced bone loss mainly by decreasing osteoclast and pro-inflammatory cytokines.[158] Another FA found in milk and dairy products, conjugated linoleic acid, also decreased bone resorption in adult rats.[159]

9.2.6 Other Compounds from Herbal Origin

Several herbs and fruits have been tested for their beneficial properties in OVX rodent models for osteoporosis: 2-methoxyestradiol decreased ovariectomy-induced bone loss in rats[160]; heated powder of *Ostreae testa* prevented ovariectomy-induced bone loss by activation of osteoblasts[161]; triterpenoids from *Cimicifugae rhizome* inhibited osteoclast formation and activity in OVX mice[162]; bean snack prevented ovariectomy-induced bone loss[163]; *Dioscorea spongiosa* prevented bone loss in both cortical and trabecular bone compartments and preserved bone strength in OVX mice and rats[164];

blueberry treatment also prevented bone loss in middle-aged SD rats[165]; citrus nobiletin inhibited osteoclast activity in DBA/1 J mice[166]; methanolic extract of *Sambucus sieboldiana* reduced bone resorption in OVX mice.[167]

9.3 OVX Rats and Mice as Models for Effects of Physical Activity and Mechanical Strain on Bone

OVX rats are also used to study the effects of physical activity on bone. Physical activity can stimulate bone formation directly by putting strain on the muscle which in turn increases the strain on the bone. Exercise can also indirectly affect bone by increasing GH and IGF-I secretion. Several studies have shown that moderate and voluntary exercise is beneficial to bone. Femur strength was increased in OVX rats by low and moderate-intensity exercise.[168] Moderate treadmill exercise increased cortical and cancellous bone mass in young adult OVX female rats.[169] Wistar rats after ovariectomy and on treadmill exercise treatment increased vertebral bone mass.[170] Voluntary running increased BMD in appendicular skeleton in OVX rats.[127] Voluntary exercise increased BMD in rats after ovariectomy.[127] Slow running induced optimal loading and strengthened bones in OVX rats.[171]

Although voluntary running and treadmill exercise are the most common types of exercises tested, recently vibration, tower climbing, and jumping have also been tested in OVX rodents: female SD rats have been used in whole-body vertical vibration and this form of physical activity increased the biomechanical properties and significantly improved bone with greater effects on the trabecular bone than the cortical bone[172]; adult OVX rats on an exercise regimen showed differential changes at the neck of the condylar process apart from long bones[173]; tower climbing exercise by OVX SD rats has both preventive and recovery effects on the strength of bone[174]; high-impact exercise (jumping) completely prevented ovariectomy-induced bone loss.[175]

Exercise treatment has been combined with hormones and other compounds to see if there is additional effect on bone. Estrogen deficiency reduced bone mass but supplementation only reduced bone resorption and did not increase bone formation; therefore, other therapies including combining estrogen with exercise were also tested in OVX rodents. When estrogen therapy was combined with treadmill exercise there were additive effects in bone turnover rates[176] and decreased bone resorption.[177-179] Young adult OVX rats given 17β-estradiol and on bipedal stance exercise showed complete reversal of bone loss.[180] In young female OVX rats, intermittent treatment with PTH followed by treadmill exercise maintained bone mass in PTM.[181] Bipedal stance exercise and prostaglandin had synergistic effects in decreasing bone resorbing.[182]

Isoflavone-supplemented soy yoghurt, in combination with resistance exercise, prevented bone loss in OVX rats.[183,184] Genestein and exercise have bone-protective properties in OVX rats[185] and mice.[186,187] Sympathetic nervous system blocker propranolol and exercise increased trabecular number and trabecular thickness and biomechanical properties but no additive effects were seen on trabecular micro-architecture, such as cortical width.[188] Bisphosphonates like alendronate and treadmill exercise decreased endocortical resorption and increased periosteal perimeter in 14-week-old rats.[189] Endurance exercise did not have any effect in combination with alendronate.[190] Combination treatment of exercise and calcium increased BMD in the lumbar vertebrae and femur of OVX old rats.[191]

In summary, OVX rats and mice are widely used animal models to study several aspects of bone loss. Young adult animals, middle-aged animals, and old animals have been used successfully to study the mechanism of bone loss as well as to understand the therapeutic properties of different agents. The advantages of using OVX rats and mice to study bone include low cost, easy handling, and the similarities they share with the human pathological condition. Many compounds tested in rats and mice have been tested in humans, and PTH has been approved by the FDA as a bone anabolic therapy for treating osteoporosis.

References

1. Matsumoto T, Ezawa I, Morita K, Kawanobe Y, Ogata E. Effect of vitamin D metabolites on bone metabolism in a rat model of postmenopausal osteoporosis. *J Nutr Sci Vitaminol.* 1985;31(Suppl):S61-S65.
2. Kalu DN. The ovariectomized rat model of postmenopausal bone loss. *Bone Miner.* 1991;15(3):175-191.

3. Takano-Yamamoto T, Rodan GA. Direct effects of 17 beta-estradiol on trabecular bone in ovariectomized rats. *Proc Natl Acad Sci USA*. 1990;87(6):2172-2176.
4. Wronski TJ, Cintron M, Doherty AL, Dann LM. Estrogen treatment prevents osteopenia and depresses bone turnover in ovariectomized rats. *Endocrinology*. 1988;123(2):681-686.
5. Orlic I, Borovecki F, Simic P, Vukicevic S. Gene expression profiling in bone tissue of osteoporotic mice. *Arh Hig Rada Toksikol*. 2007;58(1):3-11.
6. FDA. *Guidelines for Preclinical and Clinical Evaluation of Agents Used for the Prevention of Treatment of Postmenopausal Osteoporosis.*. Washington, DC: Division of Metabolism and Endocrine Drug Products, Food and Drug Administration; 1994.
7. Wronski TJ, Cintron M, Dann LM. Temporal relationship between bone loss and increased bone turnover in ovariectomized rats. *Calcif Tissue Int*. 1988;43(3):179-183.
8. Wronski TJ, Dann LM, Scott KS, Cintron M. Long-term effects of ovariectomy and aging on the rat skeleton. *Calcif Tissue Int*. 1989;45(6):360-366.
9. Li M, Shen Y, Wronski TJ. Time course of femoral neck osteopenia in ovariectomized rats. *Bone*. 1997;20(1):55-61.
10. Wronski TJ, Dann LM, Horner SL. Time course of vertebral osteopenia in ovariectomized rats. *Bone*. 1989;10(4): 295-301.
11. Danielsen CC, Mosekilde L, Svenstrup B. Cortical bone mass, composition, and mechanical properties in female rats in relation to age, long-term ovariectomy, and estrogen substitution. *Calcif Tissue Int*. 1993;52(1):26-33.
12. Ke HZ, Jee WS, Zeng QQ, Li M, Lin BY. Prostaglandin E2 increased rat cortical bone mass when administered immediately following ovariectomy. *Bone Miner*. 1993;21(3): 189-201.
13. Yamamoto N, Jee WS, Ma YF. Bone histomorphometric changes in the femoral neck of aging and ovariectomized rats. *Anat Rec*. 1995;243(2):175-185.
14. Jee WS, Yao W. Animal models of bone diseases. Introduction. *J Musculoskelet Neuronal Interact*. 2001;1(3): 183-184.
15. Dexter TM, Allen TD, Lajtha LG. Conditions controlling the proliferation of haemopoietic stem cells *in vitro*. *J Cell Physiol*. 1977;91(3):335-344.
16. Horowitz M, Jilka RL. Colony stimulating factors and bone remodeling. In: Gowen M, ed. *Cytokines and Bone Metabolism*. Boca Raton: CRC; 1992:185.
17. Mundy GR. Cytokines and local factors which affect osteoclast function. *Int J Cell Cloning*. 1992;10(4):215-222.
18. Shevde N, Anklesaria P, Greenberger JS, Bleiberg I, Glowacki J. Stromal cell-mediated stimulation of osteoclastogenesis. *Proc Soc Exp Biol Med*. 1994;205(4):306-315.
19. Shevde NK, Pike JW. Estrogen modulates the recruitment of myelopoietic cell progenitors in rat through a stromal cell-independent mechanism involving apoptosis. *Blood*. 1996; 87(7):2683-2692.
20. Zhou S, Zilberman Y, Wassermann K, Bain SD, Sadovsky Y, Gazit D. Estrogen modulates estrogen receptor alpha and beta expression, osteogenic activity, and apoptosis in mesenchymal stem cells (MSCs) of osteoporotic mice. *J Cell Biochem*. 2001;81(Suppl 36):144-155.
21. Pacifici R, Brown C, Puscheck E, et al. Effect of surgical menopause and estrogen replacement on cytokine release from human blood mononuclear cells. *Proc Natl Acad Sci USA*. 1991;88(12):5134-5138.
22. Matsuda T, Matsui K, Shimakoshi Y, Aida Y, Hukuda S. 1-Hydroxyethylidene-1, 1-bisphosphonate decreases the postovariectomy enhanced interleukin 1 secretion from peritoneal macrophages in adult rats. *Calcif Tissue Int*. 1991; 49(6):403-406.
23. Kimble RB, Vannice JL, Bloedow DC, et al. Interleukin-1 receptor antagonist decreases bone loss and bone resorption in ovariectomized rats. *J Clin Investig*. 1994;93(5): 1959-1967.
24. Kitazawa R, Kimble RB, Vannice JL, Kung VT, Pacifici R. Interleukin-1 receptor antagonist and tumor necrosis factor binding protein decrease osteoclast formation and bone resorption in ovariectomized mice. *J Clin Investig*. 1994;94(6):2397-2406.
25. Pioli G, Basini G, Pedrazzoni M, et al. Spontaneous release of interleukin-I and interleukin-6 by peripheral blood mononuclear cells after oophorectomy. *Clin Sci (Lond)*. 1992; 83(4):503-507.
26. Jilka RL, Hangoc G, Girasole G, et al. Increased osteoclast development after estrogen loss: mediation by interleukin-6. *Science (New York, NY)*. 1992;257(5066):88-91.
27. Pottratz ST, Bellido T, Mocharla H, Crabb D, Manolagas SC. 17 beta-Estradiol inhibits expression of human interleukin-6 promoter-reporter constructs by a receptor-dependent mechanism. *J Clin Investig*. 1994;93(3):944-950.
28. Shaughnessy SG, Walton KJ, Deschamps P, Butcher M, Beaudin SM. Neutralization of interleukin-11 activity decreases osteoclast formation and increases cancellous bone volume in ovariectomized mice. *Cytokine*. 2002; 20(2):78-85.
29. Gao Y, Morita I, Kubota T, Murota S, Aso T. Expression of adhesion molecules LFA-I and ICAM-I on osteoclast precursors during osteoclast differentiation and involvement of estrogen deficiency. *Climacteric*. 2000;3(4):278-287.
30. Oshima S, Onodera S, Amizuka N, et al. Macrophage migration inhibitory factor-deficient mice are resistant to ovariectomy-induced bone loss. *FEBS Lett*. 2006;580(5):1251-1256.
31. Kanematsu M, Sato T, Takai H, Watanabe K, Ikeda K, Yamada Y. Prostaglandin E2 induces expression of receptor activator of nuclear factor-kappa B ligand/osteoprotegrin ligand on pre-B cells: implications for accelerated osteoclastogenesis in estrogen deficiency. *J Bone Miner Res*. 2000; 15(7):1321-1329.
32. Cenci S, Weitzmann MN, Gentile MA, Aisa MC, Pacifici R. M-CSF neutralization and egr-1 deficiency prevent ovariectomy-induced bone loss. *J Clin Investig*. 2000;105(9): 1279-1287.
33. Bouxsein ML, Myers KS, Shultz KL, Donahue LR, Rosen CJ, Beamer WG. Ovariectomy-induced bone loss varies among inbred strains of mice. *J Bone Miner Res*. 2005; 20(7): 1085-1092.
34. Klinck J, Boyd SK. The magnitude and rate of bone loss in ovariectomized mice differs among inbred strains as determined by longitudinal *in vivo* micro-computed tomography. *Calcif Tissue Int*. 2008;83(1):70-79.
35. Li CY, Schaffler MB, Wolde-Semait HT, Hernandez CJ, Jepsen KJ. Genetic background influences cortical bone response to ovariectomy. *J Bone Miner Res*. 2005;20(12): 2150-2158.

36. Srivastava AK, Castillo G, Wergedal JE, Mohan S, Baylink DJ. Development and application of a synthetic peptide-based osteocalcin assay for the measurement of bone formation in mouse serum. *Calcif Tissue Int*. 2000;67(3):255-259.
37. Srivastava AK, Bhattacharyya S, Castillo G, Miyakoshi N, Mohan S, Baylink DJ. Development and evaluation of C-telopeptide enzyme-linked immunoassay for measurement of bone resorption in mouse serum. *Bone*. 2000; 27(4):529-533.
38. Jiang Y, Zhao J, White DL, Genant HK. Micro CT and Micro MR imaging of 3D architecture of animal skeleton. *J Musculoskelet Neuronal Interact*. 2000;1:45-51.
39. Breen SA, Loveday BE, Millest AJ, Waterton JC. Stimulation and inhibition of bone formation: use of peripheral quantitative computed tomography in the mouse *in vivo*. *Lab Anim*. 1998;32(4):467-476.
40. Gaumet N, Seibel MJ, Coxam V, Davicco MJ, Lebecque P, Barlet JP. Influence of ovariectomy and estradiol treatment on calcium homeostasis during aging in rats. *Arch Physiol Biochem*. 1997;105(5):435-444.
41. Goulding A, Gold E. Effects of chronic prednisolone treatment on bone resorption and bone composition in intact and ovariectomized rats and in ovariectomized rats receiving beta-estradiol. *Endocrinology*. 1988;122(2):482-487.
42. Verhaeghe J, Oloumi G, van Herck E, et al. Effects of long-term diabetes and/or high-dose 17 beta-estradiol on bone formation, bone mineral density, and strength in ovariectomized rats. *Bone*. 1997;20(5):421-428.
43. Modder UI, Riggs BL, Spelsberg TC, et al. Dose-response of estrogen on bone versus the uterus in ovariectomized mice. *Eur J Endocrinol*. 2004;151(4):503-510.
44. Edwards MW, Bain SD, Bailey MC, Lantry MM, Howard GA. 17 beta estradiol stimulation of endosteal bone formation in the ovariectomized mouse: an animal model for the evaluation of bone-targeted estrogens. *Bone*. 1992;13(1):29-34.
45. Garabedian M, Tanaka Y, Holick MF, Deluca HF. Response of intestinal calcium transport and bone calcium mobilization to 1,25-dihydroxyvitamin D3 in thyroparathyroidectomized rats. *Endocrinology*. 1974;94(4):1022-1027.
46. Garabedian M, Holick MF, Deluca HF, Boyle IT. Control of 25-hydroxycholecalciferol metabolism by parathyroid glands. *Proc Natl Acad Sci USA*. 1972;69(7):1673-1676.
47. Hori M, Uzawa T, Morita K, Noda T, Takahashi H, Inoue J. Effect of human parathyroid hormone (PTH(1-34)) on experimental osteopenia of rats induced by ovariectomy. *Bone Miner*. 1988;3(3):193-199.
48. Hock JM, Gera I, Fonseca J, Raisz LG. Human parathyroid hormone-(1-34) increases bone mass in ovariectomized and orchidectomized rats. *Endocrinology*. 1988;122(6):2899-2904.
49. Watson P, Lazowski D, Han V, Fraher L, Steer B, Hodsman A. Parathyroid hormone restores bone mass and enhances osteoblast insulin-like growth factor I gene expression in ovariectomized rats. *Bone*. 1995;16(3):357-365.
50. Kalu DN, Echon R, Hollis BW. Modulation of ovariectomy-related bone loss by parathyroid hormone in rats. *Mech Ageing Dev*. 1990;56(1):49-62.
51. Liu CC, Kalu DN, Salerno E, Echon R, Hollis BW, Ray M. Preexisting bone loss associated with ovariectomy in rats is reversed by parathyroid hormone. *J Bone Miner Res*. 1991;6(10):1071-1080.
52. Kimmel DB, Bozzato RP, Kronis KA, et al. The effect of recombinant human (1-84) or synthetic human (1-34) parathyroid hormone on the skeleton of adult osteopenic ovariectomized rats. *Endocrinology*. 1993;132(4):1577-1584.
53. Qi H, Li M, Wronski TJ. A comparison of the anabolic effects of parathyroid hormone at skeletal sites with moderate and severe osteopenia in aged ovariectomized rats. *J Bone Miner Res*. 1995;10(6):948-955.
54. Zhang KQ, Chen JW, Li QN, et al. Effect of intermittent injection of recombinant human parathyroid hormone on bone histomorphometry of ovariectomized rats. *Acta Pharmacol Sin*. 2002;23(7):659-662.
55. Brouwers JE, van Rietbergen B, Huiskes R, Ito K. Effects of PTH treatment on tibial bone of ovariectomized rats assessed by *in vivo* micro-CT. *Osteoporos Int*. 2009;20(11): 1823-1835.
56. Fox J, Miller MA, Newman MK, et al. Daily treatment of aged ovariectomized rats with human parathyroid hormone (1-84) for 12 months reverses bone loss and enhances trabecular and cortical bone strength. *Calcif Tissue Int*. 2006;79(4):262-272.
57. Mosekilde L, Danielsen CC, Gasser J. The effect on vertebral bone mass and strength of long term treatment with antiresorptive agents (estrogen and calcitonin), human parathyroid hormone-(1-38), and combination therapy, assessed in aged ovariectomized rats. *Endocrinology*. 1994;134(5): 2126-2134.
58. Cheng PT, Chan C, Muller K. Cyclical treatment of osteopenic ovariectomized adult rats with PTH(1-34) and pamidronate. *J Bone Miner Res*. 1995;10(1):119-126.
59. Whitfield JF, Morley P, Ross V, Isaacs RJ, Rixon RH. Restoration of severely depleted femoral trabecular bone in ovariectomized rats by parathyroid hormone-(1-34). *Calcif Tissue Int*. 1995;56(3):227-231.
60. Sogaard CH, Wronski TJ, McOsker JE, Mosekilde L. The positive effect of parathyroid hormone on femoral neck bone strength in ovariectomized rats is more pronounced than that of estrogen or bisphosphonates. *Endocrinology*. 1994; 134(2):650-657.
61. Li M, Wronski TJ. Response of femoral neck to estrogen depletion and parathyroid hormone in aged rats. *Bone*. 1995;16(5):551-557.
62. Li M, Liang H, Shen Y, Wronski TJ. Parathyroid hormone stimulates cancellous bone formation at skeletal sites regardless of marrow composition in ovariectomized rats. *Bone*. 1999;24(2):95-100.
63. Mashiba T, Tanizawa T, Takano Y, Takahashi HE, Mori S, Norimatsu H. A histomorphometric study on effects of single and concurrent intermittent administration of human PTH (1-34) and bisphosphonate cimadronate on tibial metaphysis in ovariectomized rats. *Bone*. 1995;17(4 Suppl): 273S-278S.
64. Zhou H, Iida-Klein A, Lu SS, et al. Anabolic action of parathyroid hormone on cortical and cancellous bone differs between axial and appendicular skeletal sites in mice. *Bone*. 2003;32(5):513-520.
65. Liu CC, Kalu DN. Human parathyroid hormone-(1-34) prevents bone loss and augments bone formation in sexually mature ovariectomized rats. *J Bone Miner Res*. 1990;5(9): 973-982.

66. Lane NE, Kimmel DB, Nilsson MH, et al. Bone-selective analogs of human PTH(1-34) increase bone formation in an ovariectomized rat model. *J Bone Miner Res*. 1996;11(5): 614-625.
67. Miller SC, Hunziker J, Mecham M, Wronski TJ. Intermittent parathyroid hormone administration stimulates bone formation in the mandibles of aged ovariectomized rats. *J Dent Res*. 1997;76(8):1471-1476.
68. Nakajima M, Ejiri S, Tanaka M, Toyooka E, Kohno S, Ozawa H. Effect of intermittent administration of human parathyroid hormone (1-34) on the mandibular condyle of ovariectomized rats. *J Bone Miner Metab*. 2000;18(1):9-17.
69. Hunziker J, Wronski TJ, Miller SC. Mandibular bone formation rates in aged ovariectomized rats treated with anti-resorptive agents alone and in combination with intermittent parathyroid hormone. *J Dent Res*. 2000;79(6):1431-1438.
70. Marques MR, da Silva MA, Manzi FR, Cesar-Neto JB, Nociti FH Jr, Barros SP. Effect of intermittent PTH administration in the periodontitis-associated bone loss in ovariectomized rats. *Arch Oral Biol*. 2005;50(4):421-429.
71. Kishi T, Hagino H, Kishimoto H, Nagashima H. Bone responses at various skeletal sites to human parathyroid hormone in ovariectomized rats: effects of long-term administration, withdrawal, and readministration. *Bone*. 1998;22(5): 515-522.
72. Shen V, Dempster DW, Mellish RW, Birchman R, Horbert W, Lindsay R. Effects of combined and separate intermittent administration of low-dose human parathyroid hormone fragment (1-34) and 17 beta-estradiol on bone histomorphometry in ovariectomized rats with established osteopenia. *Calcif Tissue Int*. 1992;50(3):214-220.
73. Shen V, Dempster DW, Birchman R, Xu R, Lindsay R. Loss of cancellous bone mass and connectivity in ovariectomized rats can be restored by combined treatment with parathyroid hormone and estradiol. *J Clin Investig*. 1993;91(6):2479-2487.
74. Wronski TJ, Yen CF, Qi H, Dann LM. Parathyroid hormone is more effective than estrogen or bisphosphonates for restoration of lost bone mass in ovariectomized rats. *Endocrinology*. 1993;132(2):823-831.
75. Wronski TJ, Yen CF. Anabolic effects of parathyroid hormone on cortical bone in ovariectomized rats. *Bone*. 1994; 15(1):51-58.
76. Mosekilde L. Assessing bone quality – animal models in preclinical osteoporosis research. *Bone*. 1995;17(4 Suppl): 343S-352S.
77. Baumann BD, Wronski TJ. Response of cortical bone to antiresorptive agents and parathyroid hormone in aged ovariectomized rats. *Bone*. 1995;16(2):247-253.
78. Wang L, Orhii PB, Banu J, Kalu DN. Effects of separate and combined therapy with growth hormone and parathyroid hormone on lumbar vertebral bone in aged ovariectomized osteopenic rats. *Bone*. 2001;28(2):202-207.
79. Banu MJ, Orhii PB, Wang L, Kalu DN. Separate and combined effects of growth hormone and parathyroid hormone on cortical bone osteopenia in ovariectomized aged rats. *Aging (Milano)*. 2001;13(4):282-292.
80. Wang L, Orhii PB, Banu J, Kalu DN. Bone anabolic effects of separate and combined therapy with growth hormone and parathyroid hormone on femoral neck in aged ovariectomized osteopenic rats. *Mech Ageing Dev*. 2001;122(1):89-104.
81. Mosekilde L, Tornvig L, Thomsen JS, Orhii PB, Banu MJ, Kalu DN. Parathyroid hormone and growth hormone have additive or synergetic effect when used as intervention treatment in ovariectomized rats with established osteopenia. *Bone*. 2000;26(6):643-651.
82. Zhang L, Endo N, Yamamoto N, Tanizawa T, Takahashi HE. Effects of single and concurrent intermittent administration of human PTH (1-34) and incadronate on cancellous and cortical bone of femoral neck in ovariectomized rats. *Tohoku J Exp Med*. 1998;186(2):131-141.
83. Kostenuik PJ, Capparelli C, Morony S, et al. OPG and PTH-(1-34) have additive effects on bone density and mechanical strength in osteopenic ovariectomized rats. *Endocrinology*. 2001;142(10):4295-4304.
84. Wronski TJ, Ratkus AM, Thomsen JS, Vulcan Q, Mosekilde L. Sequential treatment with basic fibroblast growth factor and parathyroid hormone restores lost cancellous bone mass and strength in the proximal tibia of aged ovariectomized rats. *J Bone Miner Res*. 2001;16(8):1399-1407.
85. Rhee Y, Won YY, Baek MH, Lim SK. Maintenance of increased bone mass after recombinant human parathyroid hormone (1-84) with sequential zoledronate treatment in ovariectomized rats. *J Bone Miner Res*. 2004;19(6):931-937.
86. Ma YL, Bryant HU, Zeng Q, et al. New bone formation with teriparatide [human parathyroid hormone-(1-34)] is not retarded by long-term pretreatment with alendronate, estrogen, or raloxifene in ovariectomized rats. *Endocrinology*. 2003;144(5):2008-2015.
87. Eschen C, Andreassen TT. Growth hormone normalizes vertebral strength in ovariectomized rats. *Calcif Tissue Int*. 1995;57(5):392-396.
88. Verhaeghe J, van Bree R, Van Herck E, et al. Effects of recombinant human growth hormone and insulin-like growth factor-I, with or without 17 beta-estradiol, on bone and mineral homeostasis of aged ovariectomized rats. *J Bone Miner Res*. 1996;11(11):1723-1735.
89. Mosekilde L, Thomsen JS, Orhii PB, Kalu DN. Growth hormone increases vertebral and femoral bone strength in osteopenic, ovariectomized, aged rats in a dose-dependent and site-specific manner. *Bone*. 1998;23(4):343-352.
90. Fritton JC, Emerton KB, Sun H, et al. Growth hormone protects against ovariectomy-induced bone loss in states of low circulating IGF-1*. *J Bone Miner Res*. 2010;25(2):235-246.
91. Sampath TK, Simic P, Sendak R, et al. Thyroid-stimulating hormone restores bone volume, microarchitecture, and strength in aged ovariectomized rats. *J Bone Miner Res*. 2007;22(6):849-859.
92. Iwamoto J, Yeh JK, Schmidt A, et al. Raloxifene and vitamin K2 combine to improve the femoral neck strength of ovariectomized rats. *Calcif Tissue Int*. 2005;77(2):119-126.
93. Folwarczna J, Sliwinski L, Cegiela U, et al. Raloxifene similarly affects the skeletal system of male and ovariectomized female rats. *Pharmacol Rep*. 2007;59(3):349-358.
94. Narayana Murthy PS, Sengupta S, Sharma S, Singh MM. Effect of ormeloxifene on ovariectomy-induced bone resorption, osteoclast differentiation and apoptosis and TGF beta-3 expression. *J Steroid Biochem Mol Biol*. 2006;100(4-5): 117-128.
95. Ammann P, Bourrin S, Brunner F, et al. A new selective estrogen receptor modulator HMR-3339 fully corrects bone

alterations induced by ovariectomy in adult rats. *Bone*. 2004;35(1):153-161.
96. Goss PE, Qi S, Cheung AM, Hu H, Mendes M, Pritzker KP. The selective estrogen receptor modulator SCH 57068 prevents bone loss, reduces serum cholesterol and blocks estrogen-induced uterine hypertrophy in ovariectomized rats. *J Steroid Biochem Mol Biol*. 2004;92(1–2):79-87.
97. Ikeno A, Minato H, Kohayakawa C, Tsuji J. Effect of OS-0544, a selective estrogen receptor modulator, on endothelial function and increased sympathetic activity in ovariectomized rats. *Vasc Pharmacol*. 2009;50(1–2):40-44.
98. Iwamoto J, Seki A, Takeda T, Sato Y, Yamada H, Yeh JK. Comparative therapeutic effects of alendronate and alfacalcidol on cancellous and cortical bone mass and mechanical properties in ovariectomized osteopenic rats. *J Nutr Sci Vitaminol*. 2006;52(1):1-8.
99. Rodan GA, Seedor JG, Balena R. Preclinical pharmacology of alendronate. *Osteoporos Int*. 1993;3(Suppl 3):S7-S12.
100. Bonjour JP, Ammann P, Barbier A, Caverzasio J, Rizzoli R. Tiludronate: bone pharmacology and safety. *Bone*. 1995; 17(5 Suppl):473S-477S.
101. Russell RG. Ibandronate: pharmacology and preclinical studies. *Bone*. 2006;38(4 Suppl 1):S7-S12.
102. Lespessailles E, Jaffre C, Beaupied H, et al. Does exercise modify the effects of zoledronic acid on bone mass, microarchitecture, biomechanics, and turnover in ovariectomized rats? *Calcif Tissue Int*. 2009;85(2):146-157.
103. Qu Q, Zheng H, Dahllund J, et al. Selective estrogenic effects of a novel triphenylethylene compound, FC1271a, on bone, cholesterol level, and reproductive tissues in intact and ovariectomized rats. *Endocrinology*. 2000;141(2):809-820.
104. Chikazu D, Shindo M, Iwasaka T, et al. A novel synthetic triazolotriazepine derivative JTT-606 inhibits bone resorption by down-regulation of action and production of bone resorptive factors. *J Bone Miner Res*. 2000;15(4):674-682.
105. Nich C, Marchadier A, Sedel L, Petite H, Vidal C, Hamadouche M. Decrease in particle-induced osteolysis in ovariectomized mice. *J Orthop Res*. 2010;28(2):178-183.
106. Caverzasio J, Higgins L, Ammann P. Prevention of trabecular bone loss induced by estrogen deficiency by a selective p38alpha inhibitor. *J Bone Miner Res*. 2008;23(9):1389-1397.
107. Strait K, Li Y, Dillehay DL, Weitzmann MN. Suppression of NF-kappaB activation blocks osteoclastic bone resorption during estrogen deficiency. *Int J Mol Med*. 2008; 21(4):521-525.
108. Kasukawa Y, Miyakoshi N, Srivastava AK, et al. The selective cyclooxygenase-2 inhibitor celecoxib reduces bone resorption, but not bone formation, in ovariectomized mice *in vivo*. *Tohoku J Exp Med*. 2007;211(3):275-283.
109. Onoe Y, Miyaura C, Ito M, Ohta H, Nozawa S, Suda T. Comparative effects of estrogen and raloxifene on B lymphopoiesis and bone loss induced by sex steroid deficiency in mice. *J Bone Miner Res*. 2000;15(3):541-549.
110. Arai C, Kohguchi M, Akamatsu S, et al. Trehalose suppresses lipopolysaccharide-induced osteoclastogenesis bone marrow in mice. *Nutr Res (New York, NY)*. 2001; 21(7):993-999.
111. Yamaza T, Miura Y, Bi Y, et al. Pharmacologic stem cell based intervention as a new approach to osteoporosis treatment in rodents. *PLoS ONE*. 2008;3(7):e2615.
112. Sasaki T, Ohyori N, Debari K, Ramamurthy NS, Golub LM. Effects of chemically modified tetracycline, CMT-8, on bone loss and osteoclast structure and function in osteoporotic states. *Ann NY Acad Sci*. 1999;878:347-360.
113. Xiang A, Kanematsu M, Kumar S, et al. Changes in micro-CT 3D bone parameters reflect effects of a potent cathepsin K inhibitor (SB-553484) on bone resorption and cortical bone formation in ovariectomized mice. *Bone*. 2007; 40(5):1231-1237.
114. Simic P, Culej JB, Orlic I, et al. Systemically administered bone morphogenetic protein-6 restores bone in aged ovariectomized rats by increasing bone formation and suppressing bone resorption. *J Biol Chem*. 2006;281(35): 25509-25521.
115. Kim D, Cho SW, Her SJ, et al. Retrovirus-mediated gene transfer of receptor activator of nuclear factor-kappaB-Fc prevents bone loss in ovariectomized mice. *Stem Cells*. 2006;24(7):1798-1805.
116. Dunstan CR, Boyce R, Boyce BF, et al. Systemic administration of acidic fibroblast growth factor (FGF-1) prevents bone loss and increases new bone formation in ovariectomized rats. *J Bone Miner Res*. 1999;14(6):953-959.
117. Yao W, Balooch G, Balooch M, et al. Sequential treatment of ovariectomized mice with bFGF and risedronate restored trabecular bone microarchitecture and mineralization. *Bone*. 2006;39(3):460-469.
118. Pierroz DD, Bouxsein ML, Rizzoli R, Ferrari SL. Combined treatment with a beta-blocker and intermittent PTH improves bone mass and microarchitecture in ovariectomized mice. *Bone*. 2006;39(2):260-267.
119. Waki Y, Horita T, Miyamoto K, Ohya K, Kasugai S. Effects of XT-44, a phosphodiesterase 4 inhibitor, in osteoblastgenesis and osteoclastgenesis in culture and its therapeutic effects in rat osteopenia models. *Jpn J Pharmacol*. 1999; 79(4):477-483.
120. Cho SW, Sun HJ, Yang JY, et al. Transplantation of mesenchymal stem cells overexpressing RANK-Fc or CXCR4 prevents bone loss in ovariectomized mice. *Mol Ther*. 2009;17(11):1979-1987.
121. Zhao Y, Zou B, Shi Z, Wu Q, Chen GQ. The effect of 3-hydroxybutyrate on the *in vitro* differentiation of murine osteoblast MC3T3-E1 and *in vivo* bone formation in ovariectomized rats. *Biomaterials*. 2007;28(20):3063-3073.
122. Kostenuik PJ, Bolon B, Morony S, et al. Gene therapy with human recombinant osteoprotegerin reverses established osteopenia in ovariectomized mice. *Bone*. 2004;34(4): 656-664.
123. Shimizu-Ishiura M, Kawana F, Sasaki T. Osteoprotegerin administration reduces femural bone loss in ovariectomized mice via impairment of osteoclast structure and function. *J Electron Microsc*. 2002;51(5):315-325.
124. Nielsen KL, Allen MR, Bloomfield SA, et al. Biglycan deficiency interferes with ovariectomy-induced bone loss. *J Bone Miner Res*. 2003;18(12):2152-2158.
125. Shahnazari M, Martin BR, Legette LL, Lachcik PJ, Welch J, Weaver CM. Diet calcium level but not calcium supplement particle size affects bone density and mechanical properties in ovariectomized rats. *J Nutr*. 2009;139(7):1308-1314.
126. Hirasawa T, Omi N, Ezawa I. Effect of 1alpha-hydroxyvitamin D3 and egg-shell calcium on bone metabolism in ovariectomized osteoporotic model rats. *J Bone Miner Metab*. 2001;19(2):84-88.
127. Omi N, Morikawa N, Ezawa I. The effect of voluntary exercise on bone mineral density and skeletal muscles in the rat

model at ovariectomized and sham stages. *Bone Miner.* 1994;24(3):211-222.

128. Chen CC, Liu MH, Wang MF, Chen CC. Effects of aging and dietary antler supplementation on the calcium-regulating hormones and bone status in ovariectomized SAMP8 mice. *Chin J Physiol.* 2007;50(6):308-314.
129. Reddy PN, Lakshmana M, Udupa UV. Effect of Praval bhasma (Coral calx), a natural source of rich calcium on bone mineralization in rats. *Pharmacol Res.* 2003;48(6): 593-599.
130. Scholz-Ahrens KE, Acil Y, Schrezenmeir J. Effect of oligofructose or dietary calcium on repeated calcium and phosphorus balances, bone mineralization and trabecular structure in ovariectomized rats*. *Br J Nutr.* 2002;88(4): 365-377.
131. Wronski TJ, Yen CF, Burton KW, et al. Skeletal effects of calcitonin in ovariectomized rats. *Endocrinology.* 1991; 129(4):2246-2250.
132. Shen Y, Li M, Wronski TJ. Skeletal effects of calcitonin treatment and withdrawal in ovariectomized rats. *Calcif Tissue Int.* 1996;58(4):263-267.
133. Nitta T, Hoshino T, Koida M, Nakamuta H. Histomorphometrical evaluation of anti-osteopenic effect of nasal salmon calcitonin in a type 1 osteoporotic model of rats. *Biol Pharm Bull.* 1996;19(2):214-216.
134. Sakai A, Nishida S, Nishida S, et al. 1alpha-Hydroxyvitamin D3 suppresses trabecular bone resorption by inhibiting osteoclastogenic potential in bone marrow cells after ovariectomy in mice. *J Bone Miner Metab.* 2001;19(5): 277-286.
135. Shibata T, Shira-Ishi A, Sato T, et al. Vitamin D hormone inhibits osteoclastogenesis *in vivo* by decreasing the pool of osteoclast precursors in bone marrow. *J Bone Miner Res.* 2002;17(4):622-629.
136. Asawa Y, Amizuka N, Hara K, et al. Histochemical evaluation for the biological effect of menatetrenone on metaphyseal trabeculae of ovariectomized rats. *Bone.* 2004;35(4): 870-880.
137. Matsumoto Y, Mikuni-Takagaki Y, Kozai Y, et al. Prior treatment with vitamin K(2) significantly improves the efficacy of risedronate. *Osteoporos Int.* 2009;20(11):1863-1872.
138. Shevde NK, Plum LA, Clagett-Dame M, Yamamoto H, Pike JW, DeLuca HF. A potent analog of 1alpha, 25-dihydroxyvitamin D3 selectively induces bone formation. *Proc Natl Acad Sci USA.* 2002;99(21):13487-13491.
139. Arjmandi BH, Alekel L, Hollis BW, et al. Dietary soybean protein prevents bone loss in an ovariectomized rat model of osteoporosis. *J Nutr.* 1996;126(1):161-167.
140. Omi N, Aoi S, Murata K, Ezawa I. Evaluation of the effect of soybean milk and soybean milk peptide on bone metabolism in the rat model with ovariectomized osteoporosis. *J Nutr Sci Vitaminol.* 1994;40(2):201-211.
141. Kim DW, Yoo KY, Lee YB, et al. Soy isoflavones mitigate long-term femoral and lumbar vertebral bone loss in middle-aged ovariectomized mice. *J Med Food.* 2009;12(3):536-541.
142. Devareddy L, Khalil DA, Korlagunta K, Hooshmand S, Bellmer DD, Arjmandi BH. The effects of fructo-oligosaccharides in combination with soy protein on bone in osteopenic ovariectomized rats (New York, NY). *Menopause.* 2006;13(4): 692-699.
143. Johnson CD, Lucas EA, Hooshmand S, Campbell S, Akhter MP, Arjmandi BH. Addition of fructooligosaccharides and dried plum to soy-based diets reverses bone loss in the ovariectomized rat. *Evid Based Complement Altern Med.* 2008 PMID: 18955356.
144. Pie JE, Park JH, Park YH, et al. Effect of genistein on the expression of bone metabolism genes in ovariectomized mice using a cDNA microarray. *J Nutr Biochem.* 2006; 17(3):157-164.
145. Erlandsson MC, Islander U, Moverare S, Ohlsson C, Carlsten H. Estrogenic agonism and antagonism of the soy isoflavone genistein in uterus, bone and lymphopoiesis in mice. *APMIS.* 2005;113(5):317-323.
146. Ishimi Y, Arai N, Wang X, et al. Difference in effective dosage of genistein on bone and uterus in ovariectomized mice. *Biochem Biophys Res Commun.* 2000;274(3):697-701.
147. Ishimi Y, Miyaura C, Ohmura M, et al. Selective effects of genistein, a soybean isoflavone, on B-lymphopoiesis and bone loss caused by estrogen deficiency. *Endocrinology.* 1999;140(4):1893-1900.
148. Li B, Yu S. Genistein prevents bone resorption diseases by inhibiting bone resorption and stimulating bone formation. *Biol Pharm Bull.* 2003;26(6):780-786.
149. Ohtomo T, Uehara M, Penalvo JL, et al. Comparative activities of daidzein metabolites, equol and O-desmethylangolensin, on bone mineral density and lipid metabolism in ovariectomized mice and in osteoclast cell cultures. *Eur J Nutr.* 2008;47(5):273-279.
150. Fonseca D, Ward WE. Daidzein together with high calcium preserve bone mass and biomechanical strength at multiple sites in ovariectomized mice. *Bone.* 2004;35(2):489-497.
151. Wang X, Wu J, Chiba H, Umegaki K, Yamada K, Ishimi Y. Puerariae radix prevents bone loss in ovariectomized mice. *J Bone Miner Metab.* 2003;21(5):268-275.
152. Ohta A, Uehara M, Sakai K, et al. A combination of dietary fructooligosaccharides and isoflavone conjugates increases femoral bone mineral density and equol production in ovariectomized mice. *J Nutr.* 2002;132(7):2048-2054.
153. Tsuji M, Yamamoto H, Sato T, et al. Dietary quercetin inhibits bone loss without effect on the uterus in ovariectomized mice. *J Bone Miner Metab.* 2009;27(6):673-681.
154. Chiba H, Uehara M, Wu J, et al. Hesperidin, a citrus flavonoid, inhibits bone loss and decreases serum and hepatic lipids in ovariectomized mice. *J Nutr.* 2003;133(6):1892-1897.
155. Zhang G, Qin L, Hung WY, et al. Flavonoids derived from herbal Epimedium Brevicornum Maxim prevent OVX-induced osteoporosis in rats independent of its enhancement in intestinal calcium absorption. *Bone.* 2006;38(6): 818-825.
156. Sun D, Krishnan A, Zaman K, Lawrence R, Bhattacharya A, Fernandes G. Dietary n-3 fatty acids decrease osteoclastogenesis and loss of bone mass in ovariectomized mice. *J Bone Miner Res.* 2003;18(7):1206-1216.
157. Fernandes G, Lawrence R, Sun D. Protective role of n-3 lipids and soy protein in osteoporosis. *Prostaglandins Leukot Essent Fatty Acids.* 2003;68(6):361-372.
158. Rahman MM, Bhattacharya A, Banu J, Kang JX, Fernandes G. Endogenous n-3 fatty acids protect ovariectomy induced bone loss by attenuating osteoclastogenesis. *J Cell Mol Med.* 2009;13(8B):1833-1844.
159. Kelly O, Cashman KD. The effect of conjugated linoleic acid on calcium absorption and bone metabolism and composition in adult ovariectomised rats. *Prostaglandins Leukot Essent Fatty Acids.* 2004;71(5):295-301.

160. Sibonga JD, Lotinun S, Evans GL, Pribluda VS, Green SJ, Turner RT. Dose-response effects of 2-methoxyestradiol on estrogen target tissues in the ovariectomized rat. *Endocrinology*. 2003;144(3):785-792.
161. Han SY, Lee JR, Kwon YK, et al. Ostreae testa prevent ovariectomy-induced bone loss in mice by osteoblast activations. *J Ethnopharmacol*. 2007;114(3):400-405.
162. Li JX, Liu J, He CC, et al. Triterpenoids from Cimicifugae rhizoma, a novel class of inhibitors on bone resorption and ovariectomy-induced bone loss. *Maturitas*. 2007;58(1): 59-69.
163. Ohtani J, Hernandez RA, Sunagawa H, et al. A newly developed snack effective for enhancing bone volume. *Nutr J*. 2009;8:30.
164. Yin J, Tezuka Y, Kouda K, et al. *In vivo* antiosteoporotic activity of a fraction of *Dioscorea spongiosa* and its constituent, 22-O-methylprotodioscin. *Planta Med*. 2004; 70(3):220-226.
165. Devareddy L, Hooshmand S, Collins JK, Lucas EA, Chai SC, Arjmandi BH. Blueberry prevents bone loss in ovariectomized rat model of postmenopausal osteoporosis. *J Nutr Biochem*. 2008;19(10):694-699.
166. Murakami A, Song M, Katsumata S, Uehara M, Suzuki K, Ohigashi H. Citrus nobiletin suppresses bone loss in ovariectomized ddY mice and collagen-induced arthritis in DBA/1 J mice: possible involvement of receptor activator of NF-kappaB ligand (RANKL)-induced osteoclastogenesis regulation. *BioFactors*. 2007;30(3):179-192.
167. Li H, Li J, Prasain JK, et al. Antiosteoporotic activity of the stems of *Sambucus sieboldiana*. *Biol Pharm Bull*. 1998; 21(6):594-598.
168. Barengolts EI, Curry DJ, Bapna MS, Kukreja SC. Effects of two non-endurance exercise protocols on established bone loss in ovariectomized adult rats. *Calcif Tissue Int*. 1993;52(3):239-243.
169. Iwamoto J, Takeda T, Sato Y. Effect of treadmill exercise on bone mass in female rats. *Exp Anim*. 2005;54(1):1-6.
170. Simoes PA, Zamarioli A, Bloes P, et al. Effect of treadmill exercise on lumbar vertebrae in ovariectomized rats: anthropometrical and mechanical analyses. *Acta Bioeng Biomech*. 2008;10(2):39-41.
171. Peng ZQ, Vaananen HK, Tuukkanen J. Ovariectomy-induced bone loss can be affected by different intensities of treadmill running exercise in rats. *Calcif Tissue Int*. 1997;60(5):441-448.
172. Sehmisch S, Galal R, Kolios L, et al. Effects of low-magnitude, high-frequency mechanical stimulation in the rat osteopenia model. *Osteoporos Int*. 2009;20(12): 1999-2008.
173. Sakakura Y, Shide N, Tsuruga E, Irie K, Yajima T. Effects of running exercise on the mandible and tibia of ovariectomized rats. *J Bone Miner Metab*. 2001;19(3):159-167.
174. Notomi T, Okimoto N, Okazaki Y, Nakamura T, Suzuki M. Tower climbing exercise started 3 months after ovariectomy recovers bone strength of the femur and lumbar vertebrae in aged osteopenic rats. *J Bone Miner Res*. 2003;18(1): 140-149.
175. Honda A, Sogo N, Nagasawa S, Shimizu T, Umemura Y. High-impact exercise strengthens bone in osteopenic ovariectomized rats with the same outcome as Sham rats. *J Appl Physiol*. 2003;95(3):1032-1037.
176. Yeh JK, Aloia JF, Barilla ML. Effects of 17 beta-estradiol replacement and treadmill exercise on vertebral and femoral bones of the ovariectomized rat. *Bone Miner*. 1994; 24(3):223-234.
177. Barengolts EI, Lathon PV, Curry DJ, Kukreja SC. Effects of endurance exercise on bone histomorphometric parameters in intact and ovariectomized rats. *Bone Miner*. 1994;26(2):133-140.
178. Yeh JK, Aloia JF, Chen MM, Tierney JM, Sprintz S. Influence of exercise on cancellous bone of the aged female rat. *J Bone Miner Res*. 1993;8(9):1117-1125.
179. Yeh JK, Liu CC, Aloia JF. Additive effect of treadmill exercise and 17 beta-estradiol replacement on prevention of tibial bone loss in adult ovariectomized rat. *J Bone Miner Res*. 1993;8(6):677-683.
180. Li CY, Jee WS, Chen JL, et al. Estrogen and "exercise" have a synergistic effect in preventing bone loss in the lumbar vertebra and femoral neck of the ovariectomized rat. *Calcif Tissue Int*. 2003;72(1):42-49.
181. Yamamoto N, Takahashi HE, Tanizawa T, Fujimoto R, Hara T, Tanaka S. Maintenance of bone mass by physical exercise after discontinuation of intermittent hPTH(1-34) administration. *Bone Miner*. 1993;23(3):333-342.
182. Mo A, Yao W, Li C, et al. Bipedal stance exercise and prostaglandin E2 (PGE2) and its synergistic effect in increasing bone mass and in lowering the PGE2 dose required to prevent ovariectomized-induced cancellous bone loss in aged rats. *Bone*. 2002;31(3):402-406.
183. Shiguemoto GE, Rossi EA, Baldissera V, Gouveia CH, de Valdez Vargas GM, Andrade Perez SE. Isoflavone-supplemented soy yoghurt associated with resistive physical exercise increase bone mineral density of ovariectomized rats. *Maturitas*. 2007;57(3):261-270.
184. Liu K, Ma G, Lv G, et al. Effects of soybean isoflavone dosage and exercise on the serum markers of bone metabolism in ovariectomized rats. *Asia Pac J Clin Nutr*. 2007;16(Suppl 1):193-195.
185. Hertrampf T, Gruca MJ, Seibel J, Laudenbach U, Fritzemeier KH, Diel P. The bone-protective effect of the phytoestrogen genistein is mediated via ER alpha-dependent mechanisms and strongly enhanced by physical activity. *Bone*. 2007;40(6):1529-1535.
186. Wu J, Wang XX, Takasaki M, Ohta A, Higuchi M, Ishimi Y. Cooperative effects of exercise training and genistein administration on bone mass in ovariectomized mice. *J Bone Miner Res*. 2001;16(10):1829-1836.
187. Wu J, Wang X, Chiba H, et al. Combined intervention of soy isoflavone and moderate exercise prevents body fat elevation and bone loss in ovariectomized mice. *Metabolism*. 2004;53(7):942-948.
188. Bonnet N, Beaupied H, Vico L, et al. Combined effects of exercise and propranolol on bone tissue in ovariectomized rats. *J Bone Miner Res*. 2007;22(4):578-588.
189. Fuchs RK, Shea M, Durski SL, Winters-Stone KM, Widrick J, Snow CM. Individual and combined effects of exercise and alendronate on bone mass and strength in ovariectomized rats. *Bone*. 2007;41(2):290-296.
190. Widrick JJ, Fuchs R, Maddalozzo GF, Marley K, Snow C. Relative effects of exercise training and alendronate treatment on skeletal muscle function of ovariectomized rats. *Menopause*. 2007;14(3 Pt 1):528-534.
191. Gala J, Diaz-Curiel M, de la Piedra C, Calero J. Short- and long-term effects of calcium and exercise on bone mineral density in ovariectomized rats. *Br J Nutr*. 2001;86(4): 521-527.

Classical Models of Senile Osteoporosis

10

Ken Watanabe

10.1 Introduction

Most vertebrates exhibit age-related decline in physiological function, particularly in locomotion. Loss of muscle volume and bone mass in late life is a hallmark of aging and resembles tissue obsolescence caused by disuse. However, some human populations lose bone mass more rapidly than would be predicted by normal aging. These individuals are diagnosed as having senile osteoporosis, one of the most prevalent geriatric disorders and one that seriously decreases quality of life in the elderly. As noted throughout this book, mice and rats are the most frequently used models to study osteoporosis, its treatment and prevention, and concomitant pathogenesis. Both mice and rats have an approximately 3-year lifespan. Bone mass peaks within the first quarter of life and then declines with age. This chapter describes age-related bone loss in laboratory rodents.

10.2 Aged Mice

Significant decreases in bone mass during the latter half of life are observed in laboratory rodents, such as mice and rats. Most studies of aged rodents focus on the anatomy and mechanism of age-related bone loss, a critical factor for senile osteoporosis, but the phenomenon can also be seen as part of the normal aging process. In most studies of senescence, mice of 18–30 months of age are used as models of aging. However, genetic manipulation of mice to study aging may require 2 years before a particular phenotype emerges, making it difficult for a postdoc to complete the study or to attain grant support. Fortunately, although the sources and strains are still limited, aged mice can be obtained from some resources, such as the National Institute on Aging (NIA, USA), which provides aged rodents only for academic and nonprofit research institutes.

Among mouse strains, C57BL/6 is most often used to study age-related bone loss. Age-related changes in bone structure and skeletal mass seen in this strain are reportedly representative of those observed in human aging.[1-4] One study showed that bone volume/tissue volume (BV/TV), trabecular number (Tb.N), and connectivity decrease with age, whereas cortical thickness increases between 6 weeks and 6 months of age and then declines.[3] In the same study, cortical area (Ct.Ar) was not markedly changed between 6 and 24 months, and skeletal tissue weight of the tibia defatted by organic solvents was maximal at 12 months of age and then the fat-free weight decreased. The male mice used in this study showed no changes in serum testosterone level, suggesting that age-related bone loss in male C57BL/6 mice is apparently independent of androgen deficiency.[3] Female mice do not appear to experience menopause but show age-related retardation of estrous cycles.[5] Age-related bone loss in trabecular bones of vertebra and femora is more pronounced in female *mice*,[2] which show decreases in trabecular bone as early as 2–6 months of age. However, age-related changes in the parameters of bone formation and resorption differ among femoral mid-diaphysis, metaphysis, and lumbar vertebrae, which also differ in composition of trabecular and cortical bones and in mechanical properties.[1,2,4] Serum markers of aged C57BL/6 mice suggest a high

K. Watanabe
Department of Bone and Joint Disease, National Center for Geriatrics and Gerontology, Obu, Aichi, Japan
e-mail: kwatanab@ncgg.go.jp

G. Duque and K. Watanabe (eds.), *Osteoporosis Research*,
DOI: 10.1007/978-0-85729-293-3_10, © Springer-Verlag London Limited 2011

turnover state of bone metabolism after 24 months of age.[4] Assessment of mechanical properties by three-point flexure tests also reveals that the long bones are maturing between 3 and 10 months of age.[1] From time points representing peak bone mass, parameters such as bone mass, whole bone stiffness, and energy to fracture decrease by 24 months of age, whereas periosteal perimeter and cross-sectional moments of inertia continue to increase until 24 months. The growing phase when bone formation predominates ends and the lacuno-canalicular network of osteocytes is well aligned by 3 months of age, corresponding to the time of mechanical maturity.[6]

Among factors regulating osteoclastogenesis, receptor activator of NF-κB ligand (RANKL) expression increases with age, but expression of osteoprotegerin (OPG), a decoy RANK inhibitor, slightly decreases. In mice, RANKL expression is inversely correlated with trabecular bone volume in terms of age-related changes.[7] Such age-related expression patterns are reproduced in *ex vivo* culture of the bone marrow adherent cell fraction within 7 days but diminish in longer-term cultures (~28 days). Expression of macrophage-colony stimulating factor, another factor critical for osteoclastogenesis, also increases in the bone marrow of aged mice.[8] When osteoclast differentiation is induced by only RANKL and M-CSF without stromal cells, a greater number of osteoclasts are generated from bone marrow of aged mice compared to younger mice, suggesting that the osteoclast precursor pool increases with age.[8] Thus, both stromal and hematopoietic factors associated with osteoclastogenesis are elevated upon aging, suggesting a correlation with age-related bone loss.

Insulin-like growth factor (IGF) is a well-known factor governing cell survival and somatic tissue growth and maintenance. IGF acts as an anabolic agent for bones as well as muscles and cartilage.[9,10] In aged C57BL/6 mice, growth stimulatory and survival activities of IGF significantly decrease.[11] Although expression of the IGF-1 receptor in aged mice is increased, receptor responsiveness, as evidenced by downstream MAPK and PI3K activation, is markedly reduced. Intermittent treatment with parathyroid hormone (PTH) is known to be a potential anabolic therapy among few other candidates.[12] Knopp et al. reported that 18-month-old C57BL/6 mice exhibit more pronounced increases in spinal bone mineral density (BMD) than do their 3-month-old counterparts in response to intermittent PTH injections, but those increases are not seen in the femur.[13] Mechanical stress plays critical roles in development and maintenance of the skeletal system, including bones. Low-magnitude cyclic loading, which stimulates bone formation in young mice, is not sufficient to initiate bone formation in 21-month-old mice.[14] Thus, either responsiveness to various anabolic stimuli is impaired or the response threshold is shifted, or both occur in the aged skeleton.

10.3 Senescence-Accelerated Mice

The senescence-accelerated mouse (SAM), developed by Takeda's Lab at Kyoto University, originated from the AKR/J strain.[15] SAM strains fall into two categories: P (senescence-prone) inbred strains, which exhibit an accelerated aging phenotype, and R (senescence-resistant) strains, which age normally. Several SAM strains are now commercially available. Among them, SAMP6 is often used as a mouse model of senile osteoporosis.[16] SAMP6 mice show frequent fractures in their tibias and exhibit low peak bone mass, which underlies the accelerated age-related osteoporotic phenotype. Jilka et al. determined the cellular basis of the SAMP6 phenotype and found that the number of osteoblast progenitors in the bone marrow was not altered in this strain at prepuberty (1 month) but decreased significantly at adult ages (~4 months).[17] Age-dependent decreases in BMD were also observed. A decline of histomorphometrical analysis parameters was pronounced not only in bone formation but also in resorption, resulting in reduced bone turnover. The number of osteoclasts in vertebra and femur was significantly reduced, and osteoclast formation in *ex vivo* bone marrow culture was markedly decreased. When bone marrow cells were cocultured with osteoblasts from wild-type mice, osteoclast formation from SAMP6 bone marrow cells was even higher than that seen in the control strain, suggesting that defects in osteoclast formation are caused by impairment in supporting roles of the osteoblast/stromal cell fraction. The authors of this study concluded that the decreased bone mass phenotype seen in SAMP6 mice was due to defects in osteoblastogenesis.[17] Such defects in SAMP6 mice also promote resistance to bone loss following sex hormone deficiency induced by gonadectomy.[18] Increased adipogenesis in the bone marrow of the SAMP6 strain has also been observed, and expression of an anti-adipogenic cytokine, interleukin-11, was decreased in bone marrow stromal cells of this strain.[19,20] Silva et al. reported that bone-forming activity of SAMP6 osteoblasts is normal, although the number of osteoblasts in the bone marrow was markedly reduced.[21-23] From 2 to 12 months of age, calcein-labeled surfaces in SAMP6 femur and tibia were significantly decreased in endocortical surfaces (inside the long bones) but not in periosteal surfaces (outside the bone), suggesting that SAMP6 mice possess a marrow defect.[23] Interestingly, bone marrow transplantation from normal to recipient SAMP6 mice resulted in a significant increase in trabecular bone and BMD.[24-26] This finding confirms that the defect in SAMP6 mice originates in bone marrow and can be rescued by normal marrow.

The SAMP6 strain has been used to conduct a whole genome scan for quantitative trait loci (QTLs) to identify determinants of bone mass.[27-29] Shimizu et al. analyzed QTLs of the F2 progeny obtained by crossing SAMP6 and SAMP2 mice, the latter of which possesses higher peak bone mass at 4 months of age.[29] In their study they determined cortical thickness of femurs and identified three *peak bone density* (*Pbd*) loci on chromosomes 11, 13, and X, corresponding to *Pbd1*, *Pbd2*, and *Pbd3*, respectively. They developed a congenic strain P6.P2-Pbd2, which possesses the genomic region from SAMP2 chromosome 13 that carries *Pbd2*, on a SAMP6 background. The congenic strain exhibited significantly higher peak bone mass than did SAMP6 mice.[28] Among the genes on the chromosome 13 locus, secreted frizzled-related protein 4 (Sfrp4) expression was significantly elevated in SAMP6 calvaria.[27] Sfrp4 is an antagonist of Wnt ligands and thus inhibits Wnt-β-catenin signaling, which plays an important role in regulating bone mass. Recombinant SFRP4 protein suppressed osteoblast proliferation *in vitro*, suggesting that elevated *Sfrp4* expression underlies decreased bone formation seen in SAMP6 mice.[27]

10.4 Rat Models of Aging

The aging rat also represents a good model to study age-related bone loss.[30-35] Like C57BL/6 mice, the rat strain F344 has often been used for aging research, although Sprague-Dawley and Wistar rats have also been analyzed. Trabecular bone volume of the vertebra of rats reportedly does not exhibit a decrease at 12 months of age, in contrast to mice[31,32,34,35]; however, although the time course and structural changes in bone aging phenotypes differ between these rodents, both experience age-related bone loss. As a system, mice are advantageous because of the availability of genetic manipulation techniques, but because of their larger size rats represent a more appropriate system to study alterations in the vascular system. It has been suggested that blood vessel aging is associated with senility and the onset of geriatric diseases, and age-related alterations in the skeletal vasculature system also likely promote decreased blood flow in bone. Prosby et al. determined age-related changes in femoral blood flow using rats of 4–6 and 24–26 months of age as models of young adult and aged animals, respectively.[36] Blood flow in aged rats was decreased to 70–80% of levels seen in young controls, and endothelial vasodilation of the principal nutrient artery was significantly reduced in aged animals relative to controls, whereas endothelium-independent vasodilation remained unchanged. The concentration of the intraluminal nitric oxide (NO), a vasodilator, was markedly decreased in the aged artery, suggesting that age-related reduction in NO signaling underlies decreased blood flow. The Louvain (LOU) rat exhibits an increased lifespan and is recognized as a model of healthy aging.[37] Duque et al. reported that aged LOU rats show low-turnover bone metabolism and an increase in bone marrow adiposity, which models the situation seen in human senile osteoporosis (Fig. 10.1).[38] Thus, rats are also useful to evaluate relationships between bone metabolism and physiological, age-related alterations.

10.5 Caloric Restriction

Caloric restriction (CR) is known to extend lifespan in flies, worms, and yeast as well as in mammals.[39,40] CR reduces body mass, which is positively correlated with bone mass. As early as 1935, McCay et al. reported that dietary restriction of laboratory rats increased their lifespan.[41] The authors also found that femoral bone density was decreased by CR, and hypothesized that this might be an indication of growth retardation. Currently, accumulated data indicate that CR delays

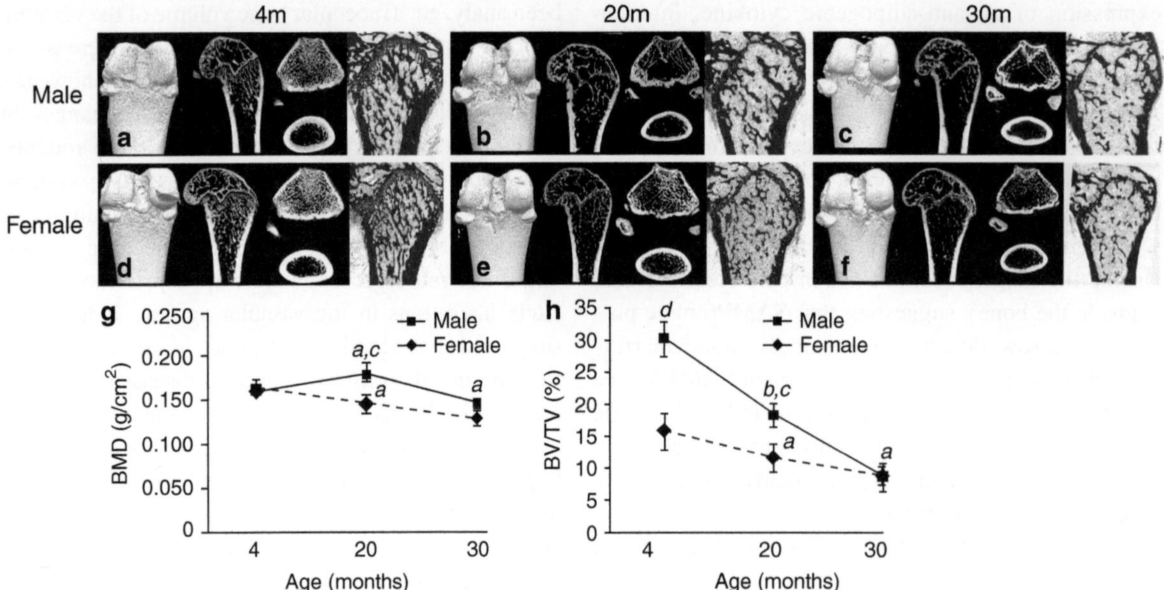

Fig. 10.1 μCT analysis (**a–f**) to evaluate bone structure and sections of undecalcified bone stained with von Kossa (**a–f**, *right panels*) (magnification ×10) to evaluate mineralized tissue (*black*) and fat volume (*white*). The figure shows 3D images of the trabecular bone and cross-sectional images of the cortical bone from rats aged 4, 20, and 30 months (**a–f**). The loss in bone volume, the reduction in both trabecular bone and cortical thickness, and the increasing cortical porosity with age are visually apparent. Age-related changes in BMD (**g**) and BV/TV (**h**) showed a significant decline in both groups matching similar levels of bone mass and bone quality at 30 months of age (*Note*: $a-p<0.01$, $b-p<0.001$ compared with 4 months, one-way ANOVA and Dunnett's test; $c-p<0.01$, $d-p<0.001$ males versus females) (From Duque et al.[38])

the progression and/or onset of age-related disorders, such as neurodegeneration, renal failure, cataracts, immune diseases, and cancer malignancy.[42,43] Thus it is plausible that CR could impact age-related bone loss.

Kalu et al. report that male F344 rats undergoing lifelong CR show reduced age-related bone loss via suppression of elevated serum PTH levels.[44] However, Sanderson et al. observed that CR starting at around 17 months of age caused femoral bone loss in Lobund-Wistar rats.[45] In another study, three mouse strains, SENCAR, C57BL/6, and DBA/2, were subjected to a 6-month period of CR, begun at 10 weeks of age.[46] CR increased vertebral BMD in SENCAR and C57BL/6 mice but decreased femoral BMD in SENCAR and DBA/2 mice, indicating that the CR effect is dependent on strain and experimental setting. Ten-week CR, started at 14 weeks of age, reduced serum leptin and IGF-1 levels, and reduced cortical bone thickness, whereas vertebral BMD and trabecular bone volume in mice were significantly increased.[47] Tatsumi et al. reported that the effects of lifelong CR, started at 12 weeks of age, are biphasic on tibial bone metabolism in C57BL/6 mice and F344 rats.[48] By 9 months of CR, trabecular bone mass was decreased compared to control ad libitum fed animals, and bone histomorphometric analyses revealed that the decrease was mainly due to reduced bone formation. However, the difference in bone mass between CR and controls was not significant with longer periods of CR, and bone mass was even higher in CR after 12 months of age, suggesting that CR delays bone aging.[48] Although overall these results differ, CR likely attenuates developmental acquisition of bone volume but delays age-related bone loss.

Recently, it has been reported that administration of rapamycin, an inhibitor of the TOR pathway that acts as nutrient sensor in cells, extends lifespan in yeast, worms, flies, and mice, mimicking CR.[49] The mammalian TOR (mTOR) pathway is known to regulate FOXO signaling, which plays important roles in osteoblast activity.[50,51] The transcription factors FOXO and ATF4 cooperatively regulate expression of osteocalcin, which in an uncarboxylated form acts as a glucose-regulating hormone.[51,52] In addition, FOXO mediates cellular defenses to oxidative stress, and ATF4 regulates expression of *Rankl*.[53,54] Thus, the mTOR pathway may directly regulate bone metabolism. Future studies should address a potential effect of rapamycin on bone metabolism, especially on age-related bone loss in senile osteoporosis.

10.6 Age-Related Bone Loss

Osteopetrotic animals constitute another classic model of bone disease. Although osteopetrosis represents an opposite phenotype of osteoporosis, age-dependent decreases in bone mass have been reported in osteopetrotic animals. In *op/op* mice, which lack functional M-CSF activity, alleviation of the osteopetrotic phenotype has been observed with age.[55] As noted, both M-CSF and RANKL are essential regulators of osteoclastogenesis, and their expression increases in the bone marrow of aged animals. The alleviation of osteopetrotic phenotypes seen in aging *op/op* mice suggests that an age-dependent factor(s), other than M-CSF and RANKL, plays a role in osteoclastogenesis and may function in age-related acceleration of bone loss, whereas we cannot rule out the possibility that unknown age- or disease-specific factors may compensate for the impairment. Development of DNA microarray techniques has led to expression profiling of various tissues in circumstances including aging. Several studies indicate that upregulation of inflammatory cytokine expression is a common feature of aged tissues and senescent cells.[56-59] Several studies suggest that the activity of nuclear factor κB (NF-κB), a transcriptional regulator of cytokine expression, increases in tissues from animals with age-related disease.[60-62] NF-κB activity, as well as the presence of inflammatory cytokines, is a critical factor in osteoclast formation.[63] Furthermore, tumor necrosis factor (TNF), a well-known inducer of NF-κB activity, is a major adipokine expressed in fat tissues whose mass is significantly reduced in adult CR animals.[64,65] TNF has also been proposed to be a cachexic hormone in various diseases.[66,67] RANKL activity is significantly increased in the presence of TNF.[68,69] Taken together, these observations suggest that age-related upregulation of the NF-κB pathway may function in age-related bone loss, although the pathway has not yet been shown to play a causative role in aging. Thus, a hypothetical aging factor, which stimulates NF-κB pathway or sensitizes cells to NF-κB signaling, may function in age-related bone loss and senile osteoporosis. Age-dependent bone loss is also caused in part by loss of responsiveness to anabolic stimuli, and the hypothetical aging factor(s) may be involved as well. The similar pathophysiology seen between human and animal models suggests that aging factor(s) functioning in senile osteoporosis identified in rodent studies could be shared by humans.

References

1. Ferguson VL, Ayers RA, Bateman TA, Simske SJ. Bone development and age-related bone loss in male C57BL/6J mice. *Bone*. 2003;33(3):387-398.
2. Glatt V, Canalis E, Stadmeyer L, Bouxsein ML. Age-related changes in trabecular architecture differ in female and male C57BL/6J mice. *J Bone Miner Res*. 2007;22(8):1197-1207.
3. Halloran BP, Ferguson VL, Simske SJ, Burghardt A, Venton LL, Majumdar S. Changes in bone structure and mass with advancing age in the male C57BL/6J mouse. *J Bone Miner Res*. 2002;17(6):1044-1050.
4. Hamrick MW, Ding KH, Pennington C, et al. Age-related loss of muscle mass and bone strength in mice is associated with a decline in physical activity and serum leptin. *Bone*. 2006;39(4):845-853.
5. Danilovich N, Sairam MR. Haploinsufficiency of the follicle-stimulating hormone receptor accelerates oocyte loss inducing early reproductive senescence and biological aging in mice. *Biol Reprod*. 2002;67(2):361-369.
6. Hirose S, Li M, Kojima T, et al. A histological assessment on the distribution of the osteocytic lacunar canalicular system using silver staining. *J Bone Miner Metab*. 2007;25(6):374-382.
7. Cao J, Venton L, Sakata T, Halloran BP. Expression of RANKL and OPG correlates with age-related bone loss in male C57BL/6 mice. *J Bone Miner Res*. 2003;18(2):270-277.
8. Cao JJ, Wronski TJ, Iwaniec U, et al. Aging increases stromal/osteoblastic cell-induced osteoclastogenesis and alters the osteoclast precursor pool in the mouse. *J Bone Miner Res*. 2005;20(9):1659-1668.
9. Giustina A, Mazziotti G, Canalis E. Growth hormone, insulin-like growth factors, and the skeleton. *Endocr Rev*. 2008; 29(5):535-559.
10. Linkhart TA, Mohan S, Baylink DJ. Growth factors for bone growth and repair: IGF, TGF beta and BMP. *Bone*. 1996; 19(1 Suppl):1S-12S.
11. Cao JJ, Kurimoto P, Boudignon B, Rosen C, Lima F, Halloran BP. Aging impairs IGF-I receptor activation and induces skeletal resistance to IGF-I. *J Bone Miner Res*. 2007;22(8): 1271-1279.
12. Hodsman AB, Bauer DC, Dempster DW, et al. Parathyroid hormone and teriparatide for the treatment of osteoporosis: a review of the evidence and suggested guidelines for its use. *Endocr Rev*. 2005;26(5):688-703.
13. Knopp E, Troiano N, Bouxsein M, et al. The effect of aging on the skeletal response to intermittent treatment with parathyroid hormone. *Endocrinology*. 2005;146(4):1983-1990.

14. Srinivasan S, Agans SC, King KA, Moy NY, Poliachik SL, Gross TS. Enabling bone formation in the aged skeleton via rest-inserted mechanical loading. *Bone*. 2003;33(6):946-955.
15. Takeda T, Hosokawa M, Takeshita S, et al. A new murine model of accelerated senescence. *Mech Ageing Dev*. 1981; 17(2):183-194.
16. Matsushita M, Tsuboyama T, Kasai R, et al. Age-related changes in bone mass in the senescence-accelerated mouse (SAM). SAM-R/3 and SAM-P/6 as new murine models for senile osteoporosis. *Am J Pathol*. 1986;125(2):276-283.
17. Jilka RL, Weinstein RS, Takahashi K, Parfitt AM, Manolagas SC. Linkage of decreased bone mass with impaired osteoblastogenesis in a murine model of accelerated senescence. *J Clin Invest*. 1996;97(7):1732-1740.
18. Weinstein RS, Jilka RL, Parfitt AM, Manolagas SC. The effects of androgen deficiency on murine bone remodeling and bone mineral density are mediated via cells of the osteoblastic lineage. *Endocrinology*. 1997;138(9):4013-4021.
19. Kodama Y, Takeuchi Y, Suzawa M, et al. Reduced expression of interleukin-11 in bone marrow stromal cells of senescence-accelerated mice (SAMP6): relationship to osteopenia with enhanced adipogenesis. *J Bone Miner Res*. 1998; 13(9):1370-1377.
20. Kajkenova O, Lecka-Czernik B, Gubrij I, et al. Increased adipogenesis and myelopoiesis in the bone marrow of SAMP6, a murine model of defective osteoblastogenesis and low turnover osteopenia. *J Bone Miner Res*. 1997; 12(11):1772-1779.
21. Silva MJ, Brodt MD. Mechanical stimulation of bone formation is normal in the SAMP6 mouse. *Calcif Tissue Int*. 2008;82(6):489-497.
22. Silva MJ, Brodt MD, Ettner SL. Long bones from the senescence accelerated mouse SAMP6 have increased size but reduced whole-bone strength and resistance to fracture. *J Bone Miner Res*. 2002;17(9):1597-1603.
23. Silva MJ, Brodt MD, Ko M, Abu-Amer Y. Impaired marrow osteogenesis is associated with reduced endocortical bone formation but does not impair periosteal bone formation in long bones of SAMP6 mice. *J Bone Miner Res*. 2005; 20(3):419-427.
24. Ichioka N, Inaba M, Kushida T, et al. Prevention of senile osteoporosis in SAMP6 mice by intrabone marrow injection of allogeneic bone marrow cells. *Stem Cells*. 2002;20(6): 542-551.
25. Takada K, Inaba M, Ichioka N, et al. Treatment of senile osteoporosis in SAMP6 mice by intra-bone marrow injection of allogeneic bone marrow cells. *Stem Cells*. 2006; 24(2):399-405.
26. Ueda Y, Inaba M, Takada K, et al. Induction of senile osteoporosis in normal mice by intra-bone marrow-bone marrow transplantation from osteoporosis-prone mice. *Stem Cells*. 2007;25(6):1356-1363.
27. Nakanishi R, Shimizu M, Mori M, et al. Secreted frizzled-related protein 4 is a negative regulator of peak BMD in SAMP6 mice. *J Bone Miner Res*. 2006;21(11):1713-1721.
28. Shimizu M, Higuchi K, Kasai S, et al. Chromosome 13 locus, Pbd2, regulates bone density in mice. *J Bone Miner Res*. 2001;16(11):1972-1982.
29. Shimizu M, Higuchi K, Bennett B, et al. Identification of peak bone mass QTL in a spontaneously osteoporotic mouse strain. *Mamm Genome*. 1999;10(2):81-87.
30. Banu J, Wang L, Kalu DN. Age-related changes in bone mineral content and density in intact male F344 rats. *Bone*. 2002;30(1):125-130.
31. Kiebzak GM, Smith R, Gundberg CC, Howe JC, Sacktor B. Bone status of senescent male rats: chemical, morphometric, and mechanical analysis. *J Bone Miner Res*. 1988;3(1): 37-45.
32. Kiebzak GM, Smith R, Howe JC, Gundberg CM, Sacktor B. Bone status of senescent female rats: chemical, morphometric, and biomechanical analyses. *J Bone Miner Res*. 1988; 3(4):439-446.
33. Turner CH, Takano Y, Owan I. Aging changes mechanical loading thresholds for bone formation in rats. *J Bone Miner Res*. 1995;10(10):1544-1549.
34. Wang L, Banu J, McMahan CA, Kalu DN. Male rodent model of age-related bone loss in men. *Bone*. 2001;29(2): 141-148.
35. Barbier A, Martel C, de Vernejoul MC, et al. The visualization and evaluation of bone architecture in the rat using three-dimensional X-ray microcomputed tomography. *J Bone Miner Metab*. 1999;17(1):37-44.
36. Prisby RD, Ramsey MW, Behnke BJ, et al. Aging reduces skeletal blood flow, endothelium-dependent vasodilation, and NO bioavailability in rats. *J Bone Miner Res*. 2007; 22(8):1280-1288.
37. Alliot J, Boghossian S, Jourdan D, et al. The LOU/c/jall rat as an animal model of healthy aging? *J Gerontol A Biol Sci Med Sci*. 2002;57(8):B312-B320.
38. Duque G, Rivas D, Li W, et al. Age-related bone loss in the LOU/c rat model of healthy ageing. *Exp Gerontol*. 2009; 44(3):183-189.
39. Mair W, Dillin A. Aging and survival: the genetics of life span extension by dietary restriction. *Annu Rev Biochem*. 2008;77:727-754.
40. Sohal RS, Weindruch R. Oxidative stress, caloric restriction, and aging. *Science*. 1996;273(5271):59-63.
41. McCay CM, Crowell MF, Maynard LA. The effect of retarded growth upon the length of life span and upon the ultimate body size. *J Nutr*. 1935;10:63-79.
42. Masoro EJ. Overview of caloric restriction and ageing. *Mech Ageing Dev*. 2005;126(9):913-922.
43. Weindruch R, Sohal RS. Seminars in medicine of the Beth Israel Deaconess Medical Center. Caloric intake and aging. *N Engl J Med*. 1997;337(14):986-994.
44. Kalu DN, Hardin RH, Cockerham R, Yu BP. Aging and dietary modulation of rat skeleton and parathyroid hormone. *Endocrinology*. 1984;115(4):1239-1247.
45. Sanderson JP, Binkley N, Roecker EB, et al. Influence of fat intake and caloric restriction on bone in aging male rats. *J Gerontol A Biol Sci Med Sci*. 1997;52(1):B20-B25.
46. Brochmann EJ, Duarte ME, Zaidi HA, Murray SS. Effects of dietary restriction on total body, femoral, and vertebral bone in SENCAR, C57BL/6, and DBA/2 mice. *Metabolism*. 2003;52(10):1265-1273.
47. Hamrick MW, Ding KH, Ponnala S, Ferrari SL, Isales CM. Caloric restriction decreases cortical bone mass but spares trabecular bone in the mouse skeleton: implications for the regulation of bone mass by body weight. *J Bone Miner Res*. 2008;23(6):870-878.
48. Tatsumi S, Ito M, Asaba Y, Tsutsumi K, Ikeda K. Life-long caloric restriction reveals biphasic and dimorphic effects on

bone metabolism in rodents. *Endocrinology*. 2008;149(2): 634-641.

49. Katewa SD, Kapahi P. Dietary restriction and aging, 2009. *Aging Cell*. 2010;9(2):105-112.
50. Ambrogini E, Almeida M, Martin-Millan M, et al. FoxO-mediated defense against oxidative stress in osteoblasts is indispensable for skeletal homeostasis in mice. *Cell Metab*. 2010;11(2):136-146.
51. Rached MT, Kode A, Xu L, et al. FoxO1 is a positive regulator of bone formation by favoring protein synthesis and resistance to oxidative stress in osteoblasts. *Cell Metab*. 2010;11(2):147-160.
52. Rached MT, Kode A, Silva BC, et al. FoxO1 expression in osteoblasts regulates glucose homeostasis through regulation of osteocalcin in mice. *J Clin Invest*. 2010;120(1): 357-368.
53. Elefteriou F, Ahn JD, Takeda S, et al. Leptin regulation of bone resorption by the sympathetic nervous system and CART. *Nature*. 2005;434(7032):514-520.
54. Manolagas SC, Almeida M. Gone with the Wnts: beta-catenin, T-cell factor, forkhead box O, and oxidative stress in age-dependent diseases of bone, lipid, and glucose metabolism. *Mol Endocrinol*. 2007;21(11):2605-2614.
55. Begg SK, Bertoncello I. The hematopoietic deficiencies in osteopetrotic (op/op) mice are not permanent, but progressively correct with age. *Exp Hematol*. 1993;21(4):493-495.
56. Blalock EM, Chen KC, Sharrow K, et al. Gene microarrays in hippocampal aging: statistical profiling identifies novel processes correlated with cognitive impairment. *J Neurosci*. 2003;23(9):3807-3819.
57. Lee CK, Klopp RG, Weindruch R, Prolla TA. Gene expression profile of aging and its retardation by caloric restriction. *Science*. 1999;285(5432):1390-1393.
58. Melov S, Hubbard A. Microarrays as a tool to investigate the biology of aging: a retrospective and a look to the future. *Sci Aging Knowl Environ*. 2004;2004(42):re7.
59. Coppe JP, Desprez PY, Krtolica A, Campisi J. The senescence-associated secretory phenotype: the dark side of tumor suppression. *Annu Rev Pathol*. 2010;5:99-118.
60. Gosselin K, Abbadie C. Involvement of Rel/NF-kappa B transcription factors in senescence. *Exp Gerontol*. 2003; 38(11–12):1271-1283.
61. Pasparakis M. Regulation of tissue homeostasis by NF-kappaB signalling: implications for inflammatory diseases. *Nat Rev Immunol*. 2009;9(11):778-788.
62. Sarkar D, Fisher PB. Molecular mechanisms of aging-associated inflammation. *Cancer Lett*. 2006;236(1):13-23.
63. Novack DV, Teitelbaum SL. The osteoclast: friend or foe? *Annu Rev Pathol*. 2008;3:457-484.
64. Hwang CS, Loftus TM, Mandrup S, Lane MD. Adipocyte differentiation and leptin expression. *Annu Rev Cell Dev Biol*. 1997;13:231-259.
65. Moller DE, Kaufman KD. Metabolic syndrome: a clinical and molecular perspective. *Annu Rev Med*. 2005;56:45-62.
66. Spiegelman BM, Hotamisligil GS. Through thick and thin: wasting, obesity, and TNF alpha. *Cell*. 1993;73(4):625-627.
67. Tracey KJ, Cerami A. Tumor necrosis factor: a pleiotropic cytokine and therapeutic target. *Annu Rev Med*. 1994;45:-491-503.
68. Chambers TJ. Regulation of the differentiation and function of osteoclasts. *J Pathol*. 2000;192(1):4-13.
69. Xing L, Schwarz EM, Boyce BF. Osteoclast precursors, RANKL/RANK, and immunology. *Immunol Rev*. 2005; 208:19-29.

11 Animal Models of Premature Aging

Wei Li and Gustavo Duque

Aging affects multiple organs and systems, which become unable to respond to stressors and environmental changes and therefore deteriorate in terms of function and structure.[1] Bone is not immune to age-related changes both in strength and cellularity. With aging, there is a progressive decrease in bone mass due to hormonal and cellular changes such as lower vitamin D, decreasing number of osteoblasts, and increasing number of osteoclasts and adipocytes.[2] In human subjects, these changes start in the third decade of life and progressively affect bone mass until the bone becomes prone to fracture.[3] In animals, as described in Chap. 10 of this book, there are significant differences in the way bone ages. Several reviews have compared changes in bone structure in mice and rats[4,5] and have found that there is a significant variability in the timing of the acquisition of their peak bone mass, variable levels of bone turnover, and higher or lower levels of marrow fat infiltration. In general, bone mass starts declining between 4 and 8 months of age in most normal animal models. However, fractures start happening only at very late ages in just a few of those models indicating that the usefulness of these "normal aging" models to assess osteoporosis mechanisms and treatment could be limited.

In this chapter, we will review a different set of models showing either premature or accelerated aging. Considering that a normal aging model takes significant time to develop and shows very variable phenotype, models of premature and accelerated aging could become a useful alternative to illustrate the mechanisms of senile osteoporosis and to develop new potential therapeutic targets for osteoporosis.

11.1 Aging Versus Ovariectomized Models of Osteoporosis

The characteristics of the ovariectomized (OVX) model of osteoporosis have been described in Chap. 9 of this book. In general, the predominant mechanism of osteoporosis in the OVX model is associated with changes in the immune system that induce an increase in RANKL and osteoclastogenesis.[6] Although estrogen deficiency has been associated with low osteoblastogenesis and high marrow adipogenesis, the predominant mechanism of osteoporosis in OVX mice are the increasing levels of osteoclastogenesis and thus bone resorption.[6]

Although the OVX model is the preferred model at many centers, this model seems to be inadequate when assessing the mechanisms of age-related bone loss and senile osteoporosis. From the drug testing point of view, and due to their higher levels of osteoclastogenesis, OVX animals are optimal when testing new anti-resorptives targeted toward osteoclast function and survival. However, it is well known that senile osteoporosis and male osteoporosis are not necessarily associated with low levels of estrogens but with changes in bone cellularity inherent to the aging process, which in most cases is independent of hormone levels. Table 11.1 describes the optimal characteristics of a good animal model of age-related bone loss and senile osteoporosis. Based on these characteristics, animal models that show high levels of adipogenesis, low levels of osteoblastogenesis,

G. Duque (✉)
Discipline of Geriatric Medicine, Ageing Bone Research Centre, Sydney Medical School – Nepean Campus, The University of Sydney, Penrith, NSW, Australia
e-mail: gustavo.duque@sydney.edu.au

G. Duque and K. Watanabe (eds.), *Osteoporosis Research*,
DOI: 10.1007/978-0-85729-293-3_11,

Table 11.1 Characteristics of animal models of age-related bone loss versus OVX mice

	OVX mice	Aged mice
Osteoblasts	Normal or low	Low
Adipocytes	High	Very high
Osteocytes	Low	Low
Osteoclasts	Very high	High

and moderately high levels of osteoclastogenesis should be the optimal approach to test anabolic compounds in bone which are considered the therapeutic choice in older individuals.[6]

11.2 Normal Aging Versus Progeria

Accelerated aging or "progeria" is characterized by the early development of multiple biological alterations normally associated with advanced age. Even though these rare and dramatic conditions only partially recapitulate normal aging, their study has the potential of rendering valuable information on the molecular mechanisms implicated in the aging process. [7] In addition, the development of animal models that mimic these syndromes can provide experimental systems useful to investigate the basis of particular pathologies associated with aging (atherosclerosis, osteoporosis, osteoarthritis, cancer) and to perform preclinical testing of therapeutic strategies against these alterations.

Table 11.2 illustrates the most common human syndromes of accelerated aging and their animal model counterparts. In terms of mechanisms of accelerated aging in these syndromes, most of them are caused by one of two major mechanisms: defects in DNA repair systems or alterations in the nuclear lamina.[8] Among the progeroid syndromes, Werner syndrome (WS) (or progeria of the adult) is the best understood syndrome and has been associated with a DNA repair defect. The typical phenotype in WS patients starts at puberty and includes early growth stop, bilateral cataracts, gray hair, scleroderma-like skin changes, subcutaneous calcification, arteriosclerosis, osteoporosis, diabetes mellitus, a prematurely aged facies, and a high incidence of cancer with high mortality at the sixth decade of life.[9] In terms of the gene involved in this progeria, typical cases of WS are caused by null mutations in *WRN*, a gene coding for a protein of the RecQ family with helicase and exonuclease activities that plays important roles in homology-dependent recombination repair and telomere maintenance.[10] A Wrn-knockout mouse model recapitulates the alterations observed in WS patients at the molecular and cellular levels but, strikingly, Wrn deficiency does not cause an accelerated aging phenotype in mice.[11] In contrast, progeroid symptoms closely recapitulating WS develop in double-mutant mice lacking both Wrn and telomerase activity, revealing the critical role of Wrn in telomere biology and its relevance for the progeroid phenotypes caused by WRN deficiency.[12,13] These findings indicate that mice and humans may show different sensitivity to progeroid-causing alterations, and these differences have to be carefully taken into consideration to interpret results derived from the use of murine models.

Another example of progeria associated with DNA damage and oxidative stress is the very rare syndrome known as ataxia telangiectasia (AT) syndrome. This human premature aging syndrome is characterized by neurodegeneration, immune defects, tumor formation, hypersensitivity to ionizing radiation, and genomic instability.[14] The responsible gene, *ATM* (AT mutated), is a large protein kinase that belongs to the PI-3 kinase family.[15] ATM functions in DNA damage checkpoint and oxidative stress responses, thereby playing a central role in the maintenance of genome stability. Mouse models for AT have been generated by knockout of the mouse Atm gene.[16] Atm knockout mice exhibit radiosensitivity, genomic instability, growth retardation, and lymphoma, recapitulating main features of human AT.[16]

Another type of progeria is the Hutchinson–Gilford progeria syndrome (HGPS) (or progeria of childhood). This progeria syndrome has been associated with defects of the nuclear envelope as its main mechanism. Patients suffering from HGPS are characterized by shortened life span, growth impairment, sclerotic skin, early hair loss, aged facies, decreased joint mobility, and cardiovascular problems.[17-19] Interestingly, this type of progeria is associated with severe osteoporosis and changes in bone structure that include micrognatia, a disproportionately large head, sculptured nose, delayed dentition, delayed closure of fontanelles, dystrophic nails, prominent joints, skeletal hypoplasia, and dysplasia.[20] Levy et al.[21] reported that most of HGPS cases are caused by a silent mutation in the *LMNA* gene. This gene encodes lamin A and C, which are two components of the nuclear envelope. Lamin A

Table 11.2 Human progeroid syndromes and their equivalent mouse model

Human progeria	Human phenotype	Mouse model
Werner syndrome	• Start at puberty • Early growth stop • Bilateral cataracts • Gray hair • Scleroderma-like skin changes • Subcutaneous calcification arteriosclerosis • Osteoporosis • Diabetes mellitus • Prematurely aged facies • Osteoporosis • High incidence of cancer with high mortality at the sixth decade of life	*Wrn*$^{-/-}$ *Terc*$^{-/-}$ *Wrn*$^{\Delta hel/\Delta hel}$
Hutchinson Gilford Progeria syndrome	• Shortened life span • Growth impairment • Sclerotic skin • Early hair loss • Aged facies • Decreased joint mobility • Cardiovascular problems • Disproportionately large head • Sculptured nose • Delayed dentition • Delayed closure of fontanelles • Dystrophic nails • Prominent joints • Skeletal hypoplasia and dysplasia	*Zmpste24*$^{-/-}$ *Lmna*$^{-/-}$
Ataxia telangiectasia	• Neurodegeneration • Immune defects • Tumor formation • Hypersensitivity to ionizing radiation • Genomic instability	*Atm*$^{-/-}$

is synthesized as a precursor known as prelamin A, which undergoes a series of posttranslational modifications including farnesylation, proteolytic removal of the C-terminal tripeptide, carboxyl methylation of the prenylated cysteine residue, and, finally, excision of the 15-residue farnesylated peptide. The mutation present in HGPS patients activates a cryptic splicing site, and leads to the synthesis of a prelamin A isoform known as progerin or LAΔ50, which lacks a 50-residue-long fragment containing the target sequence for the final proteolytic step and consequently remains constitutively farnesylated.[21,22]

The use of genetically modified mice allowed to identify the zinc metalloproteinase FACE-1 (also known as ZMPSTE24) as the enzyme responsible for the final proteolytic step during lamin A posttranslational maturation.[23] Accordingly, *Face-1/Zmpste24*-deficient mice accumulate farnesylated prelamin A at the nuclear envelope and phenocopy human HGPS, providing a valuable animal model for the study of this pathology.[23-25] Using transcriptional profiling on tissues from this knockout model, Varela et al.[26] found that hyperactivation of p53 signaling plays a key role in the accelerated aging phenotype, which is partially reversed by p53 deficiency. Moreover, the use of genetic approaches revealed that lowering the prelamin A levels results in a total rescue of this mouse model from the accelerated aging condition,[26-28] which may have an important future application in treating osteoporosis in older persons.

Although the *Face-1/Zmpste24*-deficient mice show some of the features of HGPS, this model could have a major pitfall since their phenotype could be the consequence of accumulation of unfarnesylated prelamin A at the nuclear envelope and not the typical accumulation of progerin, which seems to be more the consequence of mutations in the LMNA gene than alterations in the prelamin A processing system. Therefore, a second mouse model that could be correlated with the typical features of HGPS is the *lmna* knockout mouse. These mice, developed by Sullivan et al.,[29] develop to term with no overt abnormalities. However, their postnatal growth is severely retarded and is characterized by the appearance of muscular dystrophy. This phenotype is associated with ultrastructural perturbations to the nuclear envelope. These include the mislocalization of emerin, an inner nuclear membrane protein, defects in which are implicated in Emery–Dreifuss muscular dystrophy (EDMD), one of the three major X-linked dystrophies. Mice lacking the A-type lamins exhibit tissue-specific alterations to their nuclear envelope integrity and emerin distribution.[26] In skeletal and cardiac muscles, this is manifest as a dystrophic condition related to EDMD. In addition, these mice show the typical cardiomyopathy and valvular disease seen in patients with HGPS.

In summary, models of accelerated aging, especially the ones that show similar features of osteoporosis in humans, are pivotal to understanding the mechanisms of aging bone and to testing strategies for osteoporosis treatment in older individuals.

11.3 Wrn Mutant Mice

Mutational inactivation of the gene WRN causes WS.[12] This type of progeria is an autosomal recessive disease characterized by premature aging, elevated genomic instability, and increased cancer incidence. The capacity of enforced telomerase expression to rescue premature senescence of cultured cells from individuals with WS and the lack of a disease phenotype in Wrn-deficient mice with long telomeres implicate telomere attrition in the pathogenesis of WS.

In late-generation mice null with respect to both Wrn and Terc (encoding the telomerase RNA component), telomere dysfunction elicits a classical Werner-like premature aging syndrome typified by premature death, hair graying, alopecia, osteoporosis, type II diabetes, and cataracts. This mouse model also showed accelerated replicative senescence and accumulation of DNA-damage foci in cultured cells, as well as increased chromosomal instability and cancer, particularly nonepithelial malignancies typical of WS. These genetic data indicate that the delayed manifestation of the complex pleiotropic of Wrn deficiency relates to telomere shortening.[30]

Pignolo et al.[31] have characterized the bone phenotype of $Wrn^{-/-}$ $Terc^{-/-}$ mutant mice (Fig. 11.1). This mouse model, developed by Du et al.,[32] shows a low bone mass phenotype with impaired osteoblast differentiation in the context of intact osteoclast differentiation. Further, mesenchymal stem cells (MSCs) from single and $Wrn^{-/-}$ $Terc^{-/-}$ double mutant mice have a reduced *in vitro* life span and display impaired osteogenic potential concomitant with characteristics of premature senescence. Taking this evidence together, this mouse model could be useful to investigate the role of telomerase integrity in osteoblast function and differentiation and to understand the role of telomerase in the pathophysiology of aging bone. According to Du et al.,[32] the life span of this model seems to be longer than 14 months but their bone phenotype develops early in life, which facilitates the use of this model when looking at the mechanisms of aging bone.

The $Wrn^{\Delta hel/\Delta hel}$ mutant mouse is another model of WS largely studied by Lebel et al.[33] Although the deletion created in the Wrn gene of these mice is different from human WS mutants, there are several features that are found in this model that mimic WS such as enhanced visceral fat accumulation (but not subcutaneous fat), hypertriglyceridemia, hypercholesterolemia, and diabetes mellitus. Cardiac abnormalities include aortic stenosis and cardiac fibrosis, which are also

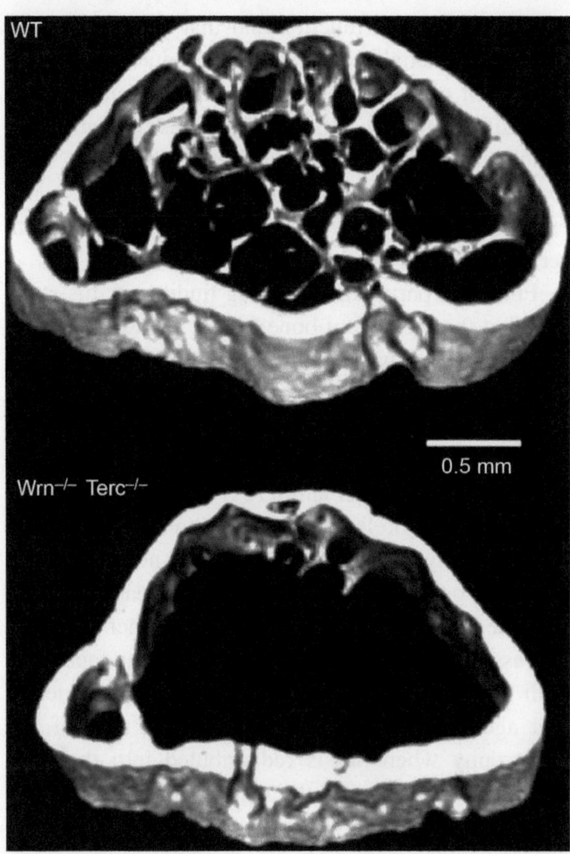

Fig. 11.1 Volume-rendered cross-sectional slabs from the distal metaphysis of two mouse femurs, revealing dramatic differences in trabecular architecture between a WT (*top*) and a $Wrn^{-/-}$ $Terc^{-/-}$ mutant (*bottom*) mouse. Quantitative analysis of these slabs shows BMD differences are trabecular rather than cortical in nature (Adapted from Pignolo et al.[31])

found in WS patients. Interestingly, and in contrast with the $Wrn^{-/-}$ $Terc^{-/-}$ model, our analysis of bone phenotype in the $Wrn^{\Delta hel/\Delta hel}$ mutant mice did not show osteoporotic changes at the structural level (Fig. 11.2). Nevertheless, due to the changes seen in fat mass and fat distribution in these mice, this model could be useful for the assessment of the relationship between fat mass and bone metabolism, a subject of growing interest closely associated with the aging process.

11.4 Zmpste-24-Deficient Mice

The zinc metalloprotease FACE-1/ZMPSTE24 is an integral membrane protein responsible for the conversion of prelamin A into lamin A/C, an important element of the nuclear envelope. Recently, we have reported that lamin A/C is required in osteoblastogenesis.[34] Our data suggest that absence of lamin A/C affects osteoblast differentiation of MSCs and facilitates adipogenesis *in vitro*. Additional evidence has shown that lamin A/C is required in MSC differentiation and could be one of the links between the aging process and the development of senile osteoporosis.

We have also reported that prelamin A accumulation due to pharmacological inhibition of prelamin A farnesylation using farnesyl transferase inhibitors (FTI-277) inhibits osteoblastogenesis and induces nuclear changes in MSCs, affecting their differentiation without affecting their survival.[35] In this context,

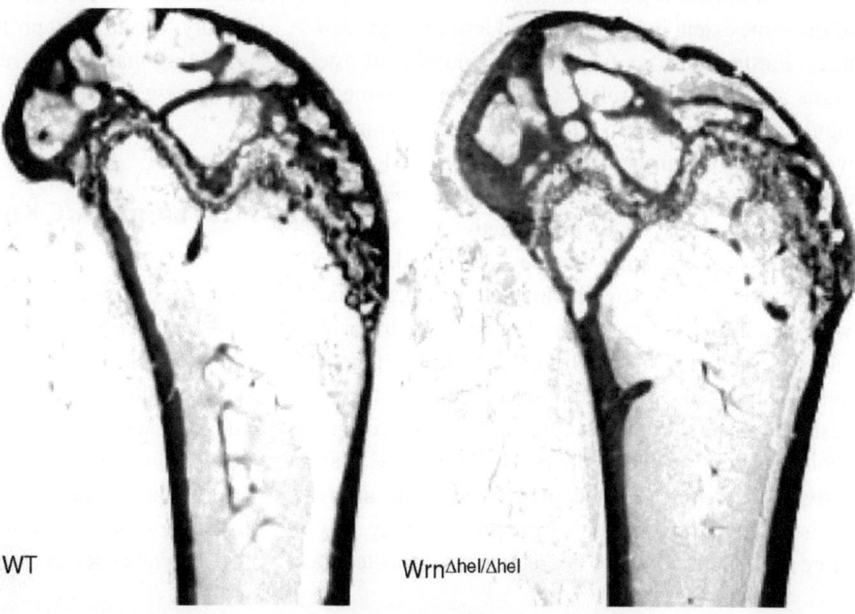

Fig. 11.2 Volume-rendered longitudinal slabs from the distal metaphysis of two mouse femurs. There are no differences in trabecular architecture between a WT and a $Wrn^{\Delta hel/\Delta hel}$ mutant mouse

the assessment of the role of FACE-1/ZMPSTE24 in bone metabolism could constitute an important approach to understand the mechanisms of senile osteoporosis.

Pendas et al.[23] used gene targeting to generate *Zmpste24* $^{-/-}$ mice. These mice are apparently normal at birth, but they show a striking accumulation of prelamin A at the nuclear envelope, which leads to frequent nuclear abnormalities at the cellular level. In turn, these molecular and cellular alterations lead to the development of severe age-related abnormalities at the organismal level, including loss of subcutaneous fat, reduced mobility due to skeletal and muscular defects, hair loss, and metabolic alterations.[23,36]

In fact, we have recently reported the bone phenotype of these mice.[37] In this study, we assessed whether the low bone mass and spontaneous fractures found in the *Zmpste24*$^{-/-}$ mice were due to the same mechanisms previously found in our experiments *in vitro*. In addition, we checked whether these abnormalities were similar in both sexes. Initially, we performed both microcomputerized tomography (μCT) and histological analyses of bones of *Zmpste24*$^{-/-}$ mice at the age of 3 months. This time point was selected due to the short life span of the homozygous mice and previous reports that, after this age, *Zmpste24*$^{-/-}$ mice start suffering spontaneous fractures. Von Kossa staining and μCT demonstrated that bone mass is significantly lower in the *Zmpste24*$^{-/-}$ mice compared with wild type (WT) control mice, leading to an osteopenic phenotype (Fig. 11.3). This bone loss is reflected by a decrease in trabecular thickness and number, which were decreased to the same extent in both male and female *Zmpste24*$^{-/-}$ mice. Furthermore, we found that the number of osteoblasts and osteoclasts relative to the bone volume was significantly reduced in *Zmpste24*$^{-/-}$ mice compared with the WT controls. This reduction in cell number correlated with serum markers of osteocalcin (OCN) and osteoclastic (C-telopeptide) activities. No difference between male and female was found. Overall, these changes in bone cellularity were not associated with changes in serum levels of either calcium or calciotropic and sex steroid hormones. Taken together, these results demonstrate that accumulation of unprocessed prelamin A induces bone loss through a significant reduction in bone turnover. However, osteoblastic activity was more affected than osteoclastic activity, suggesting that processing of prelamin A may play a more important role in the regulation of osteoblast differentiation and function and that the reduction in osteoclastic activity could be a consequence of lower number of osteoblast precursors which regulate osteoclast differentiation. In addition, MSCs obtained from bone marrow in both male and female *Zmpste24*$^{-/-}$mice lost their capacity to differentiate into osteoblasts and expressed lower levels of the osteoblastogenesis transcription factors OCN and BSPII.

Finally, a particularly striking finding of this study was that the significant bone loss in *Zmpste24*$^{-/-}$ mice was associated with higher levels of fat infiltration within the bone marrow. This evidence correlates with previous *in vitro* findings showing that lack of lamin A/C favors the differentiation of MSCs into adipocytes.[34] In fact, lack of lamin A/C and accumulation of unfarnesylated prelamin A have been associated with lipodystrophy or redistribution of fat to nonadipose tissues.[36] In our study, the abnormally increased amount of bone marrow fat correlated with higher levels of expression of proadipogenic transcription factors in both male and female *Zmpste24*$^{-/-}$ mice. Considering that age-related bone loss constitutes a type of lipodystrophy where fat is redistributed into the bone marrow compartment,[38] the regulation of the proteins of the lamina may play an important role in the prevention of this age-related phenomenon.

In summary, the *Zmpste24*$^{-/-}$ mouse is a useful model to assess the mechanisms of age-related bone loss and to test potential therapeutic targets. A potential limitation of this model is their short life span (5–6 months). A recent study using bisphosphonates and statins in these mice corrected not only their bone phenotype but also prolonged their survival rate,[6,39] suggesting that this is a reliable model to be used when testing new therapies for senile osteoporosis.

11.5 Lamin A/C Knockout (*lmna*$^{-/-}$) Mice

Using gene targeting, Sullivan et al. developed the first *lmna*$^{-/-}$ mouse model in 1999.[29] Mice lacking A-type lamins develop to term with no overt abnormalities. However, their postnatal growth is severely retarded and is characterized by the appearance of muscular dystrophy. This phenotype is associated with ultrastructural perturbations to the nuclear envelope. These include the mislocalization of emerin, an inner nuclear membrane protein, whose defects are implicated in EDMD, one of

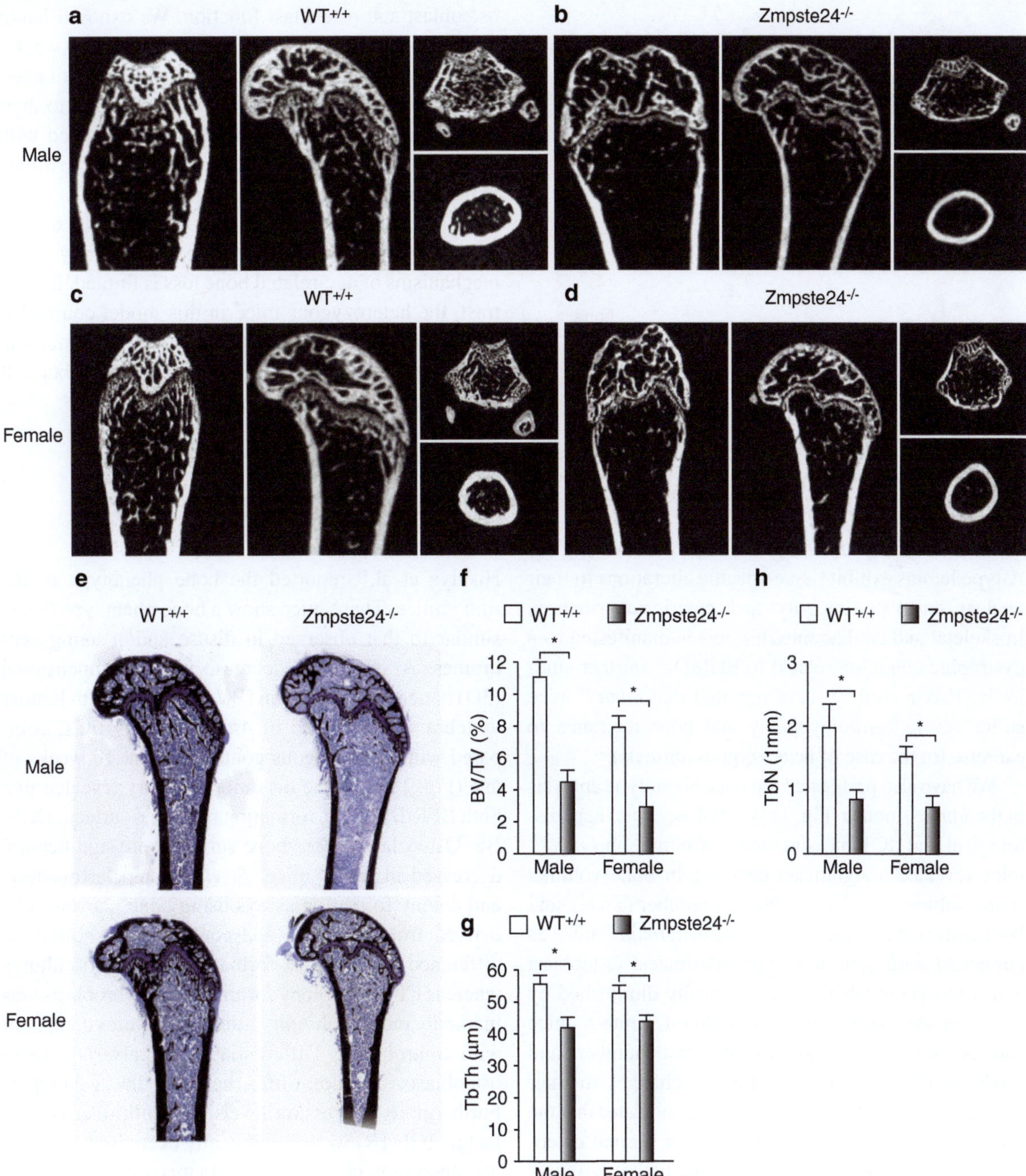

Fig. 11.3 Changes in bone architecture in male and female Zmpste24$^{-/-}$ mice. (**a–d**) µCT analysis of the distal femur of 3-month-old Zmpste24$^{-/-}$ mice and WT$^{+/+}$ littermates. Representative two-dimensional (2D) reconstructions, obtained using a Skyscan® 1,072 instrument, are shown for male and female Zmpste24$^{-/-}$ (**b**, **d**) and WT$^{+/+}$ (**a**, **c**) mice. The right upper panels are representative of the area just below the growth plate while the right lower panels show the cross-sectional (cortical) bone structure. Zmpste24$^{-/-}$ mice exhibited profound thinning of cortical bone, a reduction in platelike structures, and a lack of trabecular connectivity. These changes correlated with von Kossa staining (**e**). Quantitation of bone parameters (**f–h**) further exemplified a decrease in bone quality (BV/TV) (**f**), trabecular thickness (Tb.Th.) (**g**), and trabecular number (Tr. N.) (**h**) in the mutant femora compared with the WT$^{+/+}$ littermate controls. Results are expressed as the mean ± SD of eight independent analyses per group. Significantly different from control; $*p<0.001$ (From Rivas et al.[37])

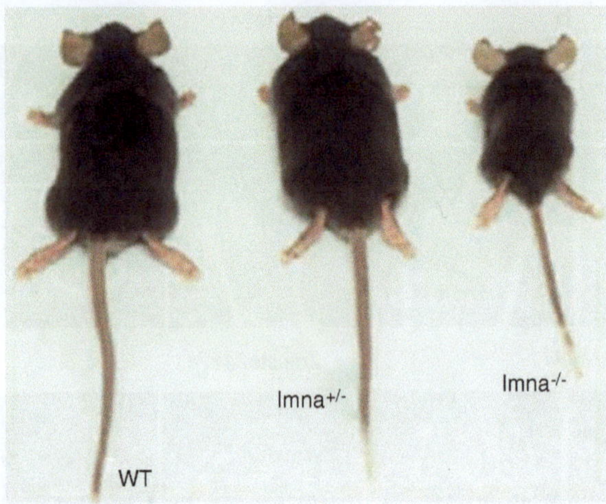

Fig. 11.4 Four-month-old *lmna*$^{-/-}$ mice. Note the differences in size between homozygous (–/–) and heterozygous (+/–) mice

the three major X-linked dystrophies. Mice lacking the A-type lamins exhibit tissue-specific alterations to their nuclear envelope integrity and emerin distribution. In skeletal and cardiac muscles, this is manifested as a dystrophic condition related to EDMD.[29] Further studies by Fatkin et al.[40,41] have reported that *lmna*$^{-/-}$ mice suffer severe cardiomyopathy and poor tolerance to exercise (in the case of heterozygous animals).[41]

We have also performed the bone phenotype analysis in the *lmna*$^{-/-}$ mouse (Fig. 11.4). At 4 weeks of age, histological and μCT measurements of femurs in *Lmna*$^{-/-}$ mice revealed a significant decrease in bone volume/tissue volume (BV/TV), trabecular number (Tb.N), and both cortical and trabecular thickness in *lmna*$^{-/-}$ mice as compared with their wild-type littermates. Osteoblast and osteocyte numbers are dramatically diminished by ~75% in the *lmna*$^{-/-}$ mice. In addition, lmna-/- mice showed significantly lower osteoclast number and eroded surfaces as well as aberrant changes in their osteoclasts (Fig. 11.5). This phenotype indicates that the presence of lamin A/C is necessary for normal osteoblast and osteoclast differentiation and activity *in vivo*, and that *lmna*$^{-/-}$ mice could constitute a useful model to assess the role of lamin A/C in bone metabolism and the mechanisms of aging bone.

As in the *Zmpste24*$^{-/-}$ mice, a potential limitation in this model is the short life span of the homozygous animals and the lack of osteoporosis in the heterozygous (*lmna*$^{+/-}$) controls. Nevertheless, we have found that mice could be useful when assessing the dynamics of bone cells and the effect of low levels of lamin A/C in osteoblast and osteoclast function. We exposed lamin *lmna*$^{+/-}$ mice to maximal strength exercise for 6 weeks. In this study we found that the beneficial effect of exercise on bone is lost in *lmna*$^{+/-}$ mice compared to their WT controls in a mechanism closely associated with the activity of β-catenin, a transcription factor involved in mechanosensing and bone formation.[42]

In summary, due to their short life span, the usefulness of homozygous *lmna*$^{+/-}$ mice for the study of the mechanisms of age-related bone loss is limited. In contrast, the heterozygous mice in this model could also be useful to assess the role of lamin A/C in multiple steps of osteoblastogenesis due to their lower but still present lamin A/C expression.

11.6 Atm Knockout (*Atm*$^{-/-}$) Mice

Hishiya et al.[43] reported the bone phenotype of the *Atm*$^{-/-}$ mice. These mice show a bone phenotype that is similar to that observed in disuse and/or aging syndromes. A significant decrease in three-dimensional (3D) bone volume fraction (BV/TV) of the fifth lumbar vertebra was observed in *Atm*$^{-/-}$ mice by μCT, compared with heterozygous control mice at 10 weeks of age (Fig. 11.6). Bone histomorphometry revealed that both BFR/BS: Bone formation rate/bone surface; Oc.S/BS: Osteoclast surface/bone surface were significantly decreased in *Atm*$^{-/-}$ mice. *In vitro* osteoclastogenesis and colony formation assays using bone marrow cells derived from knockout and control mice showed no difference in osteoclast formation in *ex vivo* cultures whereas CFU-F: Colony forming units-fybroblasts was markedly reduced in *Atm*$^{-/-}$ -derived cultures compared with control mice. Differentiation of calvaria-derived osteoblasts did not differ between the genotypes. Furthermore, expression levels of insulin-like growth factor (IGF-1R) were significantly decreased, and p38 was aberrantly phosphorylated in marrow stromal cells from *Atm*$^{-/-}$ mice. The authors conclude that the pathogenesis of the osteopenic phenotype in *Atm*$^{-/-}$ mice is similar to that of disuse and/or aging syndromes and is caused, at least in part, by a stem cell defect due to lack of IGF signaling. Since this bone phenotype starts as early as 10 weeks of age, this mouse model could be useful to identify the role of IGF in age-related bone loss and alterations in osteoblastic differentiation of MSCs associated with old age.

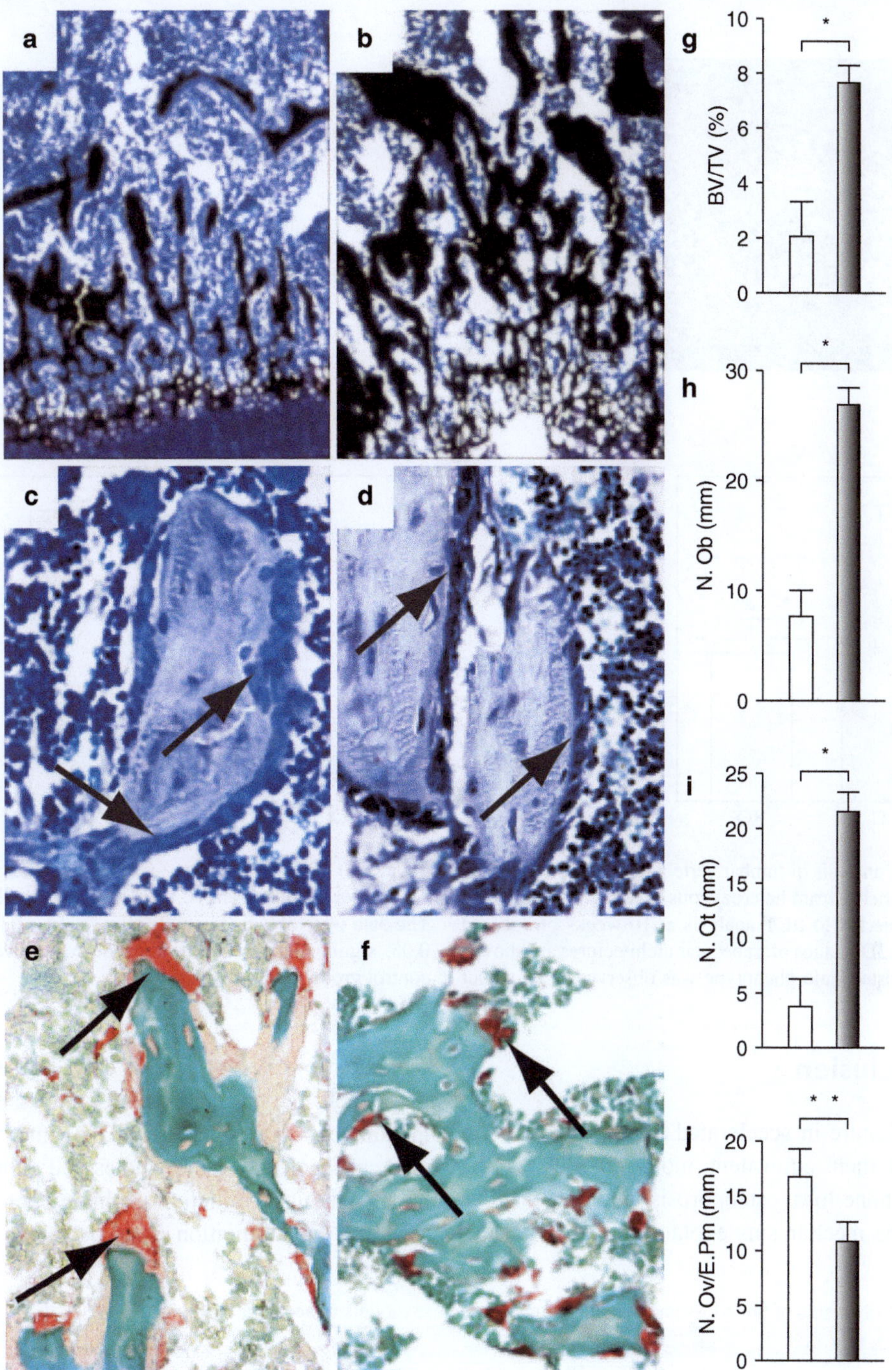

Fig. 11.5 Changes in bone architecture and cellularity in *Lmna*$^{-/-}$ mice . Von Kossa staining of distal femur obtained from female *Lmna*$^{-/-}$ mice. *Lmna*$^{-/-}$ mice (**a**) showed a profound thinning of their trabeculae compared with their WT littermates (**b**). We found a significant reduction in bone volume (BV/TV) in *Lmna*$^{-/-}$ mice as compared with their WT controls (**g**). Sections of plastic embedded femur from *Lmna*$^{-/-}$ mice (**c**, **e**) and their WT littermates (**d**, **f**) were stained sequentially for alkaline phosphatase (ALP) (osteoblasts) (**c**, **d**, *arrows*) and tartrate resistant acid phosphatase (TRAP) (osteoclasts) (**e**, **f**, *arrows*). Osteoblasts and osteocytes numbers are dramatically diminished by ~75% in the *Lmna*$^{-/-}$ mice (**c**, **h**, **i**). In contrast, *Lmna*$^{-/-}$ mice showed significantly higher osteoclast number and eroded surfaces (**e**, **j**). In addition, in *Lmna*$^{-/-}$ mice, we found aberrant forms of osteoblasts and osteoclasts including giant osteoblasts and lining cells (**c**, *arrows*) as well as "cystic" osteoclasts (**e**, *arrows*). White bars = *Lmna*$^{-/-}$ mice; gray bars = WT controls. $*p<0.001$, $**p<0.05$. Adapted from Li et al. [42]

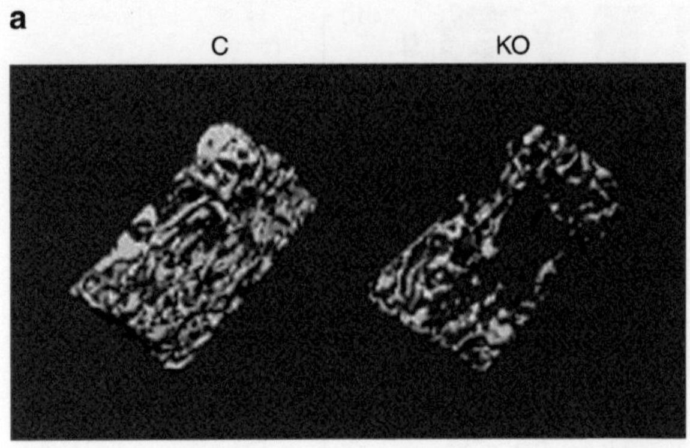

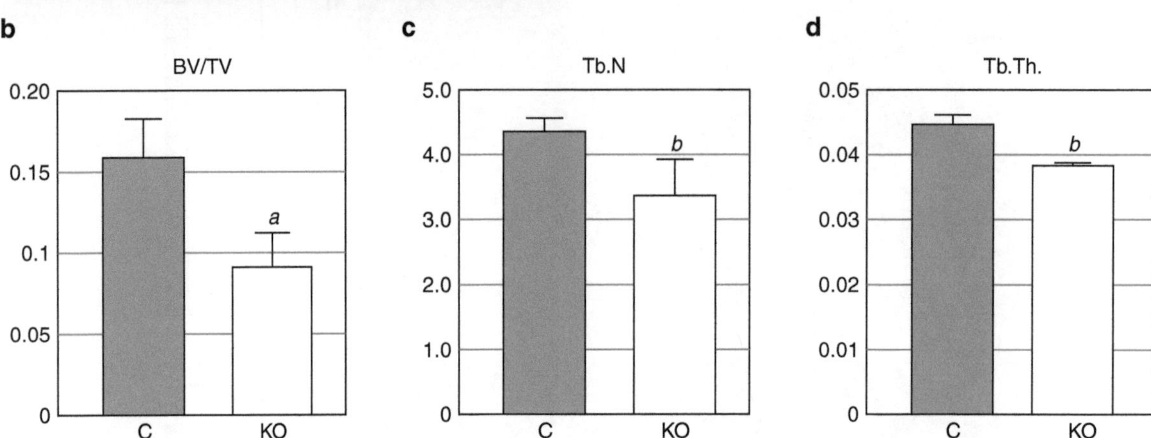

Fig. 11.6 μCT analysis of lumbar vertebrae of *Atm*$^{-/-}$ mice. The fifth lumbar vertebra from heterozygous (**c**) and knockout (KO) mice were subjected to μCT analysis at 10 weeks of age. (**a**) Representative 3D images of trabecular architectures are shown. Note that the osteopenic phenotype was observed in knockout mice. (**b**) Trabecular bone volume fraction (BV/TV). (**c**) Trabecular number (Tb.N). (**d**) Trabecular thickness (Tb.Th.). The data were obtained in male mice. $a - p < 0.005$ and $b - p < 0.05$, significantly different from the respective heterozygous control group (From Hishiya et al.[43])

11.7 Conclusion

A constant feature in accelerated aging syndromes in humans and their equivalent mouse models is the presence of bone loss, osteoporosis, and spontaneous fractures. The mechanisms explaining this bone loss seems to be different in each case (Table 11.3); however, each model could be useful in specific experimental designs when targeting into telomerases, nuclear envelope, or the wholesome aging process of bone. A typical limitation of this model is their short life span. This limitation could also be an advantage as

Table 11.3 Mechanisms of bone loss and cellular changes in mouse models of accelerated aging

Mouse model	Osteoblasts	Adipocytes	Osteocytes	Osteoclasts	Proposed mechanism
Wrn$^{-/-}$ *Terc*$^{-/-}$	Decreased number	N/A	N/A	Normal	Telomere shortening
Zmpste24$^{-/-}$	Decreased	Increased	Decreased	Decreased	• Accumulation of prelamin A • Accumulation of progerin
Lmna$^{-/-}$	Decreased and aberrant	Moderately increased	Decreased	Normal but aberrant	• Lack of lamin A/C • Nuclear changes (blebbing and vacuolization)
Atm$^{-/-}$	Decreased	N/A	N/A	Normal	• Low expression of IGFR1

N/A information not available

models of accelerated aging show the typical features of aging bone without the long experimental time and limited accessibility to the normal aging models.

Acknowledgments The experimental results reported in this chapter were obtained thanks to the support of the Australian National Health and Medical Research Council (NHMRC) and the Nepean Medical Research Foundation.

References

1. Cevenini E, Invidia L, Lescai F, et al. Human models of aging and longevity. *Expert Opin Biol Ther*. 2008;8:1393-1405.
2. Duque G, Troen BR. Understanding the mechanisms of senile osteoporosis: new facts for a major geriatric syndrome. *J Am Geriatr Soc*. 2008;56:935-941.
3. Manolagas SC, Parfitt AM. What old means to bone. *Trends Endocrinol Metab*. 2010;21:369-374.
4. Lelovas PP, Xanthos TT, Thoma SE, et al. The laboratory rat as an animal model for osteoporosis research. *Comp Med*. 2008;58:424-430.
5. Perel P, Roberts I, Sena E, et al. Comparison of treatment effects between animal experiments and clinical trials: systematic review. *BMJ*. 2007;334:197.
6. Lyritis GP, Georgoulas T, Zafeiris CP. Bone anabolic versus bone anticatabolic treatment of postmenopausal osteoporosis. *Ann NY Acad Sci*. 2010;1205:277-283.
7. Burtner CR, Kennedy BK. Progeria syndromes and ageing: what is the connection? *Nat Rev Mol Cell Biol*. 2010;11:567-578.
8. Osorio FG, Obaya AJ, López-Otín C, et al. Accelerated ageing: from mechanism to therapy through animal models. *Transgenic Res*. 2009;18:7-15.
9. Cox LS, Faragher RG. From old organisms to new molecules: integrative biology and therapeutic targets in accelerated human ageing. *Cell Mol Life Sci*. 2007;64:2620-2641.
10. Yu CE, Oshima J, Fu YH, et al. Positional cloning of the Werner's syndrome gene. *Science*. 1996;272:258-262.
11. Lombard DB, Beard C, Johnson B, et al. Mutations in the WRN gene in mice accelerate mortality in a p53-null background. *Mol Cell Biol*. 2000;20:3286-3291.
12. Chang S, Multani AS, Cabrera NG, et al. Essential role of limiting telomeres in the pathogenesis of Werner syndrome. *Nat Genet*. 2004;36:877-882.
13. Multani AS, Chang S. WRN at telomeres: implications for aging and cancer. *J Cell Sci*. 2007;120:713-721.
14. Lavin MF, Shiloh Y. The genetic defect in ataxia-telangiectasia. *Annu Rev Immunol*. 1997;15:177-202.
15. Rotman G, Shiloh Y. ATM: from gene to function. *Hum Mol Genet*. 1998;7:1555-1563.
16. Barlow C, Hirotsune S, Paylor R, et al. Atm-deficient mice: a paradigm of ataxia telangiectasia. *Cell*. 1996;86:159-171.
17. Hennekam RC. Hutchinson-Gilford progeria syndrome: review of the phenotype. *Am J Med Genet A*. 2006;140: 2603-2624.
18. Merideth MA, Gordon LB, Clauss S, et al. Phenotype and course of Hutchinson-Gilford progeria syndrome. *N Engl J Med*. 2008;358:592-604.
19. Pereira S, Bourgeois P, Navarro C, et al. HGPS and related premature aging disorders: from genomic identification to the first therapeutic approaches. *Mech Ageing Dev*. 2008; 129:449-459.
20. de Paula Rodrigues GH, das Eiras Tâmega I, et al. Severe bone changes in a case of Hutchinson-Gilford syndrome. *Ann Genet*. 2002;45:151-155.
21. De Sandre-Giovannoli A, Bernard R, Cau P, et al. Lamin A truncation in Hutchinson-Gilford progeria. *Science*. 2003; 300:2055.
22. Eriksson M, Brown WT, Gordon LB, et al. Recurrent de novo point mutations in lamin A cause Hutchinson-Gilford progeria syndrome. *Nature*. 2003;423:293-298.
23. Pendas AM, Zhou Z, Cadinanos J, et al. Defective prelamin A processing and muscular and adipocyte alterations in Zmpste24 metalloproteinase-deficient mice. *Nat Genet*. 2002;31:94-99.
24. Cadinanos J, Varela I, Lopez-Otin C, et al. From immature lamin to premature aging: molecular pathways and therapeutic opportunities. *Cell Cycle*. 2005;4:1732-1735.
25. de Carlos F, Varela I, Germana A, et al. Microcephalia with mandibular and dental dysplasia in adult Zmpste24 deficient mice. *J Anat*. 2008;213:509-519.
26. Varela I, Cadinanos J, Pendas AM, et al. Accelerated ageing in mice deficient in Zmpste24 protease is linked to p53 signalling activation. *Nature*. 2005;437:564-568.
27. Fong LG, Ng JK, Meta M, et al. Heterozygosity for Lmna deficiency eliminates the progeria-like phenotypes in Zmpste24-deficient mice. *Proc Natl Acad Sci USA*. 2004; 101:18111-18116.
28. Fong LG, Frost D, Meta M, et al. A protein farnesyltransferase inhibitor ameliorates disease in a mouse model of progeria. *Science*. 2006;311:1621-1623.
29. Sullivan T, Escalante-Alcalde D, Bhatt H, et al. Loss of A-type lamin expression compromises nuclear envelope integrity leading to muscular dystrophy. *J Cell Biol*. 1999; 147:913-920.
30. Opresko PL. Telomere ResQue and preservation–roles for the Werner syndrome protein and other RecQ helicases. *Mech Ageing Dev*. 2008;129:79-90.
31. Pignolo RJ, Suda RK, McMillan EA, et al. Defects in telomere maintenance molecules impair osteoblast differentiation and promote osteoporosis. *Aging Cell*. 2008;7:23-31.
32. Du X, Shen J, Kugan N, et al. Telomere shortening exposes functions for the mouse Werner and Bloom syndrome genes. *Mol Cell Biol*. 2004;24:8437-8446.
33. Lebel M, Spillare EA, Harris CC, et al. The Werner syndrome gene product co-purifies with the DNA replication complex and interacts with PCNA and topoisomerase I. *J Biol Chem*. 1999;274:37795-37799.
34. Akter R, Rivas D, Geneau G, et al. Effect of lamin A/C knockdown on osteoblast differentiation and function. *J Bone Miner Res*. 2009;24:283-293.
35. Duque G, Vidal C, Rivas D. Protein isoprenylation regulates osteogenic differentiation of mesenchymal stem cells: effect of alendronate, and farnesyl and geranylgeranyl transferase inhibitors. Br J Pharmacol. 2011;162:1109-1118.
36. Bergo MO, Gavino B, Ross J, et al. Zmpste24 deficiency in mice causes spontaneous bone fractures, muscle weakness, and a prelamin A processing defect. *Proc Natl Acad Sci USA*. 2002;99:13049-13054.

37. Rivas D, Li W, Akter R, et al. Accelerated features of age-related bone loss in zmpste24 metalloproteinase-deficient mice. *J Gerontol A Biol Sci Med Sci*. 2009;64:1015-1024.
38. Ng A, Duque G. Osteoporosis as a lipotoxic disease. *IBMS BoneKEy*. 2010;7:108-123.
39. Varela I, Pereira S, Ugalde AP, et al. Combined treatment with statins and aminobisphosphonates extends longevity in a mouse model of human premature aging. *Nat Med*. 2008;14:767-772.
40. Fatkin D, MacRae C, Sasaki T, et al. Missense mutations in the rod domain of the lamin A/C gene as causes of dilated cardiomyopathy and conduction-system disease. *N Engl J Med*. 1999;341:1715-1724.
41. Chandar S, Yeo LS, Leimena C, et al. Effects of mechanical stress and carvedilol in lamin A/C-deficient dilated cardiomyopathy. *Circ Res*. 2010;106:573-582.
42. Li W, Yeo LS, Vidal C, McCorquodale T, Herrmann M, et al. 2011 Decreased Bone Formation and Osteopenia in Lamin A/C-Deficient Mice. PLoS ONE 6(4): e19313. doi:10.1371/journal.pone.0019313.
43. Duque G, Li W, Yeo L, et al. Exercise has a deleterious effect on bone quality in lamin A/C happloinsuficient mice.Bone, 2011 (in press).
44. Hishiya A, Ito M, Aburatani H, et al. Ataxia telangiectasia mutated (Atm) knockout mice as a model of osteopenia due to impaired bone formation. *Bone*. 2005;37:497-503.

12 Nonhuman Primate Models of Osteoporosis

Susan Y. Smith, Aurore Varela, and Jacquelin Jolette

12.1 Introduction

This chapter reviews the use of the nonhuman primate (NHP) as an animal model for osteoporosis research. While the previous chapters have extensively covered the use of lower species, the use of a higher species such as the NHP is likely to be the ultimate, or in some cases, the only relevant species to study bone in osteoporosis research. NHPs are used extensively in osteoporosis research in the pharmaceutical industry to evaluate new drug targets and in this context have contributed much to our current understanding of the human disease. This chapter focuses on the use of the NHP in drug development, presenting practical information on model selection and current techniques used to derive the primary end points of interest. Most of the practices described are considered relevant even in a basic research laboratory setting and will hopefully prove useful to researchers outside the pharmaceutical industry.

The primary objective of any animal model of osteoporosis is to mimic as closely as possible the human disease state in order to provide translatable information on mechanistic pathways, drug safety, and efficacy, and to study factors affecting and contributing to "bone quality." The factors that define bone quality remain open to debate, but can be considered to be defined by effects on *bone dynamics*, described at the skeletal level by biochemical markers of bone turnover and at the tissue level by dynamic histomorphometry techniques; on *bone mass*, largely determined by bone densitometry techniques; on *bone architecture*, determined by histomorphometry structural parameters and research tools such as microcomputerized tomography (μCT) analysis; and on *bone strength*, determined by biomechanical tests. How to obtain accurate and precise information on each of these end points that describe indices of bone quality, as well as other tools that may be applied to this research area, is the focus of this chapter.

12.2 Selecting the Appropriate Animal Model

Selection of the NHP over other species for osteoporosis research should be based on sound scientific and ethical considerations. For a comprehensive review of other large animal species used in osteoporosis research, the reader is referred to Chap. 13 of this book and Reinwald and Burr.[1] Several monkey species have been used as models to study osteoporosis including the cynomolgus, rhesus, baboon, and African green monkeys.[2] Among these, the cynomolgus monkey is often the species of choice based on its availability, small size, and relative ease of housing and handling. There is no other higher animal species that is currently as well characterized as the cynomolgus monkey in osteoporosis research with respect to musculoskeletal biology. The fact that NHPs closely resemble human physiology with respect to several other major systems also supports the NHP as the species of choice in osteoporosis research. In addition to bone

S.Y. Smith (✉)
Department of Bone Research and General Toxicology, Charles River Preclinical Services, Montréal, Québec, Canada
e-mail: susan.smith@crl.com

G. Duque and K. Watanabe (eds.), *Osteoporosis Research*,
DOI: 10.1007/978-0-85729-293-3_12, © Springer-Verlag London Limited 2011

physiology, the NHP has close synergy with man with respect to immune, reproductive, and cardiovascular function. In drug development, these systems, as well as other major organ systems such as the kidney and liver, are evaluated for target and off-target effects, to provide a comprehensive dataset for submission to regulatory authorities worldwide that is relevant to safety in man.

The NHP has been used in osteoporosis research in short-term proof-of-concept (POC) screening studies,[3] long-term bone quality safety studies,[4] and toxicology studies,[5] in both males and females. Depending on the study objectives, young or aged monkeys can be gonadectomized (surgically or chemically) or remain intact. Examples of use of these models in the published literature are provided in Table 12.1 and are briefly discussed in the following section.

12.3 Short-Term Models

Short-term screening models, or POC studies, are used for a variety of reasons including lead-optimization and to confirm target specificity and efficacy based on the known pharmacology of the class of material under test. The primary end point in these early studies is the measurement of blood and/or urinary biochemical markers of bone formation and bone resorption. Bone anti-catabolic and anabolic molecules are expected to reduce or increase biochemical markers of bone turnover, respectively. Young intact monkeys (meaning non-gonadectomized and chemically naive animals) have relatively high levels of biochemical markers of bone turnover, providing a useful and relatively inexpensive means to compare compounds for potency and identify a lead to continue into development, and

Table 12.1 Summary of NHP models

Model	Rationale	Primary end points	Age[a] (years)	Sex	Duration[b]
Intact	POC, PK/PD	Biomarkers	≥3	♂/♀	8 Weeks
	Screening	Densitometry			
	Toxicology	Biomarkers Densitometry Histology	≥3	♂/♀	3–6 Months
Chemical: GnRh agonist	POC, PK/PD Screening	Biomarkers	Sexually mature	♂/♀	4–8 Weeks
OVX	POC	Biomarkers	Sexually mature	♀	6 Months
	Dose range finding	Densitometry Histomorphometry[c] Biomechanics+			
ORX	POC	Biomarkers	Sexually mature	♂	6 Months
	Dose range finding	Densitometry Histomorphometry Biomechanics[c]			
OVX	Bone safety	Biomarkers Densitometry Histomorphometry[c] Biomechanics[c]	≥9[d]	♀	16 Months
ORX	Bone safety	Biomarkers Densitometry Histomorphometry Biomechanics	≥9	♂	16 Months

POC Proof-of-concept, *PK/PD* pharmacokinetic/pharmacodynamic profile, *OVX* surgical ovariectomy, *ORX* surgical orchidectomy

[a]Age for cynomolgus monkeys can be variable and will depend on animal availability

[b]The duration will vary; the minimum duration is suggested for each model

[c]Optional

[d]Age ≥12 for rhesus monkeys

to confirm target activity and safety using the chosen route of administration. In older animals, which can be argued to be more representative of the age of the intended (osteoporotic) human population, chemical gonadectomy can be induced by administration of a gonadotropin-releasing hormone agonist (GnRHa) to raise turnover markers and therefore assess drug effects on markers (normally to screen for inhibitors of bone resorption). GnRHa can be discontinued to allow animals to resume normal sex hormone function and can be readministered as necessary (or appropriate) if further investigations are warranted. These models are particularly useful in establishing the pharmacokinetic/pharmacodynamic profile (PK/PD) in a relatively fast and efficient way. Markers become elevated 4 weeks after administration of GnRHa[6] and measurements of bone densitometry or other end points of interest can be obtained. Bone densitometry can be monitored every 4 weeks in short-term studies, and are routinely measured every 3 months in studies of 6 months duration or longer. It is important to obtain at least one baseline measurement, prior to the start of treatment, for these measures to be optimal. Because the number of animals in each group is usually limited in these early studies, interpretation is largely based on the change during treatment relative to baseline measures, rather than absolute values, and this response is compared with concurrent controls. When interpreted together, the biomarker and densitometry datasets usually provide solid data to assess the effects of treatment, which can be further characterized by histomorphometry evaluations. Histomorphometry evaluations provide information on dynamic parameters such as bone formation rates and mineral apposition rates. This technique is later described in more detail, but briefly requires the injection of a bone-seeking fluorochrome label, such as calcein green or tetracycline, usually on two occasions, several days apart (normally 10 days), prior to bone collection. When bones are processed to slide, exposure to fluorescent light reveals the labels captured on surfaces actively forming new bone. The derived dynamic parameters can be valuable early in compound development to provide mechanistic data which can help differentiate the effects of the compound relative to others in the same or a similar drug class.

Studies of up to 6 months duration are often performed to derive longer-term data on biochemical markers and bone densitometry, and to include important histomorphometry end points. In addition, if the in-life densitometry data show meaningful changes in treated groups relative to controls, then biomechanical testing may be appropriate. As the ultimate test of bone quality, it is important to establish as early as possible if there is a positive effect of treatment on bone biomechanical competency, or at least to verify that there is no adverse effect.

Toxicology studies performed during drug development provide an opportunity to include biomarkers and bone densitometry end points in addition to the standard toxicology end points (if appropriate for the drug class). Since dose levels are usually set higher than typically used in POC or efficacy/pharmacology studies, these studies provide a unique setting to study the potential consequences of high dose levels on bone and other organ systems, and to integrate and discriminate the effects of exaggerated pharmacology in relation to toxicologically relevant findings. Bone markers and densitometry measurements can easily be included in most toxicology study designs of usually 3 months duration or longer. Provision to obtain additional terminal end points can be added to the study design (usually in the form of blood and bone collection) and evaluations performed if, based on the results of the in-life data, it is considered that they may provide information of value to the product safety profile for regulatory submission. Table 12.2 can be used as a guideline for inclusion of appropriate tests in toxicology studies.

12.4 Long-Term Bone Safety Models

Long-term studies to provide bone safety data following exposure to a test material are required as part of the submission filing to regulatory authorities. The most important end point in these studies is the effect of treatment on biomechanical competency. This can only be achieved in a nonhuman species and for many reasons the NHP is the species of choice. The population of animals used is intended to mimic as far as possible the intended human aging population and so studies are normally conducted in older monkeys in a sex hormone–depleted state induced surgically after they are ovariectomized (OVX) or orchidectomized (ORX). Because of inter-animal variation in monkey populations, these studies need to be powered to obtain

Table 12.2 Summary of techniques for the evaluation of bone in toxicology studies

End point	Technique	*In vivo*	*Ex vivo*	Toxicology study			
				Neonatal Juvenile	Sub-chronic	Chronic	Carcinogenicity
Bone development	Clinical observations	√	–	√			
	Gait, crown-rump	√	–	√			
	Height	√	–	√			
	Body weight	√	–	√			
	Radiography	√	√	√			
Bone size/geometry	Radiography	√	√	√	√	√	√
	pQCT	√	√	√	√	√	
Bone density	DEXA	√	√	√	√	√	√
	pQCT	√	√	√	√	√	
Bone turnover	Biochemical markers	√	–	√	√	√	
	Histomorphometry	–	√			√	
Bone architecture	µCT	√	√	√		√	
	Histomorphometry	–	√	√		√	
Bone strength	Biomechanics	–	√			√	

definitive data on the biomechanics end point (the least precise end point). In order to fulfill this requirement, 15–20 monkeys per group are typically used. A standard study design includes OVX (or ORX) animals randomized to a vehicle control group and compound-treated groups. Based on current regulatory guidelines,[7-9] most often the study design includes three compound-treated groups: an optimal efficacious dose level, five times the optimal dose level, and a suboptimal dose level. Normally an intact, sham-operated control group is also included, bringing the total population to 75–100 animals on study. The duration of these studies is at least 16 months, considered the equivalent of 4 human years of exposure to test material. Depending on the class of compound (anti-catabolic or anabolic), treatment is initiated the day following surgery (an osteoporosis prevention study), or the study design may include a bone depletion period where an osteopenia is allowed to develop before the start of compound dosing (an osteoporosis intervention study). In an intervention study design, animals start dosing with compound 6–9 months following surgery.

The primary end points in the long-term bone safety studies are to assess bone mass using bone densitometry techniques, bone dynamics and architecture using histomorphometry, and bone strength by biomechanical testing. Secondary end points in these studies are the biochemical markers of bone turnover. In-life measurements of biomarkers and densitometry are obtained at baseline, prior to any surgical interventions or treatment with test material. At least duplicate measures are obtained over a 3–6-month pre-study period to ensure animals are stable with respect to bone and health parameters. During the treatment period the same measurements are obtained at generally 3–4-month intervals, ensuring final in-life data collection as close to the time of scheduled euthanasia as is feasible. Dual injection with a bone-seeking fluorochrome label is performed prior to euthanasia and bone harvesting in preparation for histomorphometry dynamic measurements. Bones are harvested at necropsy and retained for histomorphometry and biomechanical testing with additional specimens retained as backup samples for as yet undetermined additional tests. It is best to retain several long bones from the appendicular skeleton (tibiae, femurs, radii, humeri) and vertebrae from the axial skeleton (thoracic and lumbar spine vertebrae), even though initially there may be no plans to use them. Tips for specimen retention are discussed later in the chapter.

12.5 Regulatory Requirements

The regulatory authorities offer guidance for the preclinical and clinical testing of compounds intended to prevent or treat postmenopausal osteoporosis in women,[7-9] and these are also applied in principle to androgen deficiency–induced osteoporosis in men. These studies, as well as the short-term POC and screening studies, are considered pharmacology studies and as such are not subject to regulation by the Good Laboratory Practices (GLP). However, inclusion of bone end points into toxicology studies that are performed to GLP standards should also be GLP-compliant. The reader is referred to the appropriate governing body (e.g., the Federal Register of the United States Food and Drug Administration [FDA] [www.fda.gov]) for complete information on the GLP regulations that govern nonclinical toxicology studies.

12.6 Study Design Considerations

Protocols specifying use of NHPs are required to conform to the requirements of the country's governing laws and to be approved by the appropriate Animal Care and Use Authorities in the institution where experiments are to be performed. Study design and the ethical use of NHPs should be consistent, as far as possible, with the principles of initiatives such as the FDA's Critical Path Initiative and the National Toxicology Program's (NTP) plan to reduce, refine, and replace animal use. We are incumbent to exploit these animal models within well-defined and controlled boundaries to obtain as much information as is feasible that can be translated directly to clinical safety assessments and that provide information that is impossible or difficult to obtain ethically in man. The methodologies and techniques described in subsequent sections of this chapter are the same as those used in the clinic wherever possible, often with additional components that can be included because of the controlled laboratory conditions under which animal studies are performed.

12.7 Animal Selection

The objectives of the study should be clearly defined and the appropriate monkeys selected. They can be young or old, male and/or female. Neonatal and juvenile (around 12 months of age) monkeys are used specifically to assess the effects of treatment on skeletal development. This is of course of fundamental importance if the compound is intended for use in childhood diseases of bone; however, most compounds are intended for an aging population to treat or prevent osteoporosis, where the consequences of their use on skeletal development are part of the toxicology safety testing requirements for a new drug application (NDA). For most short-term POC or screening studies, young adult monkeys, male or female, are used generally in the age range of 2–6 years, with some attempt to keep the age range within a study as consistent as possible. Studies with compounds that target the hypothalamic–pituitary–gonadal axis may require sexually mature animals: 3–5-year-old females, 5–7-year-old males. For studies of 3–6 months duration with bone densitometry measurements, skeletally mature monkeys of 6 years or older are recommended in order to minimize age-related changes during the study. For the long-term bone safety studies of 16 months duration or longer, skeletally mature monkeys which have also attained peak bone mass are required. For cynomolgus monkeys peak bone mass is reported to occur around 9 years of age[10] and around 12 years of age in rhesus monkeys.[11]

Any test facility that does not breed NHPs will need to purchase animals for use. The monkey supplier should be carefully selected and approved in collaboration with the institutional veterinary staff to ensure there are appropriate breeding, housing, and testing procedures in place to assure the monkeys are maintained in a healthy environment. Where monkeys are captured for use, appropriate procedures for control of disease and age estimation should be in place. As an endangered species, NHP export and import is tightly regulated and Convention on International Trade in Endangered Species (CITES) permits are required for country-to-country shipping of animals or tissues (including slides). Violation of these procedures can lead to hefty fines and delays in receipt of animals or materials. NHPs used in pharmaceutical research most often originate from Mauritius Island and China for export to North America or Europe. The Philippines and Indonesia are less common areas for export. All monkeys are rigorously tested for known disease status and imported only if they meet all requirements and are healthy at the time of shipping. Particular emphasis is placed on use of monkeys that are Herpes B virus–negative which is relatively easy to do for young monkeys that have yet to seroconvert. However, for monkeys 6 years or older only Mauritius has maintained a closed colony of B-negative monkeys and is therefore the source of choice for studies using older animals. Housing and maintenance of NHPs is safe as long as all appropriate procedures are respected and followed.

In addition to the health requirements outlined above, for older monkeys used in the long-term studies (6–16 months), there are several other factors and requirements that are considered (Table 12.3). Because of the long-term commitment of these monkeys to these studies, up to 3 years if a bone depletion period is

Table 12.3 Selection criteria for older females for osteoporosis bone quality studies

Requirement	Specifics
X-ray films	• Ventro–dorsal of lumbar–thoracic spine • Lateral lumbar–thoracic spine • Ventro–dorsal of pelvis and femurs • Lateral of tibia (both tibias on the same film, but two different exposures) • Dorso–ventral of radius (both radii on the same film, but two different exposures)
Animal individual requirements	• Genus/species: *Macaca fascicularis* (cynomolgus macaque) • Sex: female • Feral; healthy; research naive • Each animal submitted for selection must have been exclusively housed in the facilities for the last 3 years (preferably 5 years) • Last offspring as close as possible to 2 years earlier (optimal) • Fed with a known and balanced diet for at least 3 years (preferably 5 years) • Older than 9 years at the time of delivery based on approximate age at capture and number of years since captured • Primiparous or multiparous animals • Not pregnant • No nourishing–rearing activity for at least 6 months prior to delivery • Complete and accurate breeding records • Complete and accurate medical records • Clearly visible permanent identification • Weigh within 14 days of shipment • No evidence of internal or external parasites • No congenital, hereditary, or traumatic defects • No history of chronic treatment with tetracycline since in captivity • No history of fracture (single minor, well-healed fracture might be acceptable) • Minor or no skeletal defects such as scoliosis, kyphosis, spondylitis, etc. • Minor or no evidence of degenerative joint disease • No stiffness of joints (all flexible joints should have normal movement)

included in the study design, animals are screened rigorously for any signs of physical or clinical health issues based on review of veterinary and reproductive history records, including body weights. These records are reviewed to identify animals that are "poor doers" and that may be susceptible to recurrent conditions such as chronic diarrhea and wide fluctuations in body weight. Medications used to treat these conditions are reviewed for the drug class and the period of use. For instance, the extensive and repeated use of tetracycline to control diarrhea may preclude selection because of the chance of recurrent infections, but also because tetracycline is also used as a fluorescent bone label and background labeling may interfere with the ability to perform histomorphometry measurements. Reproductive records are reviewed to determine how many pregnancies and live births female monkeys have undergone, the timing of the last birth, and weaning of the infant relative to the time of shipment. Ideally, monkeys are selected that are reproductively viable, and weaning of the last infant occurred within at least 6 months prior to their assignment to a study. Hormone analyses for estradiol (with values $\geq$20 pg/ml) and/or luteinizing hormone (LH)/follicle-stimulating hormone (FSH) can be useful to provide additional evidence that females are still reproductively viable even though menses may be less frequent. Menopaused females are not considered optimal for osteoporosis research since most study designs include intact sham-operated controls, which are used for comparison with OVX animals. For male monkey studies, veterinary examination and testes palpation are often most informative although hormone levels including testosterone and LH/FSH can be evaluated. Blood samples obtained for hormone analysis are also used to verify hematology and biochemistry parameters, particularly enzymes related to major organ function such as the liver and kidney, and blood glucose and lipid levels for any indication of diabetes.

Finally, and of paramount importance, because these monkeys are being screened for bone quality assessments, they must have a good skeleton, with few abnormalities and usually no preexisting fractures of long bones or vertebrae. Before selection for a study, radiographs are obtained at the supplier to assess the spine, hip, and long bones. All abnormalities are documented and the stage of growth plate closure recorded, along with all of the other information collected, and each animal is then either selected or rejected for shipment. Although this sounds black and white, in reality it is not and often requires a team of scientists and veterinary staff to review all of the available data and agree on the selected population. Because it is virtually impossible to select the number of animals needed for these studies (100-plus depending on study design), all with a perfect skeleton and free of age-related common diseases such as osteoarthritis or spondylosis, some compromises usually have to be made. There are many instances where animals are accepted with skeletal abnormalities that are judged not to interfere with their use on a study. Examples include the presence of osteoarthritis in one knee joint but not in the contralateral joint, which would be used for evaluations. Or there may be some vertebral abnormality in the caudal spine that would not interfere with data acquisition in the lumbar or thoracic spine. Animals with obvious old fractures are normally not considered, but when trying to complete numbers for a batch of animals they may be accepted as long as normal limb use is apparent and there are no obvious sequelae resulting from the event. Hind limbs should be fully extendable to facilitate positioning for scanning procedures. The severity of any skeletal and/or articular lesions should be carefully assessed for the animal selection. The physical examination by veterinary staff as part of the selection process is very important as not all information may get into the animal records and on examination some animals may be deemed unfit for selection or to travel. Monkeys may also be excluded based on aggressive behavior, obesity, and age, that is, too young or too old based on the age range of other animals in the population. For an aging population of monkeys, adapted to a stable environment surrounded by their "family," the transportation to another country, quarantine procedures, and finally transportation to the laboratory performing the study is stressful and may be debilitating for some animals. This is usually the time when subclinical disease will manifest itself and a parasitic or other infection may flare. A small number of additional animals are normally included in a shipment to cover for any potential losses prior to the start of treatment. Monkeys are robust animals, however, and most if not all animals recover and get back to normal social behavior once they are in a stable environment again.

12.8 Husbandry Procedures

Maintaining a stable population of physically and emotionally healthy monkeys for up to 3 years in some studies is challenging. The environment must be low stress to allow normal grooming activities and feeding to occur unheeded. Caging units built to socially house a number of monkeys together, fitted with perches, need to be carefully monitored when initially set up to ensure the hierarchy within the unit is established and allows normal grooming activities and feeding. Training staff on the rudiments of primate behavior is important in order to identify subtle signs of distress that may result from inappropriate submissive behavior or to identify changes in behavior such as depression that may result following surgical procedures. In addition to behavioral observations, monitoring body weight is an important indicator of potential problems resulting from inappropriate housing and is usually a prompt to investigate the potential reason for the change. Young monkeys adapt to social housing conditions almost without incident but older animals often need more time to accommodate and a few trials may need to be performed before optimal social conditions are established. In rooms housing multiple caging units the hierarchy within the room is seldom problematic, but occasionally units may need to be redistributed if the behavior of submissive animals is affected by the threatening behavior of a monkey across the room. Moving submissive and sensitive animals to the ends of the room, particularly away from the entrance, may prove helpful.

Although grooming is considered the most important animal enrichment activity, several other aspects of a well-designed enrichment program should be included. Human contact is important and staff working with a population of monkeys should be encouraged to bond and interact in a stimulating and positive manner. This can be aided by offering small treats such as fresh fruit or vegetables on a daily basis. The addition of uncertified dietary components such as fresh or dry fruits and vegetables should certainly be included but discretionary amounts only should be provided that will not interfere with consumption of certified laboratory chow or treats (such as Primatreats). It is important not to overfeed older monkeys to avoid excessive weight gain (it is recommended to provide fewer cookies than for young adult monkeys), and to avoid complications such as bloating. The same staff should be assigned to care for a study throughout, wherever practical and feasible. Other enrichment activities include the use of toys, foraging tools, mirrors, music, a water bucket (pool), and occasionally TV/videos. Monkeys particularly enjoy watching cartoons and nature programs – but these do need to be carefully vetted since they can become agitated if snakes appear.

Animals should also have access to diet adequately supplemented in calcium, phosphorus, and vitamin D. Recently, some NHP diets have been commercialized to minimize the presence of phytoestrogens, such as the 2056 Soy Protein-Free Primate Diet excluding alfalfa and soybean meals. Controlling phytoestrogen content in the diet is probably an important component of long-term OVX studies in NHP as use of a standard diet may attenuate the OVX response in aged monkeys.[12]

12.9 Randomization Procedures

Assignment of animals to short-term studies usually follows established procedures within the laboratory and is typically based on stratification by body weight. However, assignment of groups to long-term studies, and occasionally short-term studies where bone densitometry measurements are included, may be beneficial based on bone mass. In order to factor both bone mass and body weight, randomization is based on stratification using whole-body bone mineral content (BMC) derived from dual energy x-ray absorptiometry (DEXA) scanning (see following section). Where monkeys are socially housed in pairs, assignment is based on the average whole-body BMC for the two animals in each unit. The average BMC values are ranked from smallest to largest. Random numbers are generated for the number of groups and this is repeated until the number of animals to be assigned to each group has been achieved. For example, for a study with five treatment groups or arms, random numbers will be generated from 1 to 5 and the first five average BMC values will be assigned to the random group number. This process is repeated until all animals have been assigned to groups in equal numbers. Statistical analyses are then performed using the individual animal data to ensure that all groups are homogeneous with respect to whole body BMC. Other key parameters are analyzed to ensure homogeneity across groups, including body weight, age, and lumbar spine bone mineral density (BMD). Any imbalance in the distribution of animals can then be adjusted for prior to the start of surgery and dose administration; however, once social housing is established animals are not normally moved from their home cage.

For large studies, it is practical to perform surgery and start treatment in a staggered or replicated way. This allows completion of activities within a manageable time frame relative to the start of dose administration. For example, a study occupying three rooms with 30 animals in each room (with study arms equally represented in each room) will have surgery and the start of treatment on 3 consecutive weeks with all activities completed for each room within the designated week. This same order for activities is then applied to follow-up measurements such as sample collection for markers and bone densitometry measurements and scheduled necropsy.

12.10 Surgical Procedures

12.10.1 Ovariectomy

Surgery and anesthesia of older animals can be very challenging. Particular care in the selection of the method of anesthesia (including preanesthetic) and analgesia is needed (see Table 12.4 for guidance). It is important to ensure monitoring of vital signs and body temperature, and to provide fluid therapy during surgical procedures. Animal recovery after surgery should be closely monitored by trained veterinary staff for signs of pain, hemorrhage, or the return to a normal feeding regime to avoid bloating. The home room temperature should also be elevated a couple of degrees for a few days during recovery from surgery procedures.

The OVX NHP model of postmenopausal osteoporosis is often selected in osteoporosis drug research and has been used for many years.[13-22] The model is established by the surgical removal of both ovaries. Sham control animals can be included depending on the study design. These sham animals undergo the same surgical procedure as OVX animals but the ovaries are not cut and removed, they are examined and replaced in situ. These procedures sound straightforward but often there are complications. Adhesions between the ovaries and the uterus and/or with surrounding abdominal tissue are not uncommon in female monkeys that have had several pregnancies. These adhesions complicate the surgery and may interfere with the complete removal of ovaries. It is important to retain ovaries that are removed in order to examine them macroscopically and potentially perform histological evaluation if functional status is in question. Ovarian atrophy may indicate a menopausal or perimenopausal status of the animal, and will not be useful in these studies. Older females often have considerable body fat making location of the ovaries and their complete removal difficult. Excessive abdominal fat can also enhance wound infection. It is essential under these conditions to remove as much surrounding tissue as possible to ensure all ovarian tissue is removed. In some instances it is concluded that complete removal

Table 12.4 Formulations generally used during the conduct of an NHP osteoporosis study

Study component	Formulation used
Surgery and scanning procedures	Pre-anesthesia with glycopyrrolate (0.01 mg/kg), ketamine HCl injection, USP (10 mg/kg), and xylazine (0.6 mg/kg) and anesthesia maintained with isoflurane gas
Urine collection for bone markers	Sedated with glycopyrrolate (0.01 mg/kg), ketamine HCl injection, USP (10 mg/kg), and xylazine (0.6 mg/kg)
Surgery	Analgesic treatment (buprenorphine at 0.01 mg/kg – intramuscularly) before surgery, 8–12 h following surgery, and 24 h post surgery, then as deemed necessary. Carprofen 4 mg/kg subcutaneously on the day of surgery
Fluorochrome labeling	*Bicarbonate buffered calcein green solution*: 0.8% of calcein and 0.75% of sodium bicarbonate in 0.9% sodium chloride for injection USP *Tetracycline hydrochloride solution*: 0.25% tetracycline hydrochloride, 0.625% ascorbic acid and 5% sterile water for irrigation USP in 0.9% sodium chloride for injection USP *Alizarin complexone solution*: 2.5% of alizarin complexone and 1.4% of sodium bicarbonate in 0.9% sodium chloride for injection USP *Bicarbonate buffered xylenol orange solution*: Sodium bicarbonate 3%, 0.9% sodium chloride for injection USP, xylenol orange in 0.9% sodium chloride for injection USP

of ovarian tissue will compromise the animal health. An example is when removal of the ovaries may damage the uterus, a tissue that will bleed excessively if cut. In these instances, as long as the ovaries are intact and considered functional based on all of the available data, the animal can be reassigned to the sham control group and switched with a corresponding animal from the sham group of similar whole-body BMC, body weight, and lumbar spine BMD. The consequences of an incomplete ovariectomy may not be recognized until well into the study when it may be too late to correct the situation by additional surgery. Careful monitoring for signs of incomplete ovary removal, or the possibility that ectopic ovarian tissue may lie elsewhere (usually embedded in the uterine wall), is critical and is accomplished by a combination of several components. Physical observations of menses are looked for throughout the study, from animal arrival to euthanasia, and are recorded daily. It is normal to observe menses up to 6 weeks post surgery in a few animals, but signs after that period usually signal a problem. Supporting information is derived by measuring estradiol levels. If levels are basal on one occasion, a second measurement should be made 2 weeks later. Other parameters, such as bone marker data may also be available to help in the determination of whether the ovariectomy procedure appears to be complete or if further surgical intervention is required. Because of all of the issues discussed above associated with ovariectomy procedures, abdominal incision and the complete isolation and removal of the ovaries are necessary. The use of other less invasive techniques such as keyhole surgery results in a poor success rate due to incomplete ovariectomy resulting in unacceptable loss of study data. Open abdominal surgery also provides an opportunity to examine other organs and tissues, especially the state of the uterus, and any remarkable findings should be recorded and kept as part of the study data in case it may have an impact on later findings. Internal examinations often reveal the presence of parasitic infection, which may be dormant/no longer viable, or may indicate that medical treatment is warranted.

The incomplete removal of ovarian tissue may not manifest itself in signs of menses or quantifiable estradiol levels until late into the study when sufficient tissue from remaining follicular cells have formed a sufficient body of tissue to produce quantifiable estradiol levels and influence the appearance of menses. In this case it is often too late in the study to perform further surgical interventions and data from animals affected in this way are excluded from the study. Normally such animals continue till their schedule termination date for two reasons: (1) to maintain the social dynamics of the housing unit, and (2) for confirmation of an incomplete ovariectomy at necropsy. Gross pathology observations, organ weight data, and histopathological evaluations are used to confirm the presence/absence of functional ovarian tissue by the state of atrophy of the uterus and vagina, and by the presence/absence of corpora lutea. Pathological observations are pivotal in the final selection of animals to be included in the interpretation of the study data and further derivation of histomorphometry and biomechanics data. Histopathological evaluation of the uterus or vagina may be warranted to characterize any pathological condition that may explain why increased uterine/vaginal weights are observed. This may result in further exclusion of animals from the study data, or the findings may show that the (bone) study data will be acceptable for inclusion in data interpretation.

12.10.2 Orchidectomy

Orchidectomy procedures are less problematic than ovariectomy procedures and do not normally result in removal of animals from the study or reassignment to other groups. The only consequence of these surgeries appears to be a higher incidence of animals with abdominal hernia, which can often be easily repaired. A small median incision is made through the skin at the base of the scrotum, and each testis with the epididymis is removed after incision of each *tunica vaginalis*. For sham controls, a small median incision is made through the skin at the base of the scrotum. The scrotum skin incision is closed using a subcuticular suture. The testes with epididymides can be retained in formalin for possible future confirmation of surgical procedures.

12.11 Bone Biopsy Procedures

Biopsies of the iliac crest and/or rib are performed in long-term osteoporosis studies during the *in vivo* phase of the study to provide histomorphometry data. Biopsy of the iliac crest mimics similar collection procedures performed in human clinical trials. Optimally, biopsy procedures are performed around 6 months following the start of compound administration, which is also around 6 months post ovariectomy/orchidectomy in a prevention study design. The response to ovariectomy or orchidectomy is considered maximal at this time point with respect to bone turnover parameters, making it optimal to study the effects of treatment on bone dynamic histomorphometry parameters. Sampling is performed at the iliac crest to examine cancellous bone effects and at the rib to study cortical bone effects, following injection with a bone-seeking label such as tetracycline, calcein green, xylenol orange, or alizarin complexone. A different bone label is used when there are multiple time points in the study in order to differentiate them. For example, dual tetracycline labeling may be used to label bones collected during a 6-month bone biopsy procedure, and dual calcein green bone labeling may be used prior to bone harvesting at necropsy at the end of a 16-month treatment period. In an intervention study design, biopsy procedures can be included at the end of the bone depletion period, and again 6 months following the start of compound administration.

Bone biopsy procedures are difficult and time-consuming to perform. Often the size of the iliac crest specimen is small and contains little cancellous bone for evaluation. The rib does usually yield meaningful data on cortical bone but specimen acquisition requires a skillful surgeon practiced in resuscitation techniques should a pneumothorax develop as a complication. However, if an early readout on compound efficacy is required at a time point when the response to ovariectomy/orchidectomy is maximal, then the resulting data can be valuable. These data also provide an opportunity to study the effects of treatment on histomorphometry parameters over time if equivalent sites are retained and evaluated at the end of the treatment period. Observations can also be made on the bone-healing process following the initial biopsy sampling. Also, the dynamic histomorphometry parameters characterizing the state of bone turnover often show some waning, or decline, at the end of a 16-month period following ovariectomy/orchidectomy, making it difficult to obtain statistically significant differences between sham and OVX/ORX controls, and therefore the interpretation of the compound-treated groups equivocal.

12.12 Compound Administration

Compound administration often presents some challenges in a group-housed situation, especially if performed daily. This has resulted in some creative solutions, some of which are mentioned here. Oral dose administration can be performed traditionally by physically removing the monkey from the caging unit and intubating to deliver a measured and precise dose. Restraining chairs or the use of a pole and collar can be used to make the handling of larger NHPs more manageable. Similarly, animals can be removed and held in position for subcutaneous or intravenous bolus dosing; slings can be used for intravenous administrations up to 1 h. Periods of infusion longer than this require catheterization and permanent catheter implantation. Novel approaches to some of these routes of administration have been successful including cage-side voluntary oral dosing where monkeys are trained to come to the front of the cage to receive their dose. Training is usually achieved by initially offering a fruit-flavored drink in a syringe. The compound is subsequently formulated in the same vehicle and so compound administration becomes voluntary and an enrichment activity rather than a stressful event. Complications do arise when the compound is unpalatable, so this should be tested beforehand as well as ensuring compound formulation is unaffected. Also, some monkeys refuse to be trained or drink at a very slow pace, although these instances are rare. Cage-side oral dosing can be an extremely efficient and rewarding activity and well worth the effort of training and setup for these long-term studies. For subcutaneous or intravenous bolus administration, in some laboratories, animals have also been trained to present themselves cage-side for dosing.

12.13 Methodology to Determine End Points of Interest

Unless indicated otherwise, the methodology described in this section is suitable for all monkey models although the results refer primarily to the OVX monkey model for which most of these data have been generated and reported.

12.13.1 Assays

Evaluation of bone turnover and reproductive hormonal status can be performed throughout the course of the study (from baseline to the terminal occasion with several intermediate time points every 1 or 3 months depending on the study duration). Serum and urinary biochemical markers of bone formation and resorption provide near real-time information about bone cell activity at the whole skeletal level. Immunoassays are generally easy to perform and most of the human kits used for clinical trials generally cross-react with NHP matrices, allowing bridging of data between preclinical and clinical studies. Restrictions in the amount of blood (and urine) that can be collected from NHPs during the *in vivo* phase of the study are generally less of an issue than in lower species.

12.13.1.1 Biochemical Markers of Bone Turnover

Due to the specific bone physiology (the coupling of bone formation and resorption), it is recommended to evaluate a panel of bone markers. Typically two markers of bone formation and two markers of bone resorption (depending on the class of compound to be evaluated) are selected from commonly used markers, including the bone formation markers: bone-specific alkaline phosphatase (ALP), osteocalcin, and procollagen type I propeptide (PINP); and the bone resorption markers: C-telopeptide, N-telopeptide, TRAP-5b, and deoxypyridinoline (see Table 12.5). For the urinary markers, urinary creatinine should also be determined on the same sample to calculate the bone marker ratio for each individual. The inherent variability of bone markers should be acknowledged. The analytical

Table 12.5 Commercial biomarker assays of bone formation and resorption in serum or urine, and selected hormones

Biomarker	Assay kit	Matrix
Bone-specific alkaline phosphatase	Metra™ BAP EIA Kit, Quidel Corporation	Serum
Osteocalcin	Metra™ Osteocalcin EIA Kit, Quidel Corporation	Serum
Procollagen type-I N-Terminal Propeptide	UniQ PINP RIA kit, Orion Diagnostica	Serum
C-Telopeptides	CrossLaps TM ELISA, ImmunoDiagnostics Systems Limited (IDS Ltd.)	Serum
	Urine CrossLaps TM ELISA, IDS Ltd	Urine
N-Telopeptides	Osteomark® NTx Test ELISA kit, Wampole Laboratories®	Serum
	Osteomark® NTx Urine ELISA Kit, Wampole Laboratories®	Urine
Free deoxypyridinoline	DPD RIA kit, IDS Ltd	Urine
Hormones		
1,25-Dihydroxyvitamin D	Gamma 1,25 Dihydroxy Vitamin-D RIA kit, IDS Ltd	Serum
Parathyroid hormone	Human PTH ELISA Kit, Immutopics, Inc	
Estradiol	Ultra-Sensitive Estradiol RIA, Diagnostics Systems Laboratories Inc	Serum
Luteinizing hormone	Reagents: Recombinant Cynomolgus monkey LH antigen, Recombinant Cynomolgus Monkey LH reference preparation, and Rabbit anti-recombinant Cynomolgus monkey LH antiserum. Harbor-UCLA Medical Center (Torrance, CA)	Serum
Follicle-stimulating hormone	Reagents: Recombinant Cynomolgus monkey FSH antigen, Recombinant Cynomolgus Monkey FSH reference preparation, and Rabbit anti-recombinant Cynomolgus monkey FSH antiserum. Harbor-UCLA Medical Center (Torrance, CA)	Serum

ELISA enzyme-linked immunosorbent assay, *EIA* enzyme immunoassay, *RIA* radioimmunoassay
Alternate suppliers now required (since kits from these manufacturers are no longer available)

variability depends on the marker and the measurement method. The preanalytical variability has a strong effect on the bone markers levels, which in a laboratory environment includes the circadian variation, menses status, fasting, and intercurrent diseases (especially in older animals). The collection of blood should be performed under standardized conditions, preferably in the fasting state in the morning, and samples placed immediately on ice until processed to serum. For urine collection, the choice between a spot sampling and an overnight collection in metabolic cages should be dictated by the biological interest and the practical feasibility. Collection of a sample over several hours reflects the overall bone metabolism; however, a spot sample collected directly from the bladder (under anesthesia) is performed in a more controlled way and is generally preferred.

In general, markers of bone turnover maximally increase between two- and threefold relative to baseline levels or concurrent sham controls following OVX. The time course of the response shows a rise in formation and resorption markers that peaks 6–12 months post ovariectomy, after which the response generally shows evidence of waning.[22] Increases in biochemical markers of bone turnover are consistent with histomorphometric indices of bone turnover. Depending of the class of compound tested, different patterns of response can be expected, from an overall increase in markers to an uncoupling of the response in formation and resorption markers. Anticatabolic agents like bisphosphonates rapidly decrease bone marker levels compared to OVX controls.[4,13,16] Receptor activator of NF-κB ligand (RANKL) blockade using osteoprotegerin (OPG)-Fc showed similar effects to decrease bone markers in young intact monkeys.[5] In contrast, during bone formation–stimulating treatment, human parathyroid hormone (PTH) (1–84) induced a rapid increase in bone formation markers followed by an increase in bone resorption markers.[23]

12.13.1.2 Hormones

Additional parameters such as reproductive hormones, estradiol (or testosterone for the ORX model), LH/FSH, and/or hormones related to calcium metabolism such as PTH and 1,25-dihydroxyvitamin D, are also important parameters to characterize the ovariectomy response and the effect of treatment, depending on the pharmacology of the tested compound.

12.13.2 Bone Densitometry

BMD is evaluated *in vivo* using DEXA and/or peripheral quantitative computed tomography (pQCT). DEXA and pQCT are generally used together as they provide complementary information on the skeleton. DEXA provides a two-dimensional (2D) apparent bone density measurement while pQCT provides a volumetric bone density measurement. DEXA scanning permits evaluations of the entire body and large areas of the skeleton, whereas pQCT scans provide information from a single (or multiple) slice(s) of bone at specific skeletal areas, normally the proximal tibia and distal radius. pQCT scans allow separate evaluations of the trabecular and cortical bone compartments as well as information on bone geometry. From a practical point of view, animals are required to be anesthetized for scanning. Where possible both DEXA and pQCT scans can be performed during the same anesthesia occasion in order to limit the number of anesthesia occasions for each animal. However, it can take 1–1.5 h to scan several sites with both techniques. Again, particular care should be taken during long periods of anesthesia for older animals, their body temperature should be maintained, and the duration should never exceed 2 h on any occasion. Scans are generally acquired every 1, 3, or 6 months depending on the length of the study. Baseline data are acquired before surgery, once animals are well accustomed to the laboratory environment, to calculate individual changes over the course of the study. Individual percent changes provide more powerful data (versus absolute values at each occasion) because of the individual animal variability and the small number of animals used in some study types (e.g., toxicology studies).

Researchers need to ensure that scans are consistently and precisely performed using standardized reproducible procedures over long study periods. Instrument precision should be checked on a regular basis. As a result of using rigorous control procedures, instrument and operator precision attainable at typical scan sites for primates frequently exceed similar data obtained in a clinical setting.

12.13.2.1 Dual Energy X-Ray Absorptiometry

BMD is monitored *in vivo* using DEXA bone scanners at clinically relevant sites, that is, spine, hip, and radius. Other sites are usually scanned in order to provide supportive data. Generally, it includes scanning of the lumbar and thoracic spine, proximal femur (hip), distal femur, distal radius, proximal tibia, and a whole-body scan. The use of different sites adds perspective to data generated; similar effects observed at a comparable bone site (i.e., mainly trabecular, cortical, or mixed site) add confidence to the data compared to results from a single site. Different clinical DEXA scanners can be used to scan monkeys: DEXA DPX, GE Lunar Corp., Madison, WI, or Hologic QDR 2000 or Discovery A densitometers, Bedford, MA.

Today, DEXA is still the "gold standard" for measuring BMD clinically in humans; therefore it is important to perform *in vivo* DEXA scanning to parallel clinical trial data in nonclinical studies. There are widely acknowledged limitations and disadvantages with DEXA: 2D projection when bones are three-dimensional (3D), constraining precision for positioning over time, relatively poor image quality, no evaluation of structural properties, effects of body composition.[20,24] Standard procedures for each scan position should be established to ensure optimal precision at each site. Precision measured as a percentage coefficient of variation (CV%) should be less than 1% at the spine and approximately 3–4% at the proximal femur. Analyses of important subregions of interest at the femoral neck and greater trochanter have lower precision but are useful because of their important clinical relevance. Use of the default software analyses is recommended wherever possible since manual mapping tends to decrease the precision of the measurements. DEXA scan and analysis settings for standard sites are included in Table 12.6.

The response to ovariectomy as measured by DEXA shows decreases in areal BMD (aBMD) at the lumbar spine and the hip as early as 3–4 months post ovariectomy,[22] with a slowing of bone loss around 8–9 months post ovariectomy, when a new steady state of bone turnover is established.[15,22] Therefore, a 9-month bone depletion period is recommended for an intervention study. At 12–16 months post ovariectomy, some increase in aBMD has been observed, especially at the spine and the proximal femur[2,22] and is reported to occur in other species,[1] an effect that may be related to a dietary source of phytoestrogens, the extragonadal synthesis of estrogens,[1] or the influence of changes in body composition (fat), often associated with increased weight gains following ovariectomy.[20]

12.13.2.2 Peripheral Quantitative Computed Tomography

pQCT (XCT Research SA, Stratec Medizintechnik, Pforzheim, Germany) is an important technology used in NHP models[25,26] to provide bone densitometry data, complementary to DXA, and important geometrical information on bone size. pQCT is not influenced by changes in body composition as is DEXA.[20,24] Scanning is limited to slices at a specific region of interest, usually at the proximal tibia and distal radius metaphysis and diaphysis sites, but the special analysis software allows the separation of the trabecular and cortical bone regions, providing total slice, trabecular, cortical/subcortical measurements of area, volumetric BMC (vBMC) and volumetric BMD (vBMD), as well as geometric parameters typically measured at the diaphysis site, such as periosteal circumference, endosteal circumference, and cortical thickness. Standardized positioning and definition of the appropriate landmarks are important to obtain reproducible data at representative slices at the metaphysis and diaphysis. The position of the CT slices relative to a reference line is set as a defined distance or a percentage of the bone length. One or several slices can be acquired at the metaphysis site with usually one slice at the diaphysis. Three consecutive slices are generally obtained at the metaphysis of aged animals to obtain a good representation of the

Table 12.6 Standard DEXA[a] scan sites, type, and analysis modes using Hologic Discovery A in NHP osteoporosis studies

Scan site	Scan type	Scan mode	Analysis method	Reporting
Whole body	Infant whole body	Array	Infant whole body	Global BMC and Global BMD
Lumbar spine	AP lumbar spine	Array	Lumbar spine	Total L1-L4 BMD
Right prox. femur	Right hip	Array	Subregion array hip	BMD for Global, Neck (R1), Trochanter (R2)
Right distal radius	Right forearm	Array	Right forearm	Total, 1/3 and UD BMD

[a]Hologic Discovery A, operated with QDR for Windows XP Version 12.3

Table 12.7 Standard pQCT[a] scan sites[b] and analysis modes in NHP osteoporosis studies

Scan site[c]	Scans settings	Analysis method	Reporting
Metaphysis 10–15% of the bone length	Slice thickness: 1 mm two blocks	CONTMODE and PEELMODE with a threshold or area analysis	Total, trabecular, cortical/subcortical compartments: area, BMC, BMD
Diaphysis 20% of the bone length	Slice thickness: 1 mm two blocks	CORTMODE with a threshold analysis	Total area, cortical BMC, cortical BMD, cortical area, cortical thickness, periosteal circumference and endosteal circumference

[a]Stratec XCT Research *SA* software 5.50D
[b]Distal radius and proximal tibia
[c]Selected based on the animal population and parameters of interest

site, as there is generally less trabecular bone at these sites in older monkeys. Trabecular bone analysis parameters require the setting of specific thresholds, one to define the cortical bone edge and one to separate the trabecular compartment (see Table 12.7 for standard pQCT scan and analysis parameters).

The ability to analyze the trabecular bone compartment increases the sensitivity of *in vivo* monitoring. For example, following ovariectomy, decreases in trabecular vBMD up to 20% can be observed at the proximal tibia relative to intact animals, compared to changes up to 11% at the spine measured by DEXA (aBMD).[22] Maximizing the discrimination between the sham and the OVX groups allows optimal evaluation of any potential treatment effects. Generally, the ovariectomy response is characterized at metaphyseal sites by a decrease in total slice vBMD, primarily related to a decrease in trabecular vBMD and vBMC, associated with an increase in trabecular area (reflecting increased marrow space consistent with endosteal resorption). These changes peak around 12 months after ovariectomy. Cortical thinning is the main effect observed at diaphyseal sites with a decreased cortical area.[22] These changes are similar to the ones described in humans following menopause.[27] Cortical structural changes are usually still ongoing 16 or 18 months after ovariectomy.

12.13.2.3 High-Resolution Microcomputerized Tomographs

The recent development of high-resolution μCT has ushered in a new era of *in vivo* bone research. The XtremeCT (Scanco Medical AG, Brüttisellen, Switzerland) yields highly magnified cross-sectional images of bones in humans and also *in vivo* in NHP that can substitute for invasive surgical biopsies, at least in terms of evaluating bone architecture. Because of the high resolution, it can measure not only the vBMD (cortical and trabecular BMC and BMD), but also structural parameters of trabecular bone (trabecular thickness, trabecular separation, trabecular number, cortical thickness), promising to be a powerful new tool to assess changes in bone micro-architecture, and to provide a greater sensitivity than is possible with conventional scanning procedures to monitor effects of treatments. This technology is still finding its place among the techniques available to study bone.[28,29] These scanners remain expensive and limited in usage as of today but are very promising for usage in NHP.

12.13.2.4 Radiography

The use of standard radiography equipment has already been described as part of the skeletal evaluations for animal selection. However, this relatively low-key technology has important uses in NHP osteoporosis research. High-quality digital radiographs can be obtained of the whole body or regions of interest. It is the method of choice to identify any potential areas of bone lysis or other abnormalities that might warrant further investigation (a useful technique to perform prior to necropsy to ensure retention of any bones with abnormalities), and when obtained at intervals on growing animals, provides an accurate record from which to measure bone growth and assess epiphyseal closure.

12.13.3 Histomorphometry

Ex vivo procedures in animal models offer unique opportunities to evaluate specific parameters that are not possible *in vivo* or in human trials, such as structural and dynamic histomorphometric parameters and biomechanical strength testing. Histomorphometry is widely recognized as an indispensable tool in the study of metabolic bone disease in both clinical trials and experimental animal studies. It brings a unique contribution to the understanding of the effects of therapeutic regimens in animal models of osteoporosis. However, the strict methodology imposed in the preparation of undecalcified bone sections and the high throughput demanded by large regulatory studies are a challenge. The sites typically evaluated include the lumbar vertebral body, femoral neck, tibial shaft, and rib (Table 12.8). Image analysis systems (e.g., Bioquant R&M Biometrics, Nashville, TN, or Image-Pro Plus Media Cybernetics, Bethesda, MD, OsteoMeasure, OsteoMetrics, Inc., Decatur, GA) permit the evaluation of standard and user-defined static and dynamic measurements which should be reported to conform to established criteria.[30] Preparation of high-quality ground and thin sections of plastic-embedded tissue are required for such measurements. Structural and dynamic changes in cortical and cancellous bone can be monitored through the application of computer-assisted histomorphometry, which measures bone matrix, cells, and fluorochrome labels. Several bone-seeking fluorochrome labels, preferably calcein green, tetracycline, xylenol orange, or alizarin complexone, given at fixed intervals prior to tissue collection, are necessary to monitor the mineralizing process from undecalcified sections. Typical dual labeling schedules of 15 and 5 days (10 days apart) prior to bone harvesting for NHP provide good differentiation of label incorporation for measurement of inter-label width in bone remodeling.

Table 12.8 Preferred bone site for histomorphometry in NHP and specific cuts

Bone site	Specific cut
Vertebra L2	Transverse through middle of body
Femur neck	Frontal
Ilium[a]	Caudal to cranial dorsal iliac spine
Rib seventh[a] or ninth	Transverse
Radius mid-diaphysis	Transverse
Tibia mid-diaphysis	Transverse

[a]Suggested sites for biopsy sampling

Rigorous, standardized, and supervised sampling methods, starting with collection and fixation of the tissues and trimming of bones, especially with regard to site and plane of section, are important prerequisites to ensure successful morphometric studies. Bone marrow is exposed to optimize fixation, which is carried out firstly with 10% neutral buffered formalin refrigerated for 3 days, followed by 70% ethanol. In addition to the routine paraffin embedding, several plastic media (MMA, GMA, Araldite) are used to embed tissue specimens for sectioning or grinding. Several histochemical stains are used to differentiate calcified and non-calcified bone segments and identify bone cells: Goldner's trichrome, von Kossa tetrachrome, toluidine blue, Stevenel's blue, and Villanova bone stain. Inter- and intra-observer reliability tests can be done to ensure reproducibility during data collection. Many variables may be measured from long bones and vertebrae at study completion and even from ileum and rib biopsies in NHP; they provide an evaluation of the bone mass, structure, turnover, formation, and resorption (Table 12.9). In animal models of osteoporosis several factors influence bone structure as well as bone formation and resorption indices. These factors include the age of the animals, the interval between gonadectomy and bone sampling, the bone sampled, and the diet. As a consequence, study designs differ and reference ranges are of little value in evaluating study results.

For cancellous bone, changes in structural parameters related to the ovariectomy are generally limited, but cellular activity and turnover changes are more consistent in the response to ovariectomy in cynomolgus[14,15,19] and rhesus monkeys.[23,31] At the femoral neck and lumbar vertebral body, reductions in cancellous bone volume (BV/TV) are usually small. In contrast, bone formation variables like the osteoblast surface (Ob.S/BS), bone formation rate (BFR/BS), and activation frequency (Ac.f) are generally increased at ≥16 months post ovariectomy, indicating a high bone turnover state with increased osteoclast surface (Oc.S/BS).

In cortical bone of the tibia and rib, the ovariectomy response consists of increases in cortical porosity (%Po.Ar) and Haversian labeled surface (H.L.Pm/H.Pm), indicating an acceleration of remodeling activity, associated with increased bone formation rate (H.BFR/BS), which was greater in magnitude in the tibia.[22] Despite these dynamics changes, changes in tibial geometry parameters by ovariectomy are not detected by

Table 12.9 Structural and dynamic histomorphometry variables commonly evaluated for cancellous and cortical bone

Bone compartment	Structural	Dynamic
Cancellous bone	Tissue area (T.Ar)	Mineralizing surface (MS/BS)
	Bone volume (BV/TV)	Single label surface (sLS/BS)
	Osteoid volume (OV/BV)	Double label surface (dLS/BS)
	Osteoid thickness (O.Th)	Mineral apposition rate (MAR)
	Trabecular thickness (Tb.Th)	Adjusted apposition rate (Aj.AR)
	Trabecular number (Tb.N)	Osteoid maturation rate (Omt)
	Trabecular separation (Tb.Sp)	Mineralization lag time (Mlt)
	Osteoblast surface (Ob.S/BS)	BFR, surface referent (BFR/BS)
	Osteoclast surface(Oc.S/BS)	BFR, volume referent (BFR/BV)
	Eroded surface (ES/BS)	Activation frequency (Ac.F)
	Osteoid surface (OS/BS)	Formation period (FP)
	Wall thickness (W.Th)	Resorption period (Rs.P)
Cortical bone	Total tissue area (Tt.T.AR)	Periosteal single label surface (Ps.sL.Pm/Ps.Pm)
	Cortical area (Ct.Ar)	Periosteal double label surface (Ps.dL.Pm/Ps.Pm)
	Medullary area (Me.Ar)	Periosteal labeled surface (Ps.L.Pm/Ps.Pm)
	Cortical area, relative (%Ct.Ar)	Periosteal MAR (Ps.MAR)
	Medullary area, relative (%Me.Ar)	Periosteal BFR, surface referent (Ps.BFR/BS)
	Cortical width (Ct.Wi)	Endocortical single label surface (Ec.sL.Pm/Ec.Pm)
	Periosteal perimeter (Ps.Pm)	Endocortical double label surface (Ec.dL.Pm/Ec.Pm)
	Endocortical perimeter (Ec.Pm)	Endocortical labeled surface (Ec.L.Pm/Ec.Pm)
	Percent porosity area (%Po.Ar)	Endocortical mineral apposition rate (Ec.MAR)
	Haversian wall thickness (H.W.Th)	Endocortical BFR, surface referent (Ec.BFR/BS)
		Haversian single label surface (H.sL.Pm/H.Pm)
		Haversian double label surface (H.dL.Pm/H.Pm)
		Haversian labeled surface (H.L.Pm/H.Pm)
		Haversian mineral apposition rate (H.MAR)
		Haversian BFR, surface referent (H.BFR/BS)
		Haversian BFR, volume referent (H.BFR/BV)

BFR Bone formation rate

histomorphometry techniques. In the rib, reduction of the cortical width associated with an expansion of the medullary area suggests that endocortical bone loss occurred earlier in the non-weight-bearing rib compared to the weight-bearing tibia. At cortical sites, there is no evidence of periosteal bone formation rate in the OVX cynomolgus monkey, a site that is typically quiescent in aged monkeys, and an observation which differs from the human disease.[27]

12.13.4 Biomechanical Strength Testing

Bone strength measurements are the most critical end point in evaluating the effects of drug treatment on the integrity of bone, and are an important index of bone quality. Coupled with *in vivo* and *ex vivo* bone densitometry assessments, bone strength measurements are correlated with bone densitometry parameters to evaluate the important relationship between bone mass and strength. Strength testing is typically performed on a long bone, usually the femur (in three-point bending), at the femoral neck (shear test), and at the lumbar spine (vertebral compression test). Different bones at clinically relevant sites are evaluated (sites with mainly cortical or trabecular bone or both). Specific intrinsic material properties of trabecular and cortical bone are further assessed using vertebral cores extracted from vertebral bodies and cortical beams milled from the shaft of a long bone. Changes in intrinsic properties could indicate a compromise in bone quality.[32]

Acceptable levels of precision should be verified with known materials such as acrylic tubes and/or rods in order to evaluate biological specimens. Bone specimens are prepared with the use of diamond saws, diamond core samplers, and specialized milling equipment. Bone strength is a function of both bone mass and its geometric distribution; therefore, for a complete assessment of bone quality, pQCT and DEXA scans are performed on the prepared specimens prior to biomechanical testing. For each test, the most appropriate fixture is selected according to the size and shape of the bones. On completion of the test, the specimen is examined and observations on the fracture pattern are recorded. This is of particular importance after testing the femoral neck, to ensure the fracture occurred only at the intended site.

12.13.4.1 Three-Point Bending Tests

Three-point bending is routinely performed to determine strength parameters of intact long bones. Specimens require minimal preparation (cleaning) and testing procedures are highly reproducible. The results are sensitive to the geometry of the specimens; however, this can be normalized by using the cross-sectional moment of inertia obtained from the pQCT scans performed at the expected fracture site. Cortical beams milled from long bones (typically from the anterior humerus shaft, 35 mm long × 3 mm wide × 1 mm thick) are tested in three-point bending to assess cortical bone material properties specifically, and can only be performed for large specimens (such as bones from NHPs). Cortical beams have the same size and dimension, and therefore variation due to geometry is excluded.

12.13.4.2 Femoral Neck Shear

The femoral neck is exposed to bending loads *in vivo* and its fracture is one of the leading causes of morbidity in the elderly. Femoral neck shear testing along with DEXA scans provides a sound assessment of bone quality at this site.

12.13.4.3 Compression Tests

Vertebral compression fractures are a main cause of spine deformity in elderly osteoporotic patients. Lumbar vertebrae are routinely used for compression testing. To test the specimens, end plates and spinous processes are removed from the whole vertebra to obtain a specimen with plano parallel ends, and the dorsal elements and transverse processes are trimmed using a diamond saw. The results are influenced by both cortical and trabecular bone quality. In order to investigate trabecular bone strength only, cores can be excised from the vertebral body and tested in compression, which again can only be done for large specimens (such as bones from NHPs).

12.13.4.4 Biomechanics End-Points

Biomechanical parameters include peak load, stiffness, and work to failure (area under the curve [AUC]), the energy required to break the bone.[33] Using bone geometry parameters, these parameters can be used to derive ultimate stress (apparent strength for vertebrae), modulus, and toughness (Table 12.10). Statistical correlation analyses between bone mass and bone strength parameters are used to further interpret the biomechanical strength data. It is important to establish if any changes in bone mass (BMC and/or BMD) have a corresponding change in bone strength.

Consistent with the limited effect of ovariectomy on cortical bone mass after 16 months, changes in strength parameters of the intact femur of OVX animals tested in three-point bending are minimal.[22] Inter-animal variability also limits the ability to discriminate between OVX and sham controls. Even with these limitations, the testing of long bones and milled cortical beams is effective to quantify biomechanical effects of agents affecting bone quality.[31] At trabecular-rich sites, ovariectomy-induced bone loss results

Table 12.10 Biomechanics measured parameters

Bone and test	Parameter	Unit	Formula
Femur	Peak load	N	Measured
Three-point bending	Stiffness	N/mm	Measured
	Area under the curve (AUC)	N-mm	Measured
	Ultimate stress	MPa	Peak load × $Lc/4I$
	Modulus	MPa	$SL^3/48I$
	Toughness	MPa	$(0.75 \times \text{AUC} \times b^2)/LI$
Cortical beams	Peak load	N	Measured
Three-point bending	Stiffness	N/mm	Measured
	Area under the curve (AUC)	N-mm	Measured
	Ultimate stress	MPa	Peak load $3L/2wt^2$
	Modulus	MPa	$SL^3/4wt^3$
	Toughness	MPa	$(0.75 \times \text{AUC} \times t^2)/LI$
Femoral neck	Peak load	N	Measured
Shear	Stiffness	N/mm	Measured
	Area under the curve (AUC)	N-mm	Measured
Whole vertebra	Peak load	N	Measured
Compression	Yield load	N	Measured
	Stiffness	N/mm	Measured
	Area under the curve (AUC)	N-mm	Measured
	Apparent strength	MPa	Peak load /A
	Yield stress	MPa	Yield load/A
	Modulus	MPa	St/A
	Toughness	MPa	AUC/$(A \times t)$
Vertebral cores	Peak load	N	Measured
Compression	Yield load	N	Measured
	Stiffness	N/mm	Measured
	Area under the curve (AUC)	N-mm	Measured
	Apparent strength	MPa	Peak load/A
	Yield stress	MPa	Yield load/A
	Modulus	MPa	St/A
	Toughness	MPa	AUC/$(A \times t)$

A = area (mm^2), b = diameter of the specimen (mm), c = radius of the specimen (mm), I = moment of inertia (mm^4)[$], L = span between the two lower bending supports (mm), S = stiffness (N/mm), t = thickness of the specimen (mm), W = width (mm), AUC = area under the curve (N-mm), [$] three-point bending of long bones: derived from pQCT parameter, [$] three-point bending of cortical beams: I=0.083*(wb^3),* represents multiply in slight and variable decreases in strength parameters at the femoral neck, and often significant decreases at the spine, most notably in trabecular core specimens. Interindividual variability requires to have a sufficient number of specimens per group to detect meaningful differences with these tests.

Micro-CT scanning provides micro-architectural data as well as bone mass information, and is growing as a tool for finite element modeling. Use in NHP osteoporosis research may facilitate in the translation of indices of biomechanical competency in humans.

12.14 Major Advances Obtained from NHP Osteoporosis Models

NHPs have significantly contributed to our understanding of cortical bone remodeling in particular.[34] Rodent species are extremely important in osteoporosis research to establish new targets and mechanisms of drug action and efficacy, but rodents show little evidence of Haversian remodeling and can be of limited value in this regard. Other higher species, such as the dog and sheep, are also important in contributing to our understanding of bone biology; however, NHPs are the only Haversian remodeling species that are similar to man not only with respect to bone physiology, but with respect to many other organ systems as well, the most important being the reproductive system. The NHP models most closely mimic postmenopausal and androgen deficiency–induced osteoporosis in man and are therefore the models of choice to understand disease etiology and effects of therapeutic interventions.

The similarity in reproductive physiology makes the NHP the optimal species to study important drug classes such as selective estrogen receptor modulators (SERMs) and selective androgen receptor modulators (SARMs). Many SERM studies have proven the OVX model to be predictive of efficacy and bone safety in man[20,21,35,36] while providing important safety information on the effects of treatment on the reproductive tract[37] and in cardiovascular disease.[38]

Characterization of the ORX male model of osteoporosis has demonstrated that the etiology of this model differs from that of the female.[39] A substantial loss of lean (muscle) mass as a result of testosterone depletion has been shown to contribute to the osteopenia in this model.[39] Loss of soft tissue mass does not occur in the OVX model[22] but there is some indication that the ratio of lean mass to fat mass may change (A. Varela, personal communication 2010), with muscle mass declining at the expense of fat mass in response to estrogen loss. The quantification of the changes in lean mass by densitometry techniques means that we can successfully monitor effects of compounds on muscle as well as bone mass. The ORX monkey appears to be a sensitive model with which to evaluate the effects of potential muscle anabolics or anti-catabolics, providing new tools for drug discovery and an ideal model to further our understanding of the important relationship between muscle and bone.

In the future, the use of NHPs in osteoporosis research will likely contribute substantially to further characterize the disease process by investigations into "bone quality." Bone quality encompasses a number of bone tissue properties that govern mechanical resistance, such as bone geometry, cortical properties, trabecular micro-architecture, bone tissue mineralization, quality of collagen and bone apatite crystal, and presence of microcracks.[40] All of these properties are dependant on bone turnover and its variations. Decreases in bone resorption markers, achieved with anti-catabolics, may partly predict the decrease in fracture risk. Several osteoporosis compounds can exert favorable effects on bone size and cortical thickness including the anabolics teriparatide (PTH(1–34)) and PTH (PTH(1–84)), while the anti-catabolic bisphosphonate alendronate can increase cortical thickness by a different mechanism. Marked or prolonged secondary mineralization is a key effect of bisphosphonates and prolonged use may lead to unwanted effects related to excessive mineralization, such as the development of multiple microcracks. On the other hand, high doses of PTH(1–84) in rhesus monkeys revealed that overstimulation of bone turnover reduced bone strength parameters attributed to increases in new bone formation of lower mineralization density.[23,41] These data provided important information on the consequences of forming excessive amounts of new bone and underscored the use of optimal dose levels to achieve modest amounts of bone formation. Other data from this study provided information to enable translation of monkey data to humans by demonstrating that measures made at the lumbar spine reflected changes at the thoracic spine, a more difficult site to study in humans, yet the major site of osteoporotic fractures.[42] In addition, the evaluation of multiple bone sites showed that histomorphometry data derived from the iliac crest (the biopsy site used in human clinical trials) can be extrapolated to other cancellous bone sites such as the spine, proximal femur, and distal radius.[43] Also, μCT and histomorphometry techniques used in this rhesus monkey study showed the response to PTH(1–84) was similar to data generated using the same techniques in human iliac crest biopsies.[44]

New markers of "bone quality" are gaining recognition based on investigations into changes in bone composition in normal and diseased conditions. Fourier transform infrared microspectroscopy (FTIRM) was used to verify that differences in bone mineral quality and quantity in the vertebrae of mature intact as well as OVX monkeys were analogous to those seen in osteoporotic and nondiseased human bones.[45] This technology identified changes in bone chemistry following ovariectomy, suggesting cortical and subchondral bone was less mature due to increased remodeling that occurs after ovariectomy.[46] This study also tested the effects of nandrolone decanoate treatment in OVX animals, showing differences in bone chemistry consistent with increases in bone mass but which did not reverse decreases in bone strength due to ovariectomy. The specific role of osteonal bone mineral and matrix proprieties was recently investigated by FTIR analysis in baboons, showing for the first time that age-related changes in BMC can be explained by an alteration in the mineralization process itself and not only by an imbalance in the remodeling process.[47]

Collagen cross-links also play an important role in the expression of bone strength and the proper biological function of bone.[48] Collagen cross-link formation is affected by bone turnover rate and occurs predominantly as two types: lysyl oxidase–mediated cross-links (enzymatic immature and mature cross-links) and advanced glycation end products (AGEs; nonenzymatic cross-links, pentosidine). Recent reports[48,49] demonstrate that reduced enzymatic cross-links and excessive formation of pentosidine in bone could be important to explain the variation of fracture susceptibility in osteoporosis and diabetes and may be relevant as potential new "bone quality" markers in the assessment of fracture risk, independent of bone turnover and bone density.

Our understanding of research showing interactions between bone, fat, and sugar metabolism with common pathways involved in the diseases of osteoporosis, obesity, and diabetes suggests that bone is a potential target tissue in the evaluation of new therapeutics to treat all of these areas, not just in osteoporosis research. So the goals of osteoporosis research can be predicted to increase in scope as we understand more about how these systems interact and NHPs will become an important model relevant to man to fully appreciate this.

Information on osteocytes has mushroomed as technology has developed to facilitate our understanding of osteocyte biology and the role of osteocytes in the orchestration of osteoblast and osteoclast activity.[50] Osteocyte viability has been observed to be an indicator of bone strength, with viability as the result of maintaining physiological levels of loading and osteocyte apoptosis as the result of a decrease in loading. Osteocyte apoptosis and decrease are major factors in the bone loss and fracture associated with aging.[51] Knowledge of both the osteocyte and periosteal cell layer suggests that these cells are important in maintaining skeletal integrity and as such are targets for pharmaceutical interventions to reduce fracture especially in cortical bone. Anti-catabolics such as the bisphosphonate alendronate have positive effects on cortical bone by allowing periosteal growth while reducing the rate of endocortical bone remodeling and slowing bone loss from the endocortical surface.[51] New molecules targeting osteocyte-specific cytokines such as sclerostin are now in development. Recent results reported from a short-term study in intact NHPs show that anti-sclerostin antibody increased bone turnover markers and bone mass.[3] This sclerostin antibody monoclonal antibody and other therapeutic antibodies such as denosumab, a human monoclonal antibody that binds to RANKL,[52] are examples of highly targeted biotherapeutic molecules in development or approved, since denosumab is now approved for clinical use. Because of target specificity, the NHP is often the only relevant species that can be used to assess the safety of many biotherapeutics. Use of the NHP also allows tests of immune function to be performed as part of the study design providing important safety information before dosing in man.

In summary, NHPs are an invaluable tool in osteoporosis research that can expedite drug development and provide important bone safety data to facilitate our understanding of the disease process and predict the response to new therapies in man with a high degree of confidence. The use of NHPs in osteoporosis research, and in particular the use of the gonadectomy-induced osteoporosis models, will be pivotal to further our understanding of musculoskeletal disease. The information provided in this chapter is intended to provide an understanding of the importance and relevance of using NHPs in osteoporosis research and to serve as an introduction to some of the tools with which we can continue to use NHPs to further our understanding of osteoporosis and its treatment.

Acknowledgments The authors wish to thank the technical teams in the Imaging, Histomorphometry, Biomechanics, and Immunochemistry laboratories at Charles River that made this work possible, and to Dr Luc Chouinard and Nancy Doyle for critical review of the manuscript.

References

1. Reinwald S, Burr D. Review of nonprimate, large animal models for osteoporosis research. *J Bone Miner Res*. 2008; 23(9):1353-1368.
2. Brommage R. Perspectives on using nonhuman primates to understand the etiology and treatment of postmenopausal osteoporosis. *J Musculoskelet Neuronal Interact*. 2001;1(4): 307-325.
3. Ominsky M, Vlasseros F, Jolette J, et al. Two doses of sclerostin antibody in cynomolgus monkeys increases bone formation, bone mineral density, and bone strength. *J Bone Miner Res*. 2010,25(5):948-959 (E-Pub January 8, 2010).
4. Smith SY, Recker RR, Hannan M, et al. Intermittent intravenous administration of the bisphosphonate ibandronate prevents bone loss and maintains bone strength and quality in ovariectomized cynomolgus monkeys. *Bone*. 2003;32(1): 45-55.
5. Smith BB, Cosenza ME, Mancini A, et al. A toxicity profile of osteoprotegerin in the cynomolgus monkey. *Int J Toxicol*. 2003;22(5):403-412.
6. Stroup GB, Hoffman SJ, Vasko-Moser JA, et al. Changes in bone turnover following gonadotropin-releasing hormone (GnRH) agonist administration and estrogen treatment in cynomolgus monkeys: a short-term model for evaluation of antiresorptive therapy. *Bone*. 2001;28:532-537.
7. FDA. Guidelines for preclinical and clinical evaluation of agents used in the prevention or treatment of postmenopausal osteoporosis. In: Products DoMaED, ed. Rockville: Food and Drug Administration; 1994.
8. CHMP. *Guideline on the Evaluation of Medicinal Products in the Treatment of Primary Osteoporosis*. London: European Medicines Agency; 2006.
9. JMHW. Guideline concerning the clinical evaluation method for Anti-Osteoporosis agents, pharmaceutical examination No. 742. In: Management BoH, ed.: issued by the Prefecural Bureau Chief, Bureau of Health Management, Section of Examination and Control, Bureau of Drug Safety, Japanese Ministry of Health and Welfare, 1999.
10. Jayo M, Jerome C, Lees C, et al. Bone mass in female cynomolgus macaques: a cross-sectional and longitudinal study by age. *Calcif Tissue Int*. 1994;54(3):231-236.
11. Champ J, Binkley N, Havighurst T, et al. The effect of advancing age on bone mineral content of female rhesus monkeys. *Bone*. 1996;19(5):485-492.
12. Smith SY, Varela A. Effect of diet (phytoestrogens) on the ovariectomy response in the cynomolgus monkey model of osteoporosis. *J Bone Miner Res* 2009; 24 (Suppl 1), SU0404.
13. Balena R, Toolan B, Shea M, et al. The effects of 2-year treatment with the aminobisphosphonate alendronate on bone metabolism, bone histomorphometry, and bone strength in ovariectomized nonhuman primates. *J Clin Invest*. 1993; 92(6):2577-2586.
14. Jerome C, Turner C, Lees C. Decreased bone mass and strength in ovariectomized cynomolgus monkeys (*Macaca fascicularis*). *Calcif Tissue Int*. 1997;60(3):265-270.
15. Jerome C. Primate models of osteoporosis. *Lab Anim Sci*. 1998;48(6):618-622.
16. Binkley N, Kimmel D, Bruner J, et al. Zoledronate prevents the development of absolute osteopenia following ovariectomy in adult rhesus monkeys. *J Bone Miner Res*. 1998; 13(11):1775-1782.
17. Brommage R, Hotchkiss C, Lees C, et al. Daily treatment with human recombinant parathyroid hormone-(1-34), LY333334, for 1 year increases bone mass in ovariectomized monkeys. *J Clin Endocrinol Metab*. 1999;84(10):3757-3763.
18. Burr D, Hirano T, Turner C, et al. Intermittently administered human parathyroid hormone(1-34) treatment increases intracortical bone turnover and porosity without reducing bone strength in the humerus of ovariectomized cynomolgus monkeys. *J Bone Miner Res*. 2001;16(1):157-165.
19. Jerome C, Peterson P. Nonhuman primate models in skeletal research. *Bone*. 2001;29(1):1-6.
20. Hotchkiss C, Stavisky R, Nowak J, et al. Levormeloxifene prevents increased bone turnover and vertebral bone loss following ovariectomy in cynomolgus monkeys. *Bone*. 2001; 29(1):7-15.
21. Lees C, Register T, Turner C, et al. Effects of raloxifene on bone density, biomarkers, and histomorphometric and biomechanical measures in ovariectomized cynomolgus monkeys. *Menopause*. 2002;9(5):320-328.
22. Smith SY, Jolette J, Turner CH. Skeletal health: primate model of postmenopausal. *Am J Primatol*. 2009;71:1-14.
23. Fox J, Miller MA, Newman MK, et al. Treatment of skeletally mature ovariectomized rhesus monkeys with PTH(1-84) for 16 months increases bone formation and density and improves trabecular architecture and biomechanical properties at the lumbar spine. *J Bone Miner Res*. 2007;22(2):260-273.
24. Russo CR, Lauretani F, Bandinelli S, et al. Aging bone in men and women: beyond changes in bone mineral density. *Osteoporos Int*. 2003;14(7):531-538.
25. Hotchkiss C. Use of peripheral quantitative computed tomography for densitometry of the femoral neck and spine in cynomolgus monkeys (*Macaca fascicularis*). *Bone*. 1999;24:101-107.
26. Dickerson S, Hotchkiss C. Relationships between densitometric and morphological parameters as measured by peripheral computed tomography and the compressive behavior of lumbar vertebral bodies from macaques (*Macaca fascicularis*). *Spine*. 2008;33(4):366-372.

27. Ahlborg H, Johnell O, Turner C, et al. Bone loss and bone size after menopause. *N Engl J Med*. 2003;349(4):327-334.
28. Burghardt A, Kazakia G, Ramachandran S, et al. Age and gender related differences in the geometric properties and biomechanical significance of intra-cortical porosity in the distal radius and tibia. *J Bone Miner Res*. 2009;25(5):983-993 (Accepted article online: December 14, 2009).
29. Kazakia G, Hyun B, Burghardt J, et al. *In vivo* determination of bone structure in postmenopausal women: a comparison of HR-pQCT and High-Field MR Imaging. *J Bone Miner Res*. 2008;23:463-474.
30. Parfitt A, Drezner M, Glorieux F, et al. Bone histomorphometry: standardization of nomenclature, symbols, and units. Report of the ASBMR histomorphometry nomenclature committee. *J Bone Miner Res*. 1987;2(6):595-610.
31. Fox J, Miller M, Newman M, et al. Effects of daily treatment with parathyroid hormone 1–84 for 16 months on density, architecture and biomechanical properties of cortical bone in adult ovariectomized rhesus monkeys. *Bone*. 2007;41(3): 321-330.
32. Turner C. Biomechanics of bone: determinants of skeletal fragility and bone quality. *Osteoporos Int*. 2002;13:97-104.
33. Turner C, Burr D. Basic biomechanical measurements of bone: a tutorial. *Bone*. 1993;14:595-608.
34. Burr D. Estimated intracortical bone turnover in the femur of growing macaques: implications for their use as models in skeletal pathology. *Anat Rec*. 1992;232(2):180-189.
35. Prestwood K, Gunness M, Muchmore D, et al. A comparison of the effects of raloxifene and estrogen on bone in postmenopausal women. *J Clin Endocrinol Metab*. 2000;85(6): 2197-2202.
36. Lees C, Shen V, Brommage R. Effects of lasofoxifene on bone in surgically postmenopausal cynomolgus monkeys. *Menopause*. 2007;14(1):97-105.
37. Cline J, Botts S, Lees C, et al. Effects of lasofoxifene on the uterus, vagina, and breast in ovariectomized cynomolgus monkeys (*Macaca fascicularis*). Am J Obstet Gynecol 2008;199:158.el-8.
38. Heringa M. Review on raloxifene: profile of a selective estrogen receptor modulator. *Int J Clin Pharmacol Ther*. 2003;41(8):331-345.
39. Doyle N, Smith S, Veverka K. Male and female cynomolgus monkey models of osteoporosis: comparative *in vivo* data. *J Bone Miner Res*. 2008;23:S353.
40. Benhamou C. Effects of osteoporosis medications on bone quality. *Joint Bone Spine*. 2007;74(1):39-47.
41. Fox J, Miller M, Recker R, et al. Effects of treatment of ovariectomized adult rhesus monkeys with parathyroid hormone 1–84 for 16 months on trabecular and cortical bone structure and biomechanical properties of the proximal femur. *Calcif Tissue Int*. 2007;81(1):53-63.
42. Fox J, Newman M, Turner C, et al. Effects of treatment with parathyroid hormone 1–84 on quantity and biomechanical properties of thoracic vertebral trabecular bone in ovariectomized rhesus monkeys. *Calcif Tissue Int*. 2008;82(3):212-220.
43. Miller M, Bare S, Recker R, et al. Intratrabecular tunneling increases trabecular number throughout the skeleton of ovariectomized rhesus monkeys treated with parathyroid hormone 1–84. *Bone*. 2008;42(6):1175-1183.
44. Recker R, Bare S, Smith S, et al. Cancellous and cortical bone architecture and turnover at the iliac crest of postmenopausal osteoporotic women treated with parathyroid hormone 1â€"84. *Bone*. 2009;44(1):113-119.
45. Gadeleta S, Boskey A, Paschalis E, et al. A physical, chemical, and mechanical study of lumbar vertebrae from normal, ovariectomized, and nandrlone decanoate-treated cynomolgus monkeys (*Macaca fascicularis*). *Bone*. 2000; 27(4):541-550.
46. Huang R, Miller L, Carlson C, et al. Characterization of bone mineral composition in the proximal tibia of cynomolgus monkeys: effect of ovariectomy and nandrlone decanoate treatment. *Bone*. 2002;30(3):492-497.
47. Gourion-Arsiquaud S, Burket J, Havill L, et al. Spatial variation in osteonal bone properties relative to tissue and animal age. *J Bone Miner Res*. 2009;24(7):1271-1281.
48. Saito M. Biochemical markers of bone turnover. New aspect. Bone collagen metabolism: new biological markers for eastimation of bone quality. *Clin Calcium*. 2009;19(8):1110-1117.
49. Saito M, Fujii K, Mori Y, et al. Role of collagen enzymatic and glycation induced cross-links as a determinant of bone quality in spontaneously diabetic WBN/Kob rats. *Osteoporos Int*. 2006;17(10):1514-1523.
50. Tami A, Nasser P, Verborgt O, et al. The role of interstitial fluid flow in the remodeling response to fatigue loading. *J Bone Miner Res*. 2002;17:2030-2037.
51. Epstein S. Is cortical bone hip? What determines cortical bone properties? *Bone*. 2007;41(1 Suppl 1):S3-S8.
52. Brown J, Prince R, Deal C, et al. Comparison of the effect of denosumab and alendronate on BMD and biochemical markers of bone turnover in postmenopausal women with low bone mass: a randomized, blinded, phase 3 trial. *J Bone Miner Res*. 2010;25(5):983-993.

13 Other Large Animal Models

Susan Reinwald and David B. Burr

13.1 Introduction

Osteoporosis is a disease characterized by low bone mass and micro-architectural deterioration of bone tissue leading to skeletal fragility. Guidelines established by the United States Food and Drug Administration (FDA) stipulate that therapeutic treatments formulated to attenuate or prevent postmenopausal osteoporosis should, in the first instance, be evaluated in an ovariectomized (OVX) rodent such as the rat.[1] Despite some species-related shortcomings such as a lack of intracortical bone remodeling and comparatively small size, historically rats represent a well-characterized model from which preliminary data can be gleaned to more extensively support hypotheses and justify the involvement of larger and more expensive animal models in preclinical studies from which the likely human clinical response is able to be better predicted and validated. From this information, advancements in the design of effective and safe therapeutic treatments can emerge via subsequent clinical trials. This chapter is intended to provide an overview of the practical efficacy of using select large animal species, including rabbits, dogs, sheep, goats, and swine, to meet the obligatory requirements for an animal model of bone loss – one that is predominantly associated with estrogen deficiency and which has some useful relevance to human postmenopausal osteoporosis.

While there is no single animal model that precisely reproduces all the characteristics of human osteoporosis, of all larger mammalians, nonhuman primates (NHPs) are considered preeminent in terms of replicating many important features of human physiology and disease. However, for the vast majority of researchers NHPs are not an affordable option given the substantial investment of money, resources, and time that is required to support experiments of this caliber. Furthermore, the sentient and sensitive nature of NHPs can pose ethical and social concerns that are less likely encountered with many other alternative lower-order species of animals. For osteoporosis research, practical and cost-effective alternative large animal models can be found or established from agricultural animals such as pigs, sheep, and goats, as well as from domestic animals including rabbits and dogs. An important proviso to using a larger animal model relates to thoroughly researching candidate species to become knowledgeable of the limitations and strengths of each. It is only from a well-informed perspective that an animal's suitability as a model to answer specific questions becomes more readily apparent. Equipping oneself with a solid understanding also allows experiments to be advantageously designed to optimize any underlying potential of an animal to develop the characteristic signs of postmenopausal bone loss and/or yield information of relevance to treatment regimens.

13.2 Large Animal Models in Perspective

Ovarian estrogen production is naturally exhausted at the onset of menopause when oocyte attrition results in the cessation of reproductive cycling. This period of a woman's life coincides with an initial transient (≥5 years) acceleration of bone turnover that is simultaneously characterized by dysfunctional remodeling

S. Reinwald (✉)
Department of Anatomy and Cell Biology, Indiana University School of Medicine, Indianapolis, IN, USA
e-mail: sreinwald@drivemed.com

G. Duque and K. Watanabe (eds.), *Osteoporosis Research*,
DOI: 10.1007/978-0-85729-293-3_13, © Springer-Verlag London Limited 2011

such that bone resorption chronically exceeds bone formation and leads to a net bone loss. These metabolic changes can weaken the existing bone architecture and impose an immediate or future increase in fracture risk, particularly if the genetic potential for bone accrual was not maximized earlier in life. In osteoporosis research, the use of large non-primate animal models that can reproducibly mimic the type of increase in bone turnover leading to significant bone loss and architectural deterioration[2] is desirable but not usually possible without surgical intervention or bilateral ovariectomy to induce a postmenopausal-like state.

There are multiple factors associated with reproductive and endocrinological interspecies differences that complicate an investigator's ability to evaluate the efficacy of larger animals as a model for hormone-induced bone loss. Most large animals appear to be endowed with a robust bone-forming capacity and a skeletal fitness that is unparalleled by middle-aged women. In contrast to women, a long post-reproductive period is rare among other female mammals, occurring only in some whale and primate species.[3] While many women will live about one-third of their lives beyond menopause, nearly all animals experience a late onset in decline from fecundity; estrous cycles at the time of sexual maturation continue through to late somatic senescence, reducing the period in their life during which ovarian hormone levels are significantly diminished. Compared to canine, ovine, caprine, porcine,[4] and leporine species, peak and basal circulating estradiol levels during reproductive cycling are disproportionally higher in women. Moreover, following menopause, there is a more precipitous decline in estradiol concentrations from average basal to postmenopausal levels in women (≥72%) than from basal to castration estradiol levels in these species.[4] Female farm and domestic animals breed prolifically and naturally tend to produce multiple offspring per pregnancy. They have evolved to cope superlatively with the high-energy and endocrinological demands imposed by repeated episodes of gestation and lactation during a relatively long reproductive lifespan. Due to a combination of factors such as these and biomechanical differences, animals seldom succumb to the chronic degenerative disease of osteoporosis per se and some acute form of perturbation is generally required to precipitate osteopenia.

Osteoporosis is a chronic human disease characterized by discrete anisotropic bone loss. A net amount of bone is typically lost from endosteal surfaces and transverse trabeculae at the same time net bone accrual is preferentially occurring on periosteal surfaces and vertical trabecular thickening is taking place. Adaptive metabolic changes that are the polar opposite of each other take place simultaneously at different locations in the skeleton in the same environment of hormonal[5] and possibly calcium (Ca) deficiency.[6] This suggests that the etiology of this type of pathologic bone loss and architectural deterioration may also involve other factors unique to humans, one of which may include habitual bipedalism.

The limbs of quadrupeds are bent so that body weight is largely held in tension by muscles. Furthermore, the horizontally aligned spine of quadrupeds requires higher muscle forces and passive tension to resist extension than does the musculature of bipeds. Stabilization of the erect human skeleton requires more micro-stabilizing movements to maintain balance and the vertical weight-bearing alignment of the spine as each body segment is positioned over the next lower one.[7] An erect posture with a vertically aligned spine limits loading offsets and decreases the strains compared with those in quadruped bones.[5] During locomotion, more dynamic loading and subsequent anabolic stimulation naturally occurs in the vertebrae of quadrupeds; this results from propulsive forces that generate compressive and tensile strains that deliver loads to opposite vertebral margins.[5] The forces generated by the relatively strong and sizable musculature supporting the spine of animals such as pigs and sheep increases axial compression stresses, which contribute to vertebral bone densities that greatly exceed those of humans.[8-10] Divergences in musculoskeletal structure, size, function, posture, and biomechanics in bipeds versus quadrupeds are likely important determiners of the magnitude and location of hormone-mediated bone loss. These types of differences pose an ongoing challenge to scientists seeking a larger animal model that displays the severity of bone loss observed in osteoporotic humans.

Despite the occurrence of ovariectomy-induced bone loss in a number of laboratory animals, susceptibility to fragility fractures in quadrupeds is minimal. The combined effects of higher bone mineral density (BMD), less dangerous environments (softer surfaces, confinement with limited locomotion), a lowered center of gravity with less distance to fall,[7] a different biomechanical distribution of forces compared to bipeds and/or the lifelong nutrient-rich diets formulated for laboratory animals may be somewhat protective. At best, an osteopenic condition may develop in OVX farm and domestic animals, which can be a satisfactory state from which to extrapolate preclinical results. A distinct advantage of larger animals, particularly dogs[11-18] and sheep,[19-21] is the opportunity to biopsy the iliac crest and/or ribs at different time points to yield bilateral longitudinal histomorphometric data. In addition, the mechanical corollary of any structural or material changes in bone tissue can be assessed *ex vivo* via biomechanical testing of biopsied samples. A thoughtful experimental design in conjunction with strategic manipulation of experimental conditions can induce an osteopenic state in farm and domestic animals that can be exacerbated or prolonged in order to evaluate agents for the treatment of osteoporosis.

13.3 General Requirements

The FDA recommends ovariectomy of large animal models for preclinical postmenopausal bone loss research because it provides a reasonably similar endocrinological basis (i.e., estrogen insufficiency) from which to gauge potential treatment effects – as opposed to hindlimb unloading and peripheral nerve severance models, which are less relevant mediators of pathologic bone loss in the general population. To adequately evaluate preventative or therapeutic treatment effects in animal experiments, outcomes are best evaluated in long bones and vertebrae as recommended by the FDA and following two or more bone remodeling cycles to eliminate confounding bone remodeling transients that merely represent short-term shifts in bone metabolism.[22] The appearance of bone loss very soon after castration is desirable in any large animal model of osteoporosis and is similar to postmenopausal circumstances when the loss predominantly pertains to cancellous bone, and osteonal remodeling is evident.

The World Health Organization (WHO) classifies normal bone mass, and conditions of osteopenia and osteoporosis on the basis of diagnostic T-scores that determine how many standard deviations patients are from the average peak bone mass in young healthy women (≥−1 = normal, −1 to −2.5 = osteopenia, and ≤−2.5 = osteoporosis). It should be kept in mind that it is unrealistic to expect the T-scores designed for bipedal humans and the WHO classifications to be applicable to larger quadruped mammals.

The efficacy of a larger species of animal to serve as a preclinical model of postmenopausal bone loss is contingent upon how extensively the following broad criteria can be satisfied:

- Appropriateness as a model of estrogen deficiency (i.e., significant bone loss and a similar, if not identical, tissue level mechanism for bone loss predominantly induced by estrogen depletion)
- Specific biological and physiological characteristics (e.g., osteonal bone remodeling, reproductive physiology)
- Affordability and availability of skeletally mature animals
- Housing/spatial requirements
- Manageability during an experiment
- Minimal ethical/societal implications
- A species that satisfies the reduction principle of requiring the fewest number of animals
- Reproducible outcomes
- Time until significant bone loss
- Predictive of skeletal effects of potential osteoporosis therapies in adult humans (e.g., increased BMD)[4]

Animals raised for laboratory use often subsist on nutrient-adequate or nutrient-dense rations prior to undergoing ovariectomy. This is in stark contrast to the high numbers of women in the United States, ~85% of females after childhood, that habitually fail to meet the daily recommended intake of Ca.[23] It is well recognized that a chronic Ca deficiency resulting in suboptimal bone accrual during growth and development (and maturation), or insufficient bone maintenance from late adulthood through to middle age, in conjunction with the increased bone resorption that occurs in response to estrogen insufficiency at the time of menopause, puts women at an increased risk for fragility fractures. An underlying Ca deficiency can erode skeletal Ca reserves over time to an extent that may, at least in part, explain why estrogen diminution alone is not always sufficient to stimulate pathological bone loss in all postmenopausal women. Although there are some exceptions, more often than not women entering menopause with a good nutrition status and high bone mass are less susceptible to developing osteoporosis for a longer period of time. It may therefore be worth considering the dietary intake of Ca in relation to phosphorus and even vitamin D in mature large animal models destined for bone loss research in advance of the start of an experiment. The long-term moderation of Ca prior to and following ovariectomy may be more in keeping with the typical human experience than is currently appreciated. Low Ca diets in humans warrants the inclusion of a group of intact animals that are fed a low Ca diet to enable the skeletal effects of estrogen insufficiency and lower dietary Ca to be distinguished.

13.4 Most Common Large Animal Models

13.4.1 Rabbits

Rabbits are monogastric hindgut fermenting herbivores; they ingest additional nutrients derived from cecal microbial digestion via coprophagy which also results in the recycling of various non-fibrous substances in excreta. Rabbits do not have estrous cycles, they are reflexive ovulators in response to male copulation. Ovariectomy has been shown to reduce circulating estradiol concentrations in 9-month-old female rabbits from an average level of ~23 pg/ml to a mean of ~15 pg/ml 1 month post ovariectomy.[24] Historically, rabbits have not been extensively used as a large animal model for osteoporosis research. Although rabbits possess some attractive experimental qualities, they appear to require some additional manipulation beyond bilateral ovariectomy before bone loss[25-29] and declines in bone biomechanical properties become significant.[29]

Glucocorticoid treatment of OVX rabbits, or alternatively, a low Ca diet in conjunction with ovariectomy, has proved successful in achieving a significant reduction in cortical, trabecular, and subchondral BMD, as well as bone histological changes. Although glucocorticoid therapy induces BMD decreases in rabbits of up to 19.5% 6 weeks after ovariectomy[25] and may make rabbits a good choice for studying glucocorticoid-induced osteoporosis, the mechanism of action is not relevant to what might occur in the majority of postmenopausal women. Conversely, a reduced Ca intake by rabbits is in line with suboptimal Ca intakes in humans that can lead to a loss of bone. Ca metabolism in rabbits is distinctive; they absorb it in direct proportion to the amount ingested in the diet regardless of metabolic requirement. Rabbits maintain serum Ca levels that are 30% to >40% higher (13–15 mg/dl) than those in other mammals (e.g., normal human range is 8.4–10.2 mg/dl), and levels are regulated over an unusually wide range with as much as 60% of ingested Ca being eliminated via urinary excretion.[30] A dietary supply of 0.34–0.40% is required for maximal bone calcification in rabbits.[31] Within 4 weeks, a diet containing 0.15% Ca can result in significant bone loss (−12%) in OVX rabbits.[26] Dietary phytoestrogen exposure has been shown to be associated with elevated serum testosterone concentrations and an increased BMD in OVX rabbits[28]; therefore, it is advisable to ensure diet formulations are phytoestrogen-free and that feeding clover is avoided if bone loss is the goal.

At a young age relative to many other large animals (~6 months), and soon after sexual maturity, rabbits become skeletally mature. The larger adult size of rabbits relative to rats, yet more compact size relative to other farm animals, contributes to their economic viability as a preclinical model.[32] Secondary osteons are present in the compact bone of the femoral diaphysis of juvenile rabbits by 2–3 months age[33] and their concentrations become denser in adulthood.[34] Haversian remodeling in rabbit cortical bone occurs predominantly in the posteriomedial and posterolateral aspects of the femoral shaft.[35] Bone located in medullary and periosteal regions of the femur is lamellar, or contains primary osteonal regions with longitudinally oriented vascular canals.[35] Fibrolamellar bone tissue, common to rapidly growing large mammals, is not typically present in standard experimental rabbits.[36] Rabbit bone remodeling cycles take approximately 70 days[37] and are more rapid than in humans, and therefore it can be challenging to make inferences based on treatment effects in rabbits[38]; however, the long bones of aging rabbits are characterized by a progressive, negative endosteal balance and a positive periosteal accrual analogous to that which occurs in postmenopausal women. In terms of animal manageability, the spine of rabbits can be susceptible to handling and/or restraint injuries due to the powerful muscle mass that flanks this anatomical region. It is important to handle rabbits in a firm yet gentle manner to reduce the likelihood of sudden hindlimb kicking that can also result in scratches to handlers.

13.4.2 Dogs

The beagle is a compact, low-maintenance breed of dog routinely used in biomedical research because of well-documented physiological responses.[39] Mature dogs have a bone composition that is similar to humans[8] with similar intracortical Haversian remodeling. Cancellous remodeling in dogs is also very comparable to that of humans,[39] although remodeling cycles are ~25% shorter[40,41] and cancellous turnover is two to three times more rapid.[42] The 4:1 proportion of cortical/cancellous bone in beagles is very similar to the 5:1 ratio in humans.[43] Bone loss with advancing age is also typical in beagles[39] and humans alike, and bone turnover has been shown to increase as an acute response to the loss of ovarian estrogen in dogs due to ovariectomy or ovariohysterectomy (OHX).[13,14,18,44] Castration of dogs stimulates uterine tissue atrophy[13] and a gain in body weight[11,18,45,46] in addition to shifts in canine body fat distribution and other related metabolic changes that are not uncommon following menopause in women.[47] Although the average concentration of E2 during an estrous cycle in dogs (10–15 pg/ml) is considerably lower than that of women throughout a menstrual cycle (160 pg/ml), the magnitude of the decline in E2 levels post reproductive cycling is reported to be approximately proportional for women and dogs.[45]

Despite some favorable characteristics, the effectiveness of the beagle as a preclinical model of postmenopausal bone loss has been widely debated because bone loss experiments on OVX and OHX dogs yield inconsistent results. Acute post-castration bone loss and/or significant changes in bone remodeling, as measured by dynamic and static histomorphometry, have been documented for beagles,[12-18,44,45,48,49] although a number of early changes were considered transient[13,18,44] or were reported for a period of <2 remodeling cycles,[14-17,48] which may not represent a steady-state outcome. Beyond a 6-month period, other studies have revealed a lack of response for dynamic bone parameters[11,50] and/or a lack of sizable responses for biochemical parameters.[11] A thorough comparison of published OVX and OHX dog studies[11-18,44,45,48-54] does however reveal that experimental designs have been variable between studies.

Inconsistent bone loss results for the castrated dog model may have arisen because the age range of dogs has been wide and experimental group sizes have often been small. A low number of dogs/group becomes problematic when histomorphometric end points (e.g., ratio of bone volume to tissue volume [BV/TV]) are employed because small group sizes require very large differences given the high standard deviation (~25%) for this method of assessment.[42] Canine bone turnover rates also tend to vary considerably from site to site and are contingent upon the animal's age. Rib cortical bone turnover can reach ~18% per year versus 1% per year for cortical bone turnover at the midshaft of long bones.[44] Trabecular bone turnover rates in dogs vary by a factor of >10, being highest in vertebral bodies, the pelvis, and proximal humerus, and lowest in the ulna, skull, and bones of the feet.[42] Bone remodeling rates are also different between sites on the same bone at the rib and iliac crest such that sampling sites need to be standardized[55] to be comparable.

Canines are monoestrus. Relatively low intercycle estrogen concentrations persist in ovary-intact beagles for >6 months of the year. Overall estrogen exposure in dogs versus normally cycling premenopausal women is low[43]; a marked spike in circulating estrogen only occurs once per year on average in dogs. Following castration, a significant decline in circulating estradiol concentrations has been observed to occur by 1 month,[18,50] not at all by ~1.5 months,[44] or not until 2.3 months post surgery[12] in beagles. A routine check to confirm uterine atrophy in OVX dogs and the complete extrication of ovarian tissue at necropsy is also warranted in light of ovarian remnant syndrome reports for castrated dogs.[56] However, castration of bitches during times of peak progesterone concentrations may be confounding; this hormone can potentially attenuate bone loss from multiple sites and in some cases has actually stimulated new bone formation, particularly in cortical bone.[57] Considering the relative infrequency of estrous cycles in canines, more consistent results may be achieved with a standardized experimental approach to the timing of neutering to avoid heterogeneous hormonal profiles among dogs in shorter-term experiments.

Kimmel has hypothesized that beagles may possess a smaller estrogen-dependent compartment of bone in their skeleton compared to women.[42] This notion is supported by experiments in which castration alone failed to demonstrate significant or sustained osteopenic effects in rib cortical bone[50] and iliac crest trabecular bone via static and dynamic histomorphometry,[11,18] lumbar vertebral BMD via DEXA,[11] and vertebral bone mineral content (BMC) and mechanical strength.[51]

However, the lack of a skeletal response to estrogen diminution in dogs may be impacted to some extent by the canine diet.

The importance of diet in animal models of osteoporosis cannot be overstated. Soybean meal, an all-too-common ingredient in commercial dog chows, can impart unnecessarily high concentrations of dietary phytoestrogens[58] which are known to influence bone metabolism,[59] particularly during early estrogen depletion.[60] Habitual dietary excesses of Ca (i.e., >1% dietary Ca) are also problematic in bone loss studies not intentionally designed to restrict or control the intake of this mineral.[12,14-18,45,48,51] Dietary Ca ≤0.5% has been shown to be sufficient for maintaining Ca balance and bone mineral in dogs.[61,62] Most standard canine laboratory diets contain 1.3% to ≥1.5% Ca, although in some experiments 1.8%[18] and 2.1% dietary Ca[45] has been fed to castrated dogs. Adult beagles can consume as much as 300 g of food each day under experimental laboratory conditions,[44,49,63] which can translate to as much as ~3,900–4,500 mg Ca/day or 5,400 mg[18] and 6,300 mg Ca/day[45] for animals weighing only ~13 kg. This is in stark contrast to women weighing 60–70 kg, most of whom struggle to regularly consume recommended or adequate target Ca intakes of 1,200–1,500 mg/day. Supplemental dietary Ca has been shown to play a significant role in protecting against bone mineral loss in OVX beagles[6] and limited Ca in addition to ovariectomy has led to a marked decrease in mechanical strength of the femoral neck of dogs.[51] Other beagle experiments show that restricted Ca intakes (0.14% Ca for ≥1 year) augment castration-induced bone loss, but that dietary Ca contributes more to decrements in lumbar vertebral bone mass, mechanical strength, and turnover than do the effects of ovary ablation[46,49]; however, vertebral trabecular separation has been shown to be more adversely affected by ovariectomy than by reduced dietary Ca.[63]

Accelerated endocortical resorption leads to cortical thinning, and low-level trauma rib fractures in postmenopausal women tend to indicate a significantly elevated risk for future limb fracture(s), particularly of the hip and/or humerus.[64] Because of its high rate of bone turnover, the endocortical surface of dog ribs appears to represent a suitably responsive site for the evaluation of the acute effects of estrogen withdrawal on Haversian remodeling. The bilateral abundance of ribs provides researchers with the opportunity to sequentially biopsy bone at these sites to gauge longitudinal changes. Wilson et al. observed increases in rib medullary space and alterations in rib cortical bone formation indices BFR bone formation rate and MAR mineral aposition rate between 1 and 4 months post ovariectomy for 7–9-year-old beagles although chronological midrib biopsies revealed these changes were transient because they disappeared 8.5 months after ovariectomy.[44] Cortical porosity in the same dogs continued to increase over 8.5 months, although it was maximal 4 months post ovariectomy, and osteoid maturation progressively slowed. Karambolova et al. investigated the effects of estradiol on rib bone surfaces of 4-year-old dogs and determined that ovariectomy increased the resorptive surfaces on endocortical bone over 12 months.[54] While administration of estradiol reversed that effect, it could not correct the increase in mineralization lag time associated with ovariectomy.

Assessment of the lumbar vertebrae of castrated dogs has yielded mixed evidence of bone loss and decreases in bone mechanical strength. The areal BMD of the lumbar vertebrae of 4-year-old castrated breeder beagles fed an undisclosed amount of dietary Ca for 6 months was the same as that of sham controls.[11] Martin et al. ovariectomized 3–7-year-old dogs and determined after 48 weeks that porosity at the fifth lumbar vertebra was increased by 15%, and that structural toughness and the material strength of vertebrae were decreased compared to sham dogs, despite the dogs being fed a remarkably high Ca diet (2.1%). In contrast, Nagai and Shindo reported no effect on BMC and the mechanical strength of lumbar vertebrae in OVX dogs fed a diet containing 1.4% Ca for 8 months.[51] However, when the same investigators ovariectomized dogs and simultaneously exposed them to limited dietary Ca (0.1% Ca), a 31% decrease in vertebral BMC occurred within 7 months, in addition to a 40% decrease in OVX beagles to either 0.06% or normal dietary Ca for 7 months, and they noted that Ca-restricted dogs exhibited a relative 14.4% and 21.3% decline in areal BMD for the whole vertebra and the central region of the vertebra, respectively. Motoie et al. observed an areal BMD decline compared to baseline of 19% and 30% in the second and fourth lumbar vertebrae of OVX dogs at 2 and 17 months respectively; these dogs were fed a diet containing 0.14% Ca, or one-tenth of the standard Ca ration in commercially available canine diets.[46] The earliest signs of bone loss induced by a Ca deficiency in dogs generally become apparent in the jawbones and secondly in skull bones, followed by the ribs and vertebrae, while the long bones are usually affected last of all.[62]

Weight distribution in dog limbs is very similar to that of sheep; the mean peak vertical forces generated as a percentage of body weight in the forelimbs versus hindlimbs of dogs is ~58% and 42%, respectively.[65] Motoie et al. found that BMD reductions in the forelimbs of OVX beagles on a Ca-restricted diet were less remarkable than in the spine.[46] Martin et al. determined that the cortical bone areas of the radius, ulnae, and humerus did not respond to ovariectomy, with the exception of an increase in the number of osteonal resorption spaces on the ulnae of beagles.[45] The femur is the heaviest bone in the skeleton of dogs, and femoral mechanical changes attributable to castration effects in dogs are absent[45,66] except at the femoral neck where OVX Ca-restricted dogs exhibited structurally stronger and tougher bones than Ca-unrestricted sham dogs.[51]

A long history of domestication has imposed omnivorous traits on monogastric canines that evolved from ancestors that were primarily carnivores. Although domestic dogs retain the dentition, powerful jaw muscles, meal patterning behaviors, and the internal anatomy and physiology specific to carnivores,[67] the protein content of their diets has been significantly reduced to make way for more carbohydrates, mainly to reduce costs and for the sake of human convenience. Dogs posses a relatively sensitive gastrointestinal tract and most knowledgeable dog owners know of the danger of feeding them onions, chocolate, turkey skins, certain spices, or foods rich in caffeine. Toxicologists generally prefer to use porcine versus canine models due to the higher gastrointestinal tolerance of pigs.[68] Investigators considering the administration of any therapeutic agent to dogs, including natural or synthetic estrogens,[69,70] nonsteroidal anti-inflammatory drugs,[71,72] vitamins,[73] or vitamin analogs[74] would be well advised to thoroughly research possible side effects on the gastrointestinal tract as well as other organs in this animal model in particular.

The iliac crest is often used as a biopsy site in large animal models like dogs and sheep to evaluate changes in bone remodeling dynamics. It is a site of comparative value as postmenopausal women can be biopsied at this anatomical location. Soon after castration, canine trabeculae at this site appear to show significant signs of increased bone remodeling in a number of studies,[12-18] but not in a 6-month study by Shen et al.,[11] in which nutrient levels in the chow fed to the dogs are not disclosed. Early changes have included a 20.3% reduction in iliac crest cancellous bone mass by 4 months, as well as trabecular thinning.[17] Based on percentage changes from baseline (±SEM standard error of the mean), the histomorphometry parameters MAR and BFR/TV decrease in beagles by 12.3 ± 4.2% and 3.8 ± 4.2%, respectively, in response to oophorectomy; these changes were measured on thin sections taken from iliac crest biopsies in different studies representing a total of 12 baseline versus OVX group comparisons.[11,14,17,18,43,45,75] Elevated osteocalcin levels[12] and increased osteoblast numbers have also been identified as post-castration effects in dogs at the iliac crest, and net bone loss has been attributed to a simultaneous decrease in osteoblast function at the tissue level.[17] At this location, dogs appear to mimic the early high bone turnover that is observed at cancellous-rich sites during early postmenopause.

13.4.3 Sheep

Sheep are well domesticated, ruminating herbivores with a strong flocking instinct; they are passive and cooperative when maintained in groups and pose hardly any behavioral problems. A number of environmental factors can directly affect the bone metabolism of ewes. Depending on the breed and geographical location (higher versus lower latitudes), ruminant animals like sheep and goats may be predisposed to seasonal and photoperiod sensitivities that temporally influence hormone levels and bone BMD. Short-day breeding sheep are seasonally polyestrous and begin a 10-month period of estrous cycling as daylight hours shorten in the fall.[76] OVX ewes can exhibit a 5–12% BMD reduction[77] and bone micro-architectural changes; however, seasonal effects may account for up to 50% of any such change.[78] The BMD of sheep tends to be lower during winter, representing a transient phenomenon that should be factored in to the timing and length of an experimental design.[79,80] If sheep are left to graze in pastures containing legumes, or are fed leguminous silage or by-products such as soybean meal, the phytoestrogen content can induce changes consistent with estrous[81] and potentially affect the metabolism of estrogen-responsive tissues and organs such as bone. Phytoestrogenic compounds act as selective estrogen receptor modulators (SERMs) and ewes are sensitive to the effects of both naturally occurring[82] and pharmaceutical SERMs.[83] Interlaboratory comparisons of ovariectomy results in sheep are facilitated when the latitude, diet, reproductive history (paturational and lactational), the seasons spanned, and the breed of the animals is specified.

Other physiological factors inherent to sheep have been reported to influence bone metabolism following ovariectomy. These include the capacity to synthesize estrogen extragonadally from adipose tissue and via conversion of adrenal-derived C19 steroids and possibly confound experimental results.[20] Sheep may be more sensitive to the effects of extragonadal estrogen considering that average ovine exposure to estradiol is minimal compared to human exposures and in OVX sheep it only requires 0.4 µg E_2/kg versus 10 µg E_2/kg in OVX rodents to stimulate estrus-like responses.[84] Aside from this, as cud-chewing, polygastric animals, predigestive fermentation takes place in the rumen, or the first of the four digestive compartments. Microbial fermentation can potentially biotransform orally administered nutrients, pharmaceuticals, or other bioactive substances such as phytoestrogen-rich fodder[85] prior to absorption in their true glandular stomach and alter potency. Furthermore, the pharmacokinetics and pharmacodynamics of drugs administered orally to ruminants are very different from monogastric species,[86] and absorption characteristics may vary with the volume and nature of the ingesta.[87] Alternative strategies, such as intra-abomasal delivery (i.e., direct administration into the fourth division of a ruminant's stomach) or microencapsulation to achieve rumen bypass, may need to be used to protect the viability of orally administered therapeutic substances; or alternatively, injecting ruminants may be more reliable if comparable clinically relevant doses of a drug are able to be estimated. Bone metabolism in sheep may be incorrectly evaluated if the amount of subcutaneous fat and fleece poses body positioning challenges during *in vivo* projectional x-ray imaging (dual energy x-ray absorptiometry [DEXA]) that can lead to distortion and increase the margin for error.[20] Aside from these complicating factors, sheep are readily available, not prohibitively expensive, their physical size and weight are more comparable than dogs or rabbits to humans, their bone and joint structure has made them a reliable and attractive model for multiple aspects of orthopedic research, and their use as a model for osteoporosis continues to stimulate interest.

In the long bones of fast-growing large animals, plexiform bone is rapidly formed to keep pace with the necessary periosteal apposition to provide the mechanical support required to cope with substantial increases in body weight and size. The initial compact bone formed in sheep is predominantly plexiform, or woven-fibered and lamellar bone; it is rapidly deposited and quickly becomes highly mineralized as the animal grows and reaches skeletal maturity between 3 and 4 years of age.[38,88] Primary osteons form as a result of modeling when blood vessels on a bone surface are incorporated into new endosteal and/or periosteal bone.[89] Primary bone in large animals is strong,[89] and therefore is not typically remodeled until the animals reach a reasonably old age (7–9 years).[38,90] Haversian canal distribution in sheep is typically less dense and more irregular than in humans.[38,91] There is evidence of cortical bone changes in response to ovariectomy in a number of ewe studies. Increased bone turnover between 6 and 12 months, as well as increases in resorptive porosity and biomechanical decrements, has been observed by 12 months in the mid-diaphyseal metatarsal cortical bone of skeletally mature OVX sheep versus intact controls.[92] Cortical bone histological parameters (cross-sectional and medullary areas and periosteal and endocortical perimeters) at the mid-diaphysis of the tibia were significantly more responsive to ovariectomy than in the femur of sheep 24 months post ovariectomy.[93] BMD, but not cortical thickness, of the radius/ulna in OVX versus control sheep was reduced 12 months post ovariectomy.[76] Within 6 months, ovariectomy induced significant increases in eroded and osteoid surfaces, and therefore porosity, in the cortical bone of 8 ± 1 years retired breeder ewes.[83]

In a number of studies the deterioration in various bone parameters due to ovary ablation in sheep has been demonstrated to be significant, but not typically of the magnitude observed in women. Changes from baseline in trabecular bone at the distal radius were significant and rapid (12.7%) from 0 to 4 months post ovariectomy,[20] but subsequently rebounded toward baseline levels by 17 months post surgery, possibly due to extragonadal E2 production.[20] *In vivo* assessed BMD changes from baseline in certain regions of the lumbar spine (5%) have been shown to take up to

6 months to reach significance in 7–9-year-old ewes.[94] Histological analysis of trabecular bone from the iliac crest has revealed bone volume and thickness reductions and increases in trabecular separation in OVX sheep versus controls after 1 year.[19] Wu et al. demonstrated that 12 months after castration trabecular BMD at the femoral neck and condyle in sheep decreased by an impressive >30% compared to sham controls, micro-architectural deteriorations developed in the lumbar spine and femoral neck, and declines in bone mechanical properties were evident at these same sites.[95] The wide age range of sheep used in this study (2.5–6 years) and nondisclosure of the breed make these results difficult to compare with other studies. Giavaresi et al. determined that it took 24 months for a useful osteopenic state to develop in the fifth lumbar vertebra of OVX sheep. Collectively, the data on OVX sheep indicate that a period of ≥12 months is required to develop a reliable ovine model for postmenopausal bone loss.[96]

In an attempt to increase the magnitude of bone loss in castrated ewes Egermann et al. established a new bone loss induction regimen to be used on sheep; it entailed combining ovariectomy with daily Ca and vitamin D restriction (1.5 g versus 5 g Ca; 100 IU versus 1,000 IU vitamin D_3/day) in addition to steroid medication (methylprednisolone).[77] While the >30% reduction in BMD and decrements to bone biomechanical properties yielded outstanding changes in less than 1 year, the health-related side effects of the steroid treatment rendered this ovine model unacceptable. Not only does steroid-induced osteopenia not mimic the mechanism of action for postmenopausal bone loss, but rebound of cancellous bone loss following steroid treatment is a well-documented effect in sheep.[77,97] Ca and vitamin D restriction in OVX sheep over 6 months appeared to represent a less severe yet more physiologically relevant perturbation to cancellous and cortical BMD in Egermann's pilot study. Lill et al.[98] also determined that this type of dietary restriction in conjunction with ovariectomy imparts an additional effect on bone loss. Other investigators have accentuated bone loss in OVX sheep by inducing dietary acidosis.[99] The success of the ovine model for postmenopausal bone loss appears to depend on a well-planned experiment that takes into account transient seasonal effects, dietary factors, and a longer-term approach to achieving osteopenia.

13.4.4 Goats

Although goats are an established large animal model for orthopedic research and surgical training,[100] caprine research in the area of pathology is relatively scarce.[101] Currently, goats are not used extensively as a large model for osteopenia. Access to the osteoporosis research that does exist in goats is limited because numerous publications are unavailable in English,[102-105] protocol details are often lacking, and/or the experimental designs are not always optimal, all of which makes the results of experiments difficult to interpret. Estradiol concentrations in the estrous cycling goat range from 4.72 ± 0.44 to 14.34 ± 2.32 pg/ml in the early luteal and follicular stage, respectively.[106] One month after ovariectomy a −42.30% median percentage change from baseline serum estradiol concentrations was reported for goats, and over a subsequent 6-month period the difference steadily decreased to −52.39%. Practically all of the bone loss data in this species is based on Chinese mountain goats and suggests that a significant osteopenic condition can be routinely established within 6 months when ovariectomy is combined with the restriction of dietary Ca to 0.5%.[107-109] Under this induction regimen, significant median volumetric BMD losses have been observed in the trabeculae of OVX goats versus Ca-replete sham controls at the following sites: lumbar vertebrae −30% to −32%[107]; humeral head −23.91%[107]; calcaneus −32.84%,[107] −21.8%,[107] and −7.06%[109]; proximal tibial metaphysis −18.9%[107]; and distal tibia −9.03%.[109] Bone loss at the iliac crest among OVX goats 6 months post ovariectomy versus baseline biopsies has revealed significant BMD changes of −25%[107] and −16.3%.[108] Trabecular bone architecture at the iliac crest has also been shown to significantly deteriorate in response to ovariectomy + low Ca by 8.34% for bone volume density, 8.51% for trabecular number (Tb.N), and 18.52% for connectivity density (Conn.D), while trabecular separation (Tb.Sp) increased by 8.26%.[108] *Ex vivo* mechanical indentation tests on trabecular bone from the humeral head and calcaneus of goats respectively revealed that 52% and 54% less energy was required to displace bone 3 mm in OVX samples versus sham controls.[107] Generally, the statistics employed and presented in the analyses of OVX goat data suggest that non-normality and variability in measurements is common. It is uncertain how reliably the osteopenia generated in mountain goats is able to reflect outcomes in alternate caprine breeds common to other locations.

Other research found that goats rendered osteopenic via the same induction regimen responded osteogenically to a 9-month therapeutic biophysical intervention (extracorporeal shock wave stimulation).[109] Significantly more BMD (2.9%) was observed at the treated versus non-treated contralateral calcaneus; however, no effects of therapy were exhibited at the distal radius or femoral condyle sites that were similarly treated. Osteopenic goats have also been used to examine the effects of strontium and Ca,[110] and to test the mechanical strength of cemented screws used for implant fixation in the lumbar vertebrae.[111]

Scant attention has been given to determining whether changes occur in the cortical bone of OVX goats. Plexiform tissue predominates in the cortical bone of young goats and is remodeled to Haversian bone with advancing age. The distribution of Haversian systems in the long bones of goats has been described as heterogeneous.[91] Haversian tissue has been observed near the endocortical surface[91] and in the anterior, anterior-lateral, and medial sectors of diaphyses, whereas plexiform bone is primarily located in the posterior sector.[112] Mini- and micro-breeds of goats have yet to be explored as prospective animal models for osteoporosis research.

From a practical perspective goats are social creatures, very easily managed and trained, and readily obtainable. Temperate breeds are seasonally polyestrous and reach skeletal maturity when they are between 2 and 3 years old. As herbivorous polygastric ruminants, goats are affected by the same rumen-related complications as sheep and for the purpose of bone loss research, selectively grazing animals as well as laboratory fed animals need to be protected from ingesting phytoestrogen-containing vegetation or chaff. The shortage of data on osteopenic goats warrants further research in this model.

13.4.5 Pigs

Based on their comparative anatomy and physiology and pathophysiological responses, pigs have become a viable biomedical research model for numerous human diseases.[113] Like humans, pigs are true omnivores with a monogastric stomach and a similar digestive physiology[114] that makes them a particularly attractive model for studying metabolic diseases. It is well recognized that diet and nutrition affect bone and drug metabolism; therefore, depending on the research questions of interest, the dietary, gastrointestinal, and pharmacokinetic similarities between humans and pigs may increase the relevance of this model, over ruminant (goat and sheep) and carnivorous (dog) species.[68] To avoid obesity in a species originally bred to accumulate as much weight as possible, the diet of pigs should be appropriately regulated.[115] Pigs are sensitive, intelligent, vocal animals[116] that thrive optimally in an environment of positive social interaction. Bouts of stubborn or aggressive behavior can be minimized by establishing handling routines which lessen the stress on pigs and improve their manageability.

The utility of domestic/commercial pig breeds is somewhat limited by their rapid growth rate; by 4 months of age their body weight may reach 100–110 kg,[114] and adult weights can reach ≥200 kg.[117] From a practical and economic standpoint, such an enormous increase in size can preclude their use in longitudinal studies. Osteoporosis research necessitates animal models in which growth has plateaued, and for laboratory use the sheer bulk of mature domestic pigs creates considerable challenges. By design, varieties of miniature and micro-breeds of swine have been developed and these provide a convenient alternative. Also, the ever-increasing accessibility to genetically modified pigs only enhances their usefulness as a large animal model,[118] and continued breeding progress for the trait of low body weight in miniature pigs is anticipated.[119] Minipigs take ~2.4 times as long to grow to 40% of their mature weight as do intensely or restrictively fed fattening pigs.[120] At sexual maturity Göttingen minipigs weigh between 10 and 14 kg whereas larger breeds like the Hanford weigh 25–40 kg[114] and skeletally mature Yucatan minipigs weigh between 50 and 68 kg.[117,121] Micropigs, like the Panepinto breed, do not necessarily weigh less than minipigs. A slower growth trajectory early in life may decrease the amount of plexiform bone formed and increase the amount of osteonal bone present in mature mini-livestock, but this has yet to be confirmed. Smaller pigs have the advantage of consuming fewer resources, they require less space, yield smaller-size samples that take less time to analyze, and the amount of drugs administered to elicit an effect is less than for heavier animals.

The overall exposure of estrous cycling pigs to estrogen is higher than for many other large animal models; they are polyestrous and cycle approximately every 19.5 days. On average, circulating estradiol concentrations reach a peak of ~40 pg/ml, basal levels are between ~10–16 pg/ml, and post-ovariectomy concentrations drop to <10 pg/ml.[115,122-124] Osteonal remodeling in minipigs begins at 6 months or later and the osteons are similar in dimension to those of humans.[91,125] Skeletal maturity is attained by ~2–2.5 years of age[126] at body weights reasonably comparable to those of postmenopausal women. More morphological similarities to the human spine are evident in miniature pigs versus other species[10] and there exists a close similarity between the bone remodeling rates of pigs and humans.[127]

Most of the osteoporosis research on OVX pigs has focused on changes at the spine, a site at which the BMD of vertebral cancellous bone is substantially higher in pigs versus humans (0.39–0.43 mg/cm^3 versus 0.12–0.14 mg/cm^3). Moreover, vertebral trabecular separation in minipigs (200–300 μm) is less than that in pre- and postmenopausal women (500–700 and 700–1,000 μm, respectively), although trabeculae in this region are less thick in minipigs (~100 μm) than in humans (150–170 μm).[9] Young growing minipigs that were ovariectomized and placed on a Ca-restricted diet have been shown to exhibit thinner, yet less separated and more connected, trabeculae.[128] Gluer et al. concluded that this phenomenon was likely attributable to increased bone resorptive activity[9] whereby perforation of trabeculae plates initially converts them to more numerous rods. Based on this, minipigs may represent a good model in which to detect bone architectural deterioration.

Research on porcine models of bone loss has thus far not been consistently performed in suitably aged animals that are skeletally mature for the duration of the experiment. The age of sexual maturity in minipigs is between 6 and 10 months, whereas skeletal maturity is between ~24 and 36 months. Sinclair minipigs ovariectomized at 18 months of age and euthanized at 36 months demonstrated a lack of bone volume and/or architectural changes in L4 trabecular vertebral cores as measured by microcomputerized tomography (μCT) analysis.[129] Ongoing growth and development may have interfered with the ability to detect significant differences, although there was a definite response to the bisphosphonate therapy following ovariectomy. risedronate improved trabecular architecture and increased bone strength in OVX minipigs.

A 12-month pilot study was designed to examine the skeletal effects of diminishing Ca levels (normal Ca = 0.9% versus restricted Ca = 0.75% and 0.5% in the diet for 12 months) on sham versus OVX Sinclair minipigs.[122] The OVX pigs fed 0.75% and 0.5% dietary Ca increased endocortical resorption and decreased BMD at the midshaft of the femur and radius, although midfemur cortical bone histomorphometric parameters were not different among groups. Rib cortical bone geometry was also compromised following 0.5% and 0.75% Ca + ovariectomy. Moderate Ca restriction (0.75%) introduced 6 months prior to and continued for 6 months post ovariectomy was found to be the most effective treatment for stimulating vertebral bone loss (−10% areal BMD) and deteriorating vertebral architecture (Tb.N and Tb.Th) and mechanical strength. Ovariectomy combined with normal Ca, or ovariectomy alone, was sufficient to reduce the mineral apposition rate of cancellous bone versus sham controls, as was ovariectomy + 0.75% Ca. Limitations of this study included the use of sexually mature, rather than skeletally mature, minipigs, and feeding pigs a diet containing ~25% soymeal and alfalfa which are rich in endocrine-active phytoestrogens. Although pigs appear to show some real potential, more well-planned research is required in suitably aged animals to better determine their value as a model for osteoporosis.

Tetracycline (TC) is a veterinary agent/drug used prophylactically and/or therapeutically as a broad-spectrum antibiotic, particularly in swine production.[130] If administered for this purpose, its affinity for mineralizing bone surfaces could result in inadvertent fluorescent bands appearing in histological sections that may interfere with the interpretation of bone labels administered by investigators. Avoiding swine that have been routinely treated with TC is advisable to prevent superfluous bone labels.

13.5 Summary

The use of animals in scientific research has greatly advanced the development of medicine since ancient times.[131] To date, large animals as biomedical research models have been used by as many as 17 Nobel Prize winners, and scientists are continuing to advocate that federal agencies develop joint strategies to make economic funding allowances that further enable their use when it is appropriate.[132] NHPs are among the most relevant of large animal models in terms of mimicking human disease. However, many researchers often have to contend with budgetary and resource constraints, which usually compel them to select from agricultural and domestic species. Because no large animal can be a perfect substitute model of human disease, all anticipated limitations must be carefully considered so that the rationale for choosing the animal is an astute one that provides the researcher with the best possible opportunity to address and answer the questions being posed.

For osteoporosis research, skeletally mature animals are essential in order to avoid the numerous confounding factors that are introduced when animals are still growing and accruing bone. Significant and rapid bone loss in the event of ovary ablation and estrogen insufficiency, either with or without dietary/nutrition perturbations, are among the fundamental coveted traits. The extent to which the tissue-level mechanisms of bone loss in larger animals are similar to those of humans also deserves careful consideration. Moreover, it is important that researchers are able to intelligently and effectively manage larger animals in such a way that they become the source of highly reproducible data upon which reliable predictions relevant to prevention and therapeutic treatments can be made. Regardless of the large animal model selected, meticulous attention needs to be placed on nutritious and nonnutritious contents of diets in relation to the impact they may have on the experimental model because osteoporosis is a chronic disease that in general is both hormone- and nutrition-dependent. In the current financial climate in which funding is becoming increasingly limited, careful planning is paramount to both the conservation of resources and the acquisition of meaningful data from large animal models that will result in the advancements toward clinical trials.

References

1. Food and Drug Administration. Guidelines for preclinical and clinical evaluation agents used in the prevention or treatment of postmenopausal osteoporosis. In: Division of Metabolic and Endocrine Drug Products, ed. Rockville: Food and Drug Administration; 1994.
2. Wehrli FW, Ladinsky GA, Jones C, et al. *In vivo* magnetic resonance detects rapid remodeling changes in the topology of the trabecular bone network after menopause and the protective effect of estradiol. *J Bone Miner Res*. 2008;23:730-740.
3. Cohen AA. Female post-reproductive lifespan: a general mammalian trait. *Biol Rev*. 2004;79:733-750.
4. Reinwald S, Burr DB. Review of nonprimate, large animal models for osteoporosis research. *J Bone Miner Res*. 2008; 23:1353-1368.
5. Alexander C. Idiopathic osteoporosis: an evolutionary dysadaptation? *Ann Rheum Dis*. 2001;60:554-558.
6. Shih MS, Dixon J, Anderson C. The effects of chronic dietary calcium supplementation on bone mineral density in ovariectomized beagles. *Calcif Tissue Int*. 1988;43:122-124.
7. Skoyles JR. Human balance, the evolution of bipedalism and dysequilibrium syndrome. *Med Hypotheses*. 2006;66: 1060-1068.
8. Aerssens J, Boonen S, Lowet G, Dequeker J. Interspecies differences in bone composition, density, and quality: potential implications for *in vivo* bone research. *Endocrinology*. 1998;139:663-670.
9. Gluer CC, Scholz-Ahrens KE, Helfenstein A, et al. Ibandronate treatment reverses glucocorticoid-induced loss of bone mineral density and strength in minipigs. *Bone*. 2007;40:645-655.
10. McLain RF, Yerby SA, Moseley TA. Comparative morphometry of L4 vertebrae. *Spine*. 2002;27:E200-E206.
11. Shen V, Dempster DW, Birchman R, et al. Lack of changes in histomorphometric, bone mass, and biomechanical parameters in ovariohysterectomized dogs. *Bone*. 1992;13:311-316.
12. Dannucci G, Martin RB, Patterson-Buckendahl P. Ovariectomy and trabecular bone remodeling in the dog. *Calcif Tissue Int*. 1987;40:194-199.
13. Nakamura T, Nagai Y, Yamato H, Suzuki K, Orimo H. Regulation of bone turnover and prevention of bone atrophy in ovariectomized beagle dogs by the administration of 24R,25$(OH)_2D_3$. *Calcif Tissue Int*. 1992;50:221-227.
14. Faugere M-C, Friedler RM, Fanti P, Malluche HH. Bone changes occurring early after cessation of ovarian function in beagle dogs: a histomorphometric study employing sequential biopsies. *J Bone Miner Res*. 1990;5:263-272.
15. Monier-Faugere M-C, Friedler PM, Bauss F, Malluche HH. A new bisphosphonate, BM 21.0955, prevents bone loss associated with cessation of ovarian function in experimental dogs. *J Bone Miner Res*. 1993;8:1345-1355.
16. Monier-Faugere M-C, Geng Z, Qi Q, Arnala I, Malluche HH. Calcitonin prevents bone loss but decreases osteoblastic activity in ovariohysterectomized beagle dogs. *J Bone Miner Res*. 1996;11:446-453.
17. Malluche HH, Faugere MC, Rush M, Friedler R. Osteoblastic insufficiency is responsible for maintenance of osteopenia after loss of ovarian function in experimental beagle dogs. *Endocrinology*. 1986;119:2649-2654.
18. Boyce RW, Franks AF, Jankowsky ML, et al. Sequential histomorphometric changes in cancellous bone from ovariohysterectomized dogs. *J Bone Miner Res*. 1990;5:947-953.
19. Newton BI, Cooper RC, Gilbert JA, Johnson RB, Zardiackas LD. The ovariectomized sheep as a model for human bone loss. *J Comp Pathol*. 2004;130:323-326.
20. Sigrist HM, Gerhardt C, Alini M, Schneider E, Egermann M. The long-term effects of ovariectomy on bone metabolism in sheep. *J Bone Miner Metab*. 2007;25(1):28-35.

21. Pogoda P, Egermann M, Schnell JC, et al. Leptin inhibits bone formation not only in rodents but also in sheep. *J Bone Miner Res*. 2006;21:1591-1599.
22. Frost HM. The regional acceleratory phenomenon. *Henry Ford Hosp Med J*. 1983;31:3-9.
23. Heaney RP. Bone health. *Am J Clin Nutr*. 2007;85(1): 300S-303S.
24. Slauterbeck J, Clevenger C, Lundberg W, Burchfield DM. Estrogen level alters the failure load of the rabbit anterior cruciate ligament. *J Orthop Res*. 1999;17:405-408.
25. Castañeda S, Calvo E, Largo R, et al. Characterization of a new experimental model of osteoporosis in rabbits. *J Bone Miner Metab*. 2008;26(1):53-59.
26. Mori H, Manabe M, Kurachi Y, Nagumo M. Osseointegration of dental implants in rabbit bone with low mineral density. *J Oral Maxillofac Surg*. 1997;55:351-361.
27. Castañeda S, Largo R, Calvo E, et al. Bone mineral measurements of subcholndral and trabecular bone in healthy and osteoporotic rabbits. *Skeletal Radiol*. 2006;35:34-41.
28. Adaikan PG, Srilatha B, Wheat AJ. Efficacy of red clover isoflavones in the menopausal rabbit model. *Fertil Steril*. 2009;92(6):2008-2013.
29. Saito M, Marumo K, Soshi S, Kida Y, Ushiku C, Shinohara A. Raloxifene ameliorates detrimental enzymatic and nonenzymatic collagen cross-links and bone strength in rabbits with hyperhomocysteinemia. *Osteoporos Int*. 2010;21(4):655-666.
30. Eckermann-Ross C. Hormonal regulation and calcium metabolism in the rabbit. *Vet Clin North Am Exot Anim Pract*. 2008;11(1):139-152.
31. Committee on Animal Nutrition, National Research Council (U.S.). *Nutrient Requirements for Rabbits*. 2nd revised edition. Washington, DC: National Academies Press; 1977.
32. Stoker NG, Epker BN. Age changes in endosteal bone remodeling and balance in the rabbit. *J Dent Res*. 1970; 50:1570-1574.
33. Martiniaková M, Omelka R, Grosskopf B, Sirotkin A, Chrenek P. Sex-related variation in compact bone microstructure of the femoral diaphysis in juvenile rabbits. *Acta Vet Scand*. 2008;50(1):15.
34. Martiniaková M, Omelka R, Chrenek P, Vondráková M, Buauerová M. Age-related changes in histological structure of the femur in juvenile and adult rabbits. *Bull Vet Inst Pulawy*. 2005;49:227-230.
35. Martiniaková M, Vondráková M, Fabiš M. Investigation of the microscopic structure of rabbit compact bone tissue. *Scripta Med (BRNO)*. 2003;76:215-220.
36. Martiniaková M, Omelka R, Ryban L, et al. Comparative study of compact bone tissue microstructure between nontransgenic and transgenic rabbits with WAP-hFVIII gene construct. *Anat Histol Embryol*. 2006;35(5):310-315.
37. Mashiba T, Burr DB, Turner CH, Sato M, Cain RL, Hock JM. Effects of human parathyroid hormone (1–34), LY333334, on bone mass, remodeling, and material properties of cortical bone during the first remodeling cycle in rabbits. *Bone*. 2001;28:538-547.
38. Pearce AI, Richards RG, Milz S, Schneider E, Pearce SG. Animal models from implant biomaterial research in bone: a review. *Eur Cell Mater*. 2007;13:1-10.
39. Martin RK, Albright JP, Jee WSS, Taylor GN, Clarke WR. Bone loss in the beagle tibia: influence of age, weight, and sex. *Calcif Tissue Int*. 1981;33:233-238.
40. Boyce RW, Paddock CL, Gleason JR, Sletsema WK, Eriksen EF. The effects of risedronate on canine cancellous bone remodeling: three-dimensional kinetic reconstruction of the remodeling site. *J Bone Miner Res*. 1995;10:211-221.
41. Kimmel DB, Moran EL, Bogoch ER. Animal models of osteopenia or osteoporosis. In: Yuehuei HA, Friedman RJ, eds. *Animal Models in Orthopaedic Research*. Boca Raton: CRC; 1999:280-305.
42. Kimmel DB, Jee WSSS. A quantitative histologic study of bone turnover in young adult beagles. *Anat Rec*. 1982;203: 31-45.
43. Kimmel DB. The oophorectomized beagle as an experimental model for estrogen-deplete bone loss in the adult human. *Eur Cell Mater*. 1991;suppl 1:75-84.
44. Wilson AK, Bhattacharyya MH, Miller S, Mani A, Sacco-Gibson N. Ovariectomy-induced changes in aged beagles: histomorphometry of rib cortical bone. *Calcif Tissue Int*. 1998;62:237-243.
45. Martin RB, Butcher RL, Sherwood LL, et al. Effects of ovariectomy in beagle dogs. *Bone*. 1987;8:23-31.
46. Motoie H, Kanoh H, Ogata S, Kawamuki K, Shikama H, Fujikura T. Prevention of bone loss by bisphosphonate YM175 in ovariectomized dogs with dietary calcium restriction. *Jpn J Pharmacol*. 1996;71(3):239-246.
47. Martin RB, Chow BD, Lucas PA. Bone marrow fat content in relation to bone remodeling and serum chemistry in intact and ovariectomized dogs. *Calcif Tissue Int*. 1990;46:189-194.
48. Monier-Faugere M-C, Geng Z, Paschalis E, et al. Intermittent and continuous administration of the bisphosphonate ibandronate in ovariohysterectomized beagle dogs: effects on bone morphometry and mineral properties. *J Bone Miner Res*. 1999;14:1768-1778.
49. Yoshida Y, Moriya A, Kitamura K, et al. Responses of trabecular and cortical bone turnover and bone mass and strength to bisphosphonates YH529 in ovariectomized beagles with calcium restriction. *J Bone Miner Res*. 1998;13(6): 1011-1022.
50. Snow GR, Cook MA, Anderson C. Oophorectomy and cortical bone remodeling in the beagle. *Calcif Tissue Int*. 1984;36:586-590.
51. Nagai S, Shindo H. Mechanical strength of bone in canine osteoporosis model: relationship between bone mineral content and bone fragility. *J Orthop Sci*. 1997;2(6):428-433.
52. Ekici H, Sontas BH, Toydemir TSF, Senmevsim O, Kabasakal L, Imre Y. The effect of prepubertal ovariohysterectomy on spine mineral density and mineral content of puppies: a preliminary study. *Res Vet Sci*. 2007;82:105-109.
53. Cook SD, Skinner HB, Haddad RJ. A quantitative histologic study of osteoporosis produced by nutritional secondary hyperparathyroidism in dogs. *Clin Orthop Relat Res*. 1982; 175:105-120.
54. Karambolova KK, Snow GR, Anderson C. Effects of continuous 17β-estradiol administration on the periosteal and corticoendosteal envelope activity in spayed beagles. *Calcif Tissue Int*. 1987;40:12-15.
55. Anderson C. Bone remodeling rates of the beagle: a comparison between different sites on the same rib. *Am J Vet Res*. 1978;39:1763-1765.
56. Van Goethem B, Schaefers-Okkens A, Kirpensteijn J. Making a rational choice between ovariectomy and ovariohysterectomy in the dog: a discussion of the benefits of either technique. *Vet Surg*. 2006;35:136-143.
57. Snow GR, Anderson C. The effects of continuous progestogen treatment on cortical bone remodeling activity in beagles. *Calcif Tissue Int*. 1985;37(3):282-286.

58. Cerundolo R, Court MH, Hao Q, Michel KE. Identification and concentration of soy phytoestrogens in commercial dog foods. *Am J Vet Res*. 2004;65(5):592-596.
59. Brown NM, Setchell KDR. Animal models impacted by phytoestrogens in commercial chow: implications for pathways influenced by hormones. *Lab Invest*. 2001;81: 735-747.
60. Reinwald S, Weaver CM. Soy isoflavones and bone health: a double-edged sword? *J Nat Prod*. 2006;69:450-459.
61. Gershoff SN, Legg MA, Hegsted DM. Adaptation to different calcium intakes in dogs. *J Nutr*. 1958;64(2):303-312.
62. Subcommittee on Dog Nutrition, Committee on Animal Nutrition, Board on Agriculture, National Research Council. Nutrient requirements and signs of deficiency. In: *Nutrient Requirements of Dogs* Revised 1985. Washington, DC: National Academy Press; 1985.
63. Motoie H, Nakamura T, O'uchi N, Nishikawa H, Kanoh H, Kawashima H. Effects of bisphosphonate YM175 on bone mineral density, strength, structure, and turnover in ovariectomized beagles on concommitant dietary calcium restriction. *J Bone Miner Res*. 1995;10(6):910-920.
64. Ismail AA, Silman AJ, Reeve J, Kaptope S, O'Neill TW. Rib fractures predict incident limb fractures: results from the European prospective osteoporosis study. *Osteoporos Int*. 2006;17:41-45.
65. Kim J, Breur GJ. Temporospatial and kinetic characteristics of sheep walking on a pressure sensing walkway. *Can J Vet Res*. 2008;72:50-55.
66. Yamaura M, Nakamura T, Nagai Y, Yoshihara A, Suzuki K. Reduced mechanical competence of bone by ovariectomy and its preservation with 24R, 25-dihydroxyvitamin D3 administration in beagles. *Calcif Tissue Int*. 1993; 52:49-56.
67. Bradshaw JWS. The evolutionary basis for the feeding behavior of domestic dogs (*Canis familiaris*) and cats (*Felis catus*). *J Nutr*. 2006;136(suppl 7):1927S-1931S.
68. Lehmann H. The minipig in general toxicology. *Scand J Lab Anim*. 1998;25:59-62.
69. Acke E, Mooney CT, Jones BR. Oestrogen toxicity in a dog. *Ir Vet J*. 2003;56:465-468.
70. Zayed I, van Esch E, McConnel RF. Systemic and histopathologic changes in beagle dogs after chronic daily oral administration of synthetic (ethinyl estradiol) or natural (estradiol) estrogens, with special reference to the kidney and thyroid. *Toxicol Pathol*. 1998;26:730-741.
71. Dunayer E, Volmer PA. Ibuprofen toxicosis in dogs, cats, and ferrets. *Vet Med*. 2004;99:580-586.
72. Villar D, Buck WB, Gonzalez JM. Ibuprofen, aspirin and acetaminophen toxicosis and treatment in dogs and cats. *Vet Hum Toxicol*. 1998;40:156-162.
73. Chung J-Y, Choi J-H, Hwang C-Y, Youn H-Y. Pyridoxine induced neuropathy by subcutaneous administration in dogs. *J Vet Sci*. 2008;9:127-131.
74. Baroni E, Camisa B, D'Ambrosio D. Inter-species differences in sensitivity to the calcemic activity of the novel 1,25-dihydroxyvitamin D3 analog BXL746. *Regul Toxicol Pharmacol*. 2008;52:332-341.
75. Malluche HH, Faugere MC, Friedler RM, Fanti P. 1,25-dihydroxyvitamin D3 corrects bone loss but suppresses bone remodeling in ovariohysterectomized beagle dogs. *Endocrinology*. 1988;122:1998-2006.
76. Johnson RB, Gilbert JA, Cooper RC, et al. Effect of estrogen deficiency on skeletal and alveolar bone density in sheep. *J Periodontol*. 2002;73:383-391.
77. Egermann M, Goldhahn J, Holz R, Schneider E, Lill CA. A sheep model for fracture treatment in osteoporosis: benefits of the model versus animal welfare. *Lab Anim*. 2008;42: 453-464.
78. Arens D, Sigrist I, Alini M, Schawalder P, Schneider E, Egermann M. Seasonal changes in bone metabolism in sheep. *Vet J*. 2007;174:585-591.
79. Turner SA. Seasonal changes in bone metabolism in sheep: further characterization of an animal model for human osteoporosis. *Vet J*. 2007;174:460-461.
80. Hornby SB, Ford SL, Mase CA, Evans GP. Skeletal changes in the ovariectomized ewe and subsequent response to treatment with 17β oestradiol. *Bone*. 1995;17: 389S-394S.
81. Lans C, Khan TE, Curran MM, McCorkle CM. Plant chemistry in veterinary medicine: medicinal constituents and their mechanisms of action. In: Wynn SG, Fougere B, eds. *Veterinary Herbal Medicine*. USA: Elsevier Health Sciences; Mosby, Inc. St. Louis, Missouri, 2007:159-182.
82. Croker K, Nichols P, Barbetti M, Adams N. Sheep infertility from pasture legumes. In: Department of Agriculture Farmnote; 2005 http://www.agric.wa.gov.au/objtwr/imported_assets/content/aap/sl/hea/sheepinfertfarmnote.pdf.
83. Chavassieux P, Garnero P, Duboeuf F, et al. Effects of a new selective estrogen receptor modulator (MDL 103,323) on cancellous and cortical bone in ovariectomized ewes: a biochemical, histomorphometric, and densitometric study. *J Bone Miner Res*. 2001;16:89-96.
84. Fabre-Nys C, Gelez H. Sexual behavior in ewes and other domestic ruminants. *Horm Behav*. 2007;52:18-25.
85. Wilkinson JM. Silage and animal health. *Nat Toxins*. 1999; 7:221-232.
86. Page S, Hennessy D. Pharmacology and therapeutics. In: Aitken ID, ed. *Diseases of Sheep*. 4th ed. Oxford: Blackwell; 2007: 544-572.
87. Radostits OM, Gay CC, Blood DC, Arundel JH, Hinchcliff KW. Practical usage of antimicrobial drugs. In: *Veterinary Medicine*. 9th ed. Philadelphia: W.B. Saunders; 2000:159.
88. Martini L, Fini M, Giavaresi G, Giardino R. Sheep model in orthopaedic research: a literature review. *Comp Med*. 2001; 51:292-299.
89. Martin RB, Burr, DB, Sharkey NA. Skeletal *Tissue Mechanics*. New York: Springer; 1998.
90. Turner AS. The sheep as a model for osteoporosis in humans. *Vet J*. 2002;163:232-239.
91. Hillier ML, Bell LS. Differentiating human bone from animal bone: a review of histological methods. *J Forensic Sci*. 2006;52:249-263.
92. Kennedy OD, Brennan O, Rackard SM, et al. Effects of ovariectomy on bone turnover, porosity, and biomechanical properties in ovine compact bone 12 months postsurgery. *J Orthop Res*. 2009;27:303-309.
93. Rocca M, Fini M, Giavaresi G, Aldini NN, Giardino R. Osteointegration of hydroxyapatite-coated and uncoated titanium screws in long-term ovariectomized sheep. *Biomaterials*. 2002;23:1017-1023.
94. Turner AS, Alvis M, Myers W, Stevens ML, Lundy MW. Changes in bone mineral density and bone-specific alkaline

phosphate in ovariectomized ewes. *Bone*. 1995;17: 395S-402S.

95. Wu Z-X, Lei W, Hu Y-Y, et al. Effect of ovariectomy on BMD, micro-architecture and biomechanics of cortical and cancellous bones in a sheep model. *Med Eng Phys*. 2008;30:1112-1118.
96. Giavaresi G, Fini M, Torricelli P, Giardino R. The ovariectomized ewe model in the evaluation of biomaterials for prosthetic devices in spinal fixation. *Int J Artif Organs*. 2001;24:814-820.
97. Goldhahn J, Jenet A, Schneider E, Techn D, Christoph AL. Slow rebound of cancellous bone after mainly steroid-induced osteoporosis in ovariectomized sheep. *J Orthop Trauma*. 2005;19:23-28.
98. Lill CA, Fluegel AK, Schneider E. Effect of ovariectomy, malnutrition and glucocorticoid application on bone properties in sheep: a pilot study. *Osteoporos Int*. 2002;13: 480-486.
99. MacLeay JM, Olson JD, Turner AS. Effect of dietary-induced metabloic acidosis and ovariectomy on bone mineral density and markers of bone turnover. *J Bone Miner Metab*. 2004;22:561-568.
100. Fulton LK, Clarke MS, Farris HE. The goat as a research model for biomedical research and teaching. *ILAR J*. 1994;36(2):21-29.
101. Morand-Fehr P, Lebbie SHB. Proposals for improving the research efficiency in goats. *Small Rumin Res*. 2004;51: 145-153.
102. Li L, Chen H, Wu W, Chen M, Weng L, Zheng H. Biomechanical property changes of long bone in ovariectomized goats. *Sheng Wu Yi Xue Gong Cheng Xue Za Zhi = Journal of Biomedical Engineering Perhaps it can be abbreviated to: J Biomed Eng*. 1998;15:101-115.
103. Li L, Wu W, Chen H, Tan J, Zheng H, Weng L. Bone histomorphometric changes in ovariectomized goat at different time courses. *Hua xi yi ke da xue xue bao = Journal of West China University of Medical Sciences*. Perhaps it can be abbreviated to: *J West China Uni Med Sci. Acronym = WCUMS*. 1997;28:398-400.
104. He C, Chen H, Li L, Chen M, Chen Y, Wu W. Changes of biomedical properties in goats at different times after ovariectomy. *Sheng Wu Yi Xue Gong Cheng Xue Za Zhi = Journal of Biomedical Engineering Perhaps it can be abbreviated to: J Biomed Eng*. 1999;16:295-299.
105. He Y, Sun XC, Chen HQ, Weng LL, Zheng H, Qui MC. Bone histomorphometry study on lumbar vertebrae microstructure of ovariectomized goats. *Zhonghua Fu Chan Ke Za Zhi*. 2003;38:405-408.
106. Yonezawa T, Mogi K, Li JY, Sako R, Yamanouchi K, Nishihara M. Modulation of growth hormone pulsatility by sex steroids in female goats. *Endocrinology*. 2005;146: 2736-2743.
107. Leung KS, Siu WS, Cheung NM, et al. Goats as an osteopenic animal model. *J Bone Miner Res*. 2001;16: 2348-2355.
108. Siu WS, Qin L, Cheung WH, Leung KS. A study of trabecular bones in ovariectomized goats with micro-computed tomography and peripheral quantitative computed tomography. *Bone*. 2004;35:21-26.
109. Tam KF, Cheung WH, Lee KM, Qin L, Leung KS. Shockwave exerts osteogenic effect on osteoporotic bone in an ovariectomized goat model. *Ultrasound Med Biol*. 2009;35:1109-1118.
110. Li Z, Lu WW, Chiu PKY, et al. Strontium-calcium coadministration stimulates bone matrix osteogenic factor expression and new bone formation in a large animal model. *J Orthop Res*. 2008;27:758-762.
111. Leung KS, Siu WS, Li SF, et al. An *in vitro* optimized injectable calcium phosphate cement for augmenting screw fixation in osteopenic goats. *J Biomed Mater Res B Appl Biomater*. 2005;78B:153-160.
112. Qin L, Mak ATF, Cheng CW, Hung LK, Chan KM. Histomorphological study on pattern of fluid movement in cortical bone in goats. *Anat Rec*. 1999;255:380-387.
113. Almond GW. Research applications using pigs. *Vet Clin North Am Food Anim Pract*. 1996;12:707-716.
114. Smith AC, Swindle MM. Preparation of swine for the laboratory. *ILAR J*. 2006;47:358-363.
115. Laber KE, Whary MT, Bingel SA, Goodrich JA, Smith AC, Swindle MM. Biology and diseases in swine. In: Fox JG, Anderson LC, Loew FM, Quimby FW, eds. *Laboratory Animal Medicine*. 2nd ed. San Diego: Academic; 2002: 615-673.
116. Kattelmann L, Epperson W, Chase C. Swine veterinarians and hearing loss: summary of results of audiology testing at the 2002 AASV annual meeting. *J Swine Health Prod*. 2005;13:34-37.
117. Estrada JL, Collins B, York A, et al. Successful cloning of the Yucatan minipig using commercial/occidental breeds as oocyte donors and embryo recipients. *Cloning Stem Cells*. 2008;10:287-297.
118. Dehoux JP, Gianello P. The importance of large animal models in transplantation. *Front Biosci*. 2007;12:4864-4880.
119. Kohn F, Sharifi AR, Malovrh S, Simianer H. Estimation of genetic parameters for body weight of the Goettingen minipig with random regression models. *J Anim Sci*. 2007;85:2423-2428.
120. Kohn F, Sharifi AR, Simianer H. Modeling the growth of the Göettingen minipig. *J Anim Sci*. 2007;85:84-92.
121. Muehleman AC, Li AJ, Abe AY, et al. Effect of risedronate in a minipig cartilage defect model with allograft. *J Orthop Res*. 2009;27:360-365.
122. Mosekilde L, Weisbrode SE, Safron JA, et al. Evaluation of the skeletal effects of combined mild dietary calcium restriction and ovariectomy in Sinclair S-1 minipigs: a pilot study. *J Bone Miner Res*. 1993;8:1311-1321.
123. Howard PK, Chakraborty PK, Camp JC, Stuart LD, Wildt DE. Pituitary-ovarian relationships during the estrous cycle and the influence of parity in an inbred strain of miniature swine. *J Anim Sci*. 1983;57:1517-1524.
124. Keaney JFJ, Shwaery GT, Xu A, et al. Lipids:17 beta-estradiol preserves endothelial vasodilator function and limits low-density lipoprotein oxidation in hypercholesterolemic swine. *Circulation*. 1994;85:2251-2259.
125. Martiniakova M, Grosskopf B, Omelka R, Vondrakova M. Differences among species in compact bone tissue microstructure of mammalian skeleton: use of a discriminant function analysis for species identification. *J Forensic Sci*. 2006;51:1235-1239.
126. Larsen MO, Rolin B. Use of the Göttingen minipig as a model of diabetes with special focus on type 1 diabetes research. *ILAR J*. 2004;45:303-313.

127. Martínez-González JM, Cano-Sánchez J, Campo-Trapero J, Gonzalo-Lafuente JC, Díaz-Reganon J, Vázquez-Pineiro MT. Evaluation of minipigs as an animal model for alveolar distraction. *Oral Surg Oral Med Oral Pathol Oral Radiol Endod*. 2005;99:11-16.
128. Boyce RW, Ebert DC, Youngs TA, et al. Unbiased estimation of vertebral trabecular connectivity in calcium-restricted ovariectomized minipigs. *Bone*. 1995;16:637-642.
129. Borah B, Dufresne TE, Chmielewski PA, Gross GJ, Prenger MC, Phipps RJ. Risedronate preserves trabecular architecture and increases bone strength in vertebra of ovariectomized minipigs as measured by three-dimensional microcomputed tomography. *J Bone Miner Res*. 2002; 17:1139-1147.
130. Mackie RI, Koike S, Krapac I, Chee-Sanford J, Maxwell S, Aminov RI. Tetracycline residues and tetracycline resistance genes in groundwater impacted by swine production facilities. *Anim Biotechnol*. 2006;17:157-176.
131. Baumans V. Use of animals in experimental research: an ethical dilemma? *Gene Ther*. 2004;11:S64-S66.
132. Roberts RM, Smith GW, Bazer FW, et al. Farm animal research in crisis. *Science*. 2009;324:468-469.

Mouse Models for the Study of Fracture Healing and Bone Regeneration

14

Joerg H. Holstein, Patric Garcia, Tina Histing, Moritz Klein, Steven C. Becker, Michael D. Menger, and Tim Pohlemann

14.1 Introduction

Fragility fractures represent one of the major problems associated with osteoporosis. While in the mid-1990s about half a million hospital admissions in the United States were due to osteoporotic fractures, this number will triple until 2040. Of interest, already in 1995, the direct costs produced by osteoporotic fractures were more than US$14 billion, whereas the indirect costs are estimated to be up to five times higher.[1] These alarming numbers highlight the enormous relevance of osteoporotic fractures for our society.

One objective of research on osteoporosis must be identifying ways to reduce the incidence of fragility fractures. Besides, however, there is also an essential need to improve the outcome of the treatment of osteoporotic fractures. So far, 20% of patients with osteoporotic fractures do not survive the first year after trauma, mostly because of secondary complications related to long-term hospitalization.[2,3] This poor outcome is at least partially a result of two still not satisfactorily solved issues. The first issue is the high failure rate of implants in osteoporotic bones.[4,5] The reduced bone mineral density (BMD) and the altered microarchitecture of osteoporotic bone lead to a reduced primary stability of the osteosynthesis and hence an increased risk for a secondary "cutout" or "pullout" of the implant. The diminished stability of an osteosynthesis in osteoporotic bone delays the mobilization of mostly older patients and raises the risk of implant loosening. The second challenge in the treatment of osteoporotic fractures derives from the reduced healing capacity of osteoporotic bone.[6-9] So far, there is only very limited information on the reasons for the difference between bone regeneration in osteoporotic and non-osteoporotic bone. However, *in vitro* studies have demonstrated changes in the remodeling cycle, and the sensitivity of osteoblasts to cyclic strains related to osteoporosis.[6] Additional animal studies have indicated an altered callus formation associated with osteoporosis.[7-9]

Although *in vitro* studies provide valuable information on cellular behavior related to osteoporosis, only animal models allow the investigation of the complex mechanisms involved in fracture healing and the impact of osteoporosis on bone repair. Besides, animal models serve as an important tool for the development and evaluation of new implants for an improved fixation of fractures in osteoporotic bones.

This chapter focuses on the values and limitations of mouse models for the study of fracture healing in osteoporotic bone. An additional objective of this chapter is to provide an overview of different murine fracture models and to evaluate the applicability of these models for research on the regeneration of osteoporotic bone.

14.2 The Value of Mouse Models for the Study of Fracture Healing in Osteoporotic Bone

Numerous animal models have been introduced to study fracture healing and bone regeneration.[10-16] When using animal models, however, differences in

J.H. Holstein (✉)
Department of Trauma, Hand and Reconstructive Surgery, University of Saarland, Saarland, Germany
e-mail: joerg.holstein@uks.eu

G. Duque and K. Watanabe (eds.), *Osteoporosis Research*,
DOI: 10.1007/978-0-85729-293-3_14,

size, anatomy, bone morphology, and metabolism between animals and humans have to be addressed in the experimental setup and interpretation of the experimental data.[17]

With regard to the applicability of an animal model to develop and evaluate new implants designed for fracture stabilization in humans, the skeletal size, anatomy, and morphology of the animal must be comparable to that of humans.[17,18] Because only large animals fulfill these requirements, small animals such as mice are inappropriate to serve as a model for human implant testing.[18]

Osteoporosis is characterized by altered biomechanical bone properties, which are caused by a decreased BMD, an impaired micro-architecture of cancellous bone, and a thinning and increased porosity of cortical bone.[19,20] Of interest, all of these parameters have been demonstrated to determine the stability of the bone–implant compound. While the quality of an osteosynthesis for metaphyseal or spinal fractures strongly depends on BMD and trabecular architecture, cortical thickness and porosity affect the stability of an osteosynthesis for diaphyseal fractures.[18] Tables 14.1–14.4 show differences of biomechanical properties, BMD, trabecular micro-architecture, and cortical thickness and porosity between osteoporotic and non-osteoporotic bones in humans and different animals. Studies that are designed to analyze human implants for the fixation of metaphyseal fractures should use animal models that show BMD and trabecular micro-architecture comparable to that of humans. In contrast, implants for the fixation of cortical bone should be tested in animals with human-like values of cortical thickness and porosity.

Differences in bone properties between osteoporotic animals and controls have to be considered both when evaluating implants for the fixation of osteoporotic bones and when investigating the biology of fracture healing in osteoporotic bones. Of interest, animal-specific alterations of bone parameters associated with osteoporosis show a huge variation without significant differences between large animals and mice (Tables 14.1–14.4). From this point of view, mouse models are not less appropriate to analyze fracture repair in osteoporotic bone than are large animal models.

With regard to bone morphology, it has to be considered that a Haversian system is lacking in mice. However, resorption cavities, which are used for bone remodeling during fracture healing in mice, have been shown to be very similar to the Haversian remodeling in larger animals.[17] Therefore, the common argument that mice are inappropriate for studies on bone healing because they lack a Haversian system is not correct. Moreover, there are several reasons why mice have become models of increasing interest for fracture healing studies. Of utmost importance, a broad spectrum of antibodies is available for mice, and they are gene-targeted animals, which both allow studies on molecular mechanisms of bone healing.[21-23] In addition, the expenses for purchase, breeding, and holding of mice are relatively low.

Table 14.1 Biomechanical bone properties in humans and different animal species

Species	Parameter	Δ	Region	Method	Model
Human[73]	3.3 MPa	−24%	Femur head	Compression	
Human[74]	0.1 MPa	−18%	Femur shaft	Tension	
Primate[75]	1.4 kN	−12%	Femur head	Compression	OVX
Primate[76]	3.8 Nm	−28%	Tibia shaft	Torsion	OVX
Primate[75]	2.6 kN	−18%	Spine	Compression	OVX
Sheep[77]	3.2 kN	−40%	Spine	Compression	OVX + steroid
Rat[78]	78 Nm	−7%	Femur shaft	Torsion	ORCH
Rat[79]	330 N	−36%	Spine	Compression	OVX
Rat[80]	86 N	−16%	Femur neck	Failure load	OVX
Mice[81]	80 N	±0%	Spine	Compression	SAMP6
Mice[82]	34 Nm	−37%	Femur shaft	Torsion	SAMP6

Δ mean difference of biomechanical bone properties between osteoporotic and non-osteoporotic humans/animals, *OVX* ovariectomy, *ORCH* orchidectomy, *SAMP6* senescence-accelerated mouse prone 6

Table 14.2 Bone mineral density (BMD) in humans and different animal species

Species	BMD	Δ	Region	Method	Model
Human[73]	0.47 g/cm³	−19%	Femur head	Wet weight	
Human[83]	0.16 g/cm³	−42%	Distal radius	pQCT	
Human[84]	1.08 g/cm²	−26%	Spine	DEXA	
Primate[76]	1.33 g/cm³	−2%	Femur head	Wet weight	OVX
Primate[85]	1.14 g/cm²	−11%	Spine	DEXA	OVX
Sheep[77]	0.63 g/cm³	−33%	Radius	pQCT	OVX+steroids
Sheep[77]	0.62 g/cm³	−13%	Spine	pQCT	OVX+steroids
Dog[86]	0.58 g/cm²	±0%	Spine	DEXA	OVX
Rat[87]	0.25 g/cm²	−7%	Femur	DEXA	OVX
Mice[88]	0.07 g/cm²	−14%	Whole body	DEXA	SAMP6

Δ mean difference of BMD between osteoporotic and non-osteoporotic humans/animals, *pQCT* peripheral quantitative computed tomography, *DEXA* dual energy x-ray absorptiometry, *OVX* ovariectomy, *SAMP6* senescence-accelerated mouse prone 6

Table 14.3 Histomorphometric parameters of cancellous bone in humans and different animal species

Species	BV/TV (%)	Tb.N (mm⁻¹)	Tb.Th (μm)	Tb.Sp (μm)	Model
Human (iliac crest)[89]	21 (−34%)	1.5 (−27%)	138 (−10%)	654 (+11%)	
Sheep (Iliac crest)[90]	25 (−12%)	2.0 (−5%)	127 (−7%)	381 (+14%)	OVX
Sheep (iliac crest)[77]	21 (−57%)	1.6 (−25%)	140 (−50%)	521 (+48%)	OVX+steroids
Rat (tibia)[91]	24 (−63%)	5.8 (−41%)	69 (−28)	178 (+67%)	OVX
Mice (spine)[81]	21 (−34%)	4.3 (−19%)	73 (−8%)	241(+23%)	SAMP6

BV/TV bone volume density, *Tb.N* trabecular number, *Tb.Th* trabecular thickness, *Tb.Sp* trabecular spacing, *OVX* ovariectomy, *SAMP6* senescence-accelerated mouse prone 6

Table 14.4 Cortical thickness and porosity in humans and different animal species

Species	Thickness (μm)	Porosity (%)	Region	Model
Human[92]	Not reported	4.5 (+113%)	Femur	
Human[20]	1,100 (−32%)	2.8 (+121%)	Iliac crest	
Human[93]	290 (−30%)	Not reported	Spine	
Primate[94]	1,750 (−9%)	1.3 (+100%)	Humerus	OVX
Sheep[95]	487 (−9%)	1.0 (+180%)	Iliac crest	OVX
Dog[96]	Not reported	2.2 (+132%)	Rib	OVX
Rat[97]	560 (+1%)	0.7 (+86%)	Femur	OVX
Mice[98]	182 (−4%)	Not reported	Femur	SAMP6
Mice[98]	161 (−5%)	Not reported	Tibia	SAMP6

OVX ovariectomy, *SAMP6* senescence-accelerated mouse prone 6

Thus, the implementation of larger groups in the experimental study design is more feasible. An additional advantage of mouse models when compared to larger animals is the reduced time course of fracture healing.[24]

Because of the small size of mice, the manufacturing of implants is technically demanding and the surgery requires sophisticated skills. Highly sensitive testing devices are necessary to detect minor differences in the biomechanical properties of the small and fragile mouse bones. The implementation of biomechanical testing is also challenging because minor deviations in the testing setup may significantly affect the test results.[24]

For studies on fracture healing, only animals with growth plate closure (in mice >5 months of age) should be used, since the age of the animals critically affects bone regeneration.[25] Of interest, the ratio of age at growth plate closure and life expectancy is quite comparable in mice and humans (about 20%), while it markedly differs in other species such as rats (30%), rabbits, dogs, and sheep (5–10%).[26]

14.3 Anatomical and Surgical Considerations in Mouse Models for the Study of Fracture Healing in Osteoporotic Bone

Technically and surgically, the small size of mice is challenging (length of femur: 15 mm, outer diameter of femur: 1.5 mm). Therefore, large long bones, such as the femur and the tibia (Fig. 14.1), are most suitable for studies on bone repair.[14,27] The rib, radius, ulna, mandible, and calvarium have been used for studies on bone repair as well.[28-33] However, fracture stabilization or biomechanical testing is so far not applicable in those small and irregularly shaped bones.

In most mouse models, midshaft fractures are used to analyze bone repair. As osteoporosis leads to an increased porosity and thinning of cortical bone, these models are appropriate to investigate the effect of osteoporosis on cortical bone repair. The tibia fracture model, described by Hiltunen and coworkers, has been one of the first diaphyseal fracture models in mice.[14] Because the diameter of the tibia decreases from proximal to distal, callus size is larger in the proximal than in the distal tibia. This anatomical condition is disadvantageous when using closed fracture models, in which the fracture localization cannot be determined exactly. Thus, different fracture sites resulting in markedly different callus sizes limit the standardization and comparability of bone repair in closed tibia fracture models.[24]

Further anatomical drawbacks of the tibia are its triangular cross section and bent longitudinal axis (Fig. 14.1), which demand a more sophisticated design for implants and limit biomechanical test accuracy. Because of its thin soft tissue cover, the tibia is relatively easy to fracture. However, this anatomical condition is disadvantageous when analyzing the role of soft tissue in bone repair. A further issue that has to be addressed is the role of the fibula (Fig. 14.1). To induce a closed tibial midshaft fracture, the fibula may also break, which results in either two different calluses or one combined callus, and thus limits the comparability of bone repair between different animals (Fig. 14.2). In accordance, we recommend using only open tibia fracture models, in which an additional fibular fracture can be avoided and an exact definition of the fracture localization is possible.[24]

The mouse femur has a circular cross section with a relatively consistent inner and outer diameter and a straight longitudinal axis (Fig. 14.1). Therefore, different fracture sites of the diaphysis induce comparable callus responses (Fig. 14.2). Because of its favorable anatomy, biomechanical testing is also more feasible in the femur than in the tibia. The thick muscle layer covering the femur makes the production of a fracture technically and surgically more difficult, but is on the other hand an essential anatomical condition to investigate the role of soft tissue during bone repair. In conclusion, the femur is – from the anatomical and surgical viewpoint – the most suitable bone to study the effect of osteoporosis on cortical fracture healing in mice.

Diaphyseal fracture models, which are most established in mice, are appropriate for studies on cortical bone healing. However, only metaphyseal fracture models are suitable to investigate the impact of osteoporosis on cancellous bone healing.[18] In 2001, Uusitalo and

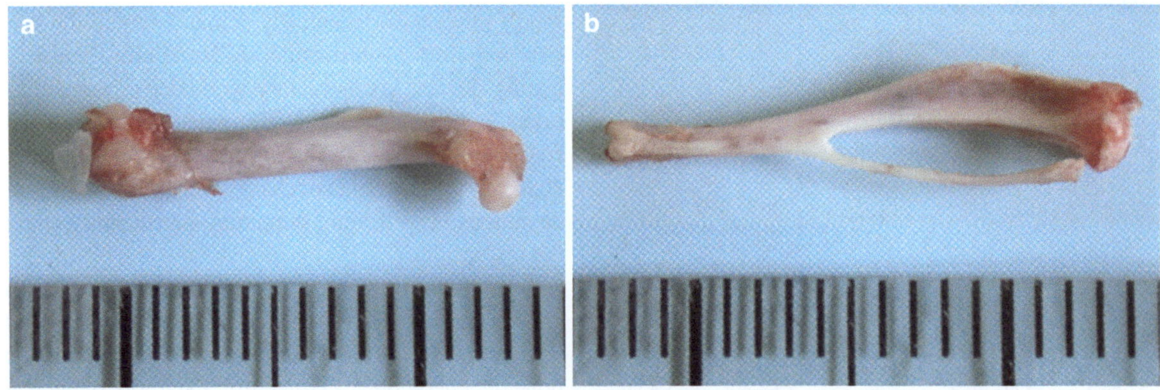

Fig. 14.1 The mouse femur (**a**) and the mouse tibia with fibula (**b**).[24] The mouse femur has a circular and consistent diameter, while the diameter of the tibia is triangular and decreases from proximal to distal

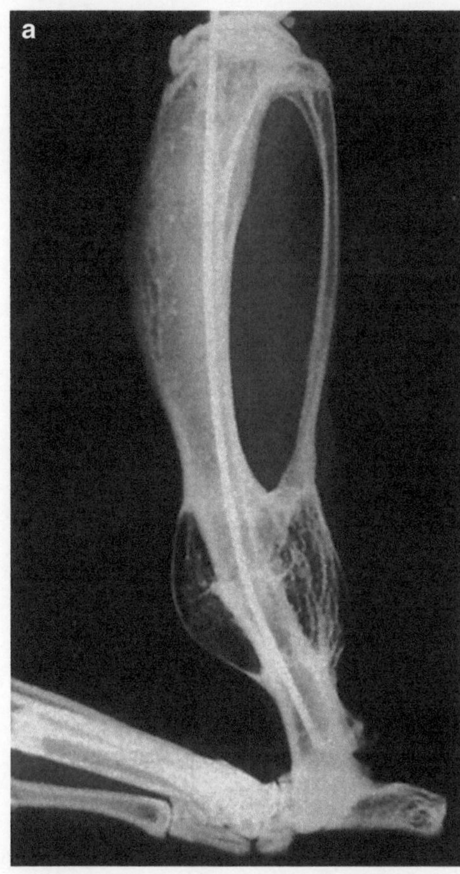

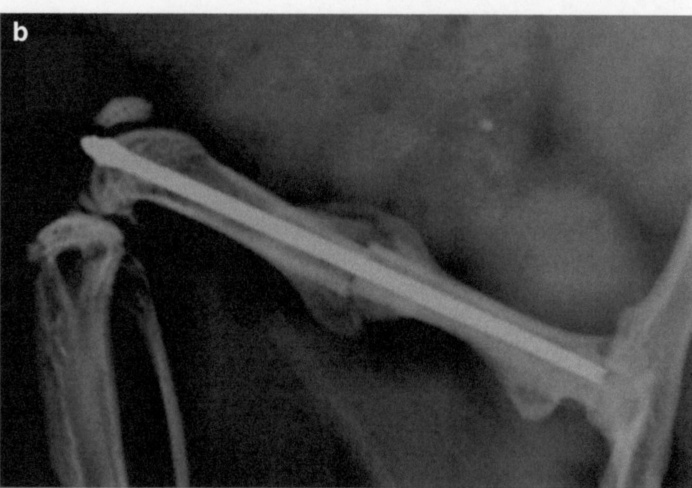

Fig. 14.2 X-ray of a mouse tibia (**a**) at day 28[14] and a mouse femur (**b**) at day 14 after closed fracture. To induce a closed tibial midshaft fracture, the fibula may also break, which results in either two different calluses or one combined callus, and thus limits the comparability of bone repair between different animals. In contrast, different fracture sites of the femur diaphysis induce comparable callus responses

coworkers developed a metaphyseal defect model for the mouse femur.[34] In this model, a hole is drilled into the anterolateral aspect of the distal femoral metaphysis. Histomorphometric analyses demonstrated a secondary fracture healing–like bone formation within the defect showing components of intramembranous and endochondral ossification. With the limitation that drilling a defect does not represent a clinical trauma scenario, this model can be used for studies on cancellous bone repair in osteoporotic mice. A different approach of developing a metaphyseal fracture model, which reflects a clinical situation of fracture healing more closely, is to osteotomize and fix the metaphysis. One major limitation of both metaphyseal models is that biomechanical testing is extremely challenging. Thus, it is nearly impossible to fix only the very distal part of a mouse femur in a biomechanical testing device.

Murine fracture models include open and closed models. Closed femur fracture models in mice have been developed in accordance to the rat femur fracture model reported by Bonnarens and Einhorn.[11] In this model, a closed fracture is produced by a three-point bending device and stabilized by an intramedullary nail, which is inserted retrograde at the intercondylar notch. In contrast to open models, closed models require only a small surgical approach, which is related to minor soft tissue injury. In open models, the lateral muscle layer has to be split to expose the femur for an osteotomy under vision.[35] While intramedullary nails, which are mostly used in closed models, injure the endosteum and the bone marrow, extramedullary plates, which are commonly used in open models, affect periosteal bone healing. The use of an external fixator for fracture stabilization is related to only a marginal disturbance of endosteal and periosteal bone repair. However, the external fixator also has to be implanted by a traumatizing surgical approach to the femur, as a closed insertion of the fixator pins is so far technically not possible in mice.[36]

Because the development of stable osteosynthesis is technically challenging, most of the former studies on bone healing in mice were conducted by using an unstable intramedullary pin fixation[27] or even without fracture stabilization.[37] However, numerous studies have shown that the course and outcome of fracture healing is critically dependent on the stability of the osteosynthesis.[38-42] Thus, interfragmentary motion has been demonstrated to promote the formation of fibrocartilage and to inhibit bone formation and angiogenesis.[40,43,44] While shear stress impairs bone regeneration, axial compression is capable of increasing bone mineral density and bending rigidity of the callus.[38,39] Fracture studies in mice have indicated that mechanical factors affect chondrogenic and osteogenic cytokine induction, the differentiation of mesenchymal cells, and the size and tissue composition of the callus.[35,42,45] While stable osteosyntheses that provide standardized biomechanical conditions for research on bone repair are mandatory in large animal models,[46] it is often argued that there is no need for biomechanical standardization in mouse models, because mouse models are predominately used for research on molecular aspects of fracture healing. This argumentation, however, is not correct, as the cellular and molecular mechanisms of fracture healing in particular are affected by the mechanical environment in the fracture gap.

During the last few years, several implants have been developed that allow a stable fixation of femur fractures in mice. Recently, the rotational stability of osteotomized cadaver femora, which were fixed by those implants, has been analyzed.[47] In addition, axial testing has been performed for some intramedullary implants.[48] Of interest, these studies revealed highly significant differences in the stability of the different osteosyntheses.

So far, there is no information on the primary and long-term stability of osteosyntheses in osteoporotic mice. However, basic considerations on the quality of human implants used for the fixation of osteoporotic bones can be transferred to the situation in mice. A diminished screw-holding power, as observed in osteoporotic bone, has less impact on the stability of a plate osteosynthesis when using interlocking screws than when using non-interlocking screws.[49] Therefore, angularly stable plates show a decreased failure rate in osteoporotic bone compared to conventional plates. In contrast to plate osteosyntheses, intramedullary nailing is not as dependent on the cortical hold of the interlocking bolts, since the bolts are not primarily responsible for the entire stability of the osteosynthesis.[49] Comparably to locking plates, the framework of an external fixator represents an angularly stable construct, which is less dependent on the holding power of the pins.[49] With regard to these principles, interlocking plates, intramedullary locking nails, and external fixators are recommended for osteosyntheses of osteoporotic bones in mice.

14.4 Murine Fracture Models and Their Applicability for Research on the Regeneration of Osteoporotic Bone

Within the last years, several mouse models have been introduced for studies on bone repair.[27,33,35,48,50-55] Implants that enable a mechanically standardized fixation of fractures or segmental bone defects in mice have been developed particularly for the femur. Femur fracture models in mice include both diaphyseal and metaphyseal models, although most models have been reported for diaphysis.

14.4.1 Closed Diaphyseal Models

14.4.1.1 Intramedullary Pin

A simple but not standardized fracture fixation is achieved by using an intramedullary pin (Fig. 14.3).[27] After the creation of a closed midshaft fracture by a three-point bending device (Fig. 14.4), the pin (e.g., a 0.25 mm stainless-steel wire) is inserted retrogradely into the intramedullary canal. For this, a

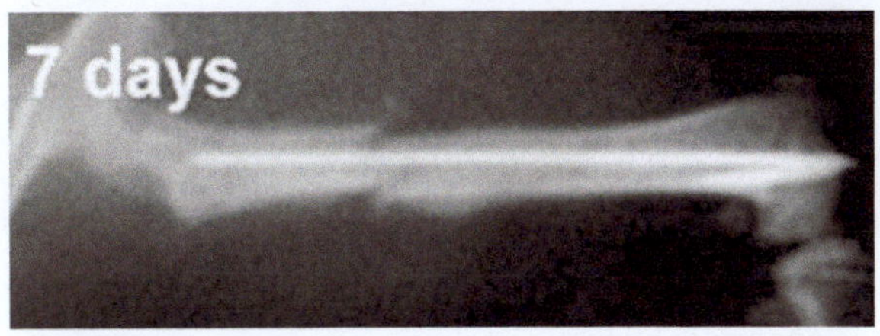

Fig. 14.3 X-ray of a fractured mouse femur at 7 days after stabilization with an intramedullary pin.[27] Migration of the pin can be prevented, for example, by wedging a second pin into the distal end of the intramedullary canal

medial parapatellar incision is performed to dislocate the patella and ream the intramedullary canal at the intercondylar notch. Migration of the pin can be prevented, for example, by wedging a second pin into the distal end of the intramedullary canal. This ordinary closed fracture model does not include biomechanically standardized fracture stabilization. Therefore, we do not recommend the use of a simple pin neither for the fixation of osteoporotic bones nor for the stabilization of non-osteoporotic bones.

14.4.1.2 Closed Intramedullary Locking Nail

In contrast to the pin fixation method, the use of a locking nail provides rotational stability after closed fixation of a femur midshaft fracture (Fig. 14.5).[50] The stability of this osteosynthesis is achieved by the flattened proximal and distal ends of the nail. Using a parapatellar surgical approach, a tungsten guide wire (diameter 0.1 or 0.2 mm) is inserted retrogradely into the intramedullary canal. After the production of a closed diaphyseal fracture (as described above), a modified injection needle (diameter 0.55 mm) is inserted over the guide wire. With the use of a guide wire, the

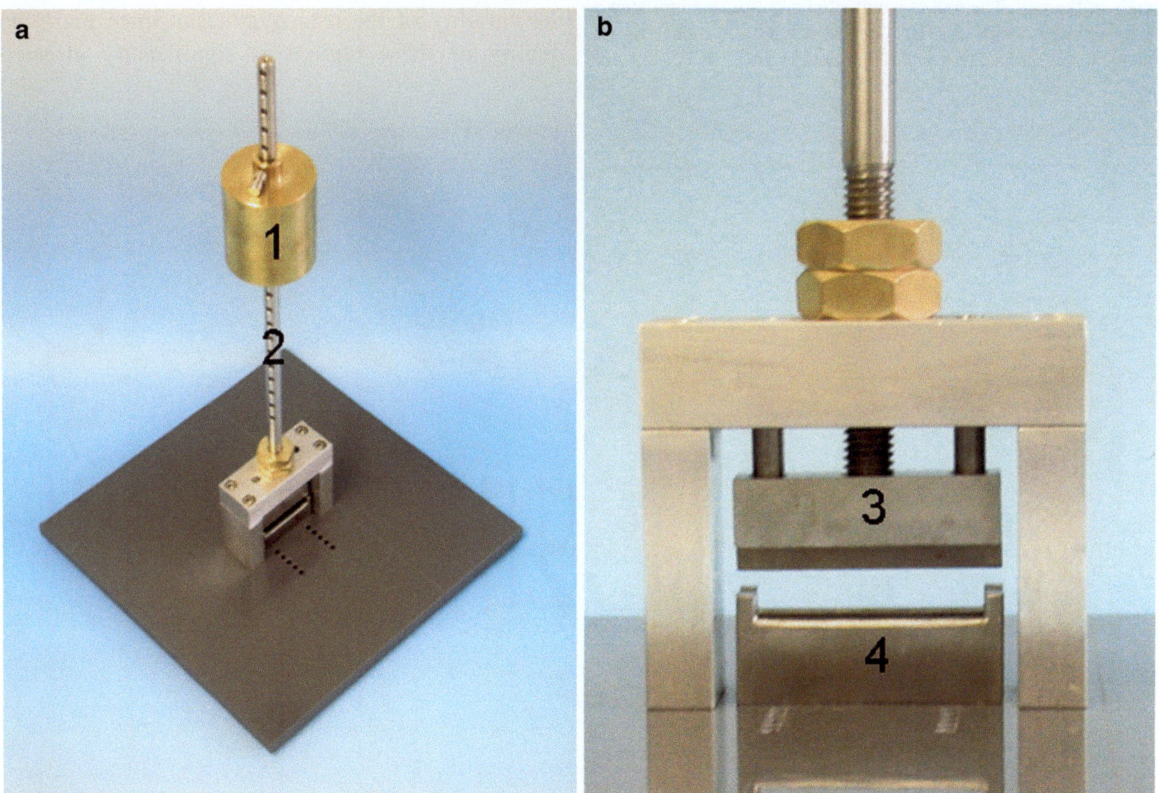

Fig. 14.4 (**a**, **b**) A closed midshaft fracture can be created by a three-point bending device: drop weight (*1*); guide bar (*2*); blunt guillotine (*3*); support anvil (*4*)

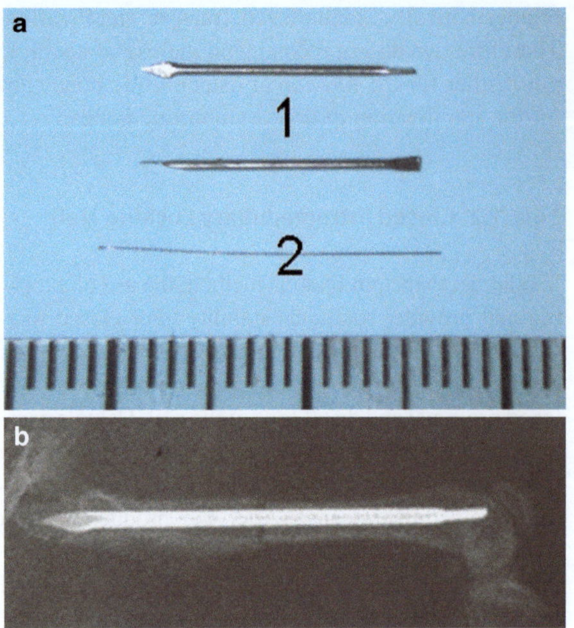

Fig. 14.5 (**a**) Closed intramedullary locking nail (*1*).[50] The stability of the nail is achieved by the flatted proximal and distal ends of the nail. The nail is cannulated and inserted by using a tungsten guide wire (*2*). (**b**) X-ray of a fractured mouse femur after closed stabilization with the locking nail[50]

femur can be fractured without pre-nailing the bone. The rotational stability of this implant depends on the bone quality of the proximal and distal metaphyses, in which the flattened ends of the nail are anchored. In accordance, the stability of an osteosynthesis with the herein introduced locking nail might be reduced in osteoporotic bones.

14.4.1.3 Intramedullary Compression Screw

To overcome the lacking axial stability of the closed locking nail, an intramedullary compression screw (diameter 0.5 mm) has been developed (Fig. 14.6).[48] Using a comparable technique as described above, the screw is implanted over a pre-positioned guide wire. An interfragmentary compression by the screw leads to a rotational and axial stability of the osteosynthesis. The bone quality of the distal femur, which bears the screw head, and the proximal femur, which holds the screw thread, determine the stability of the osteosynthesis. Since the bone quality of these regions is significantly affected

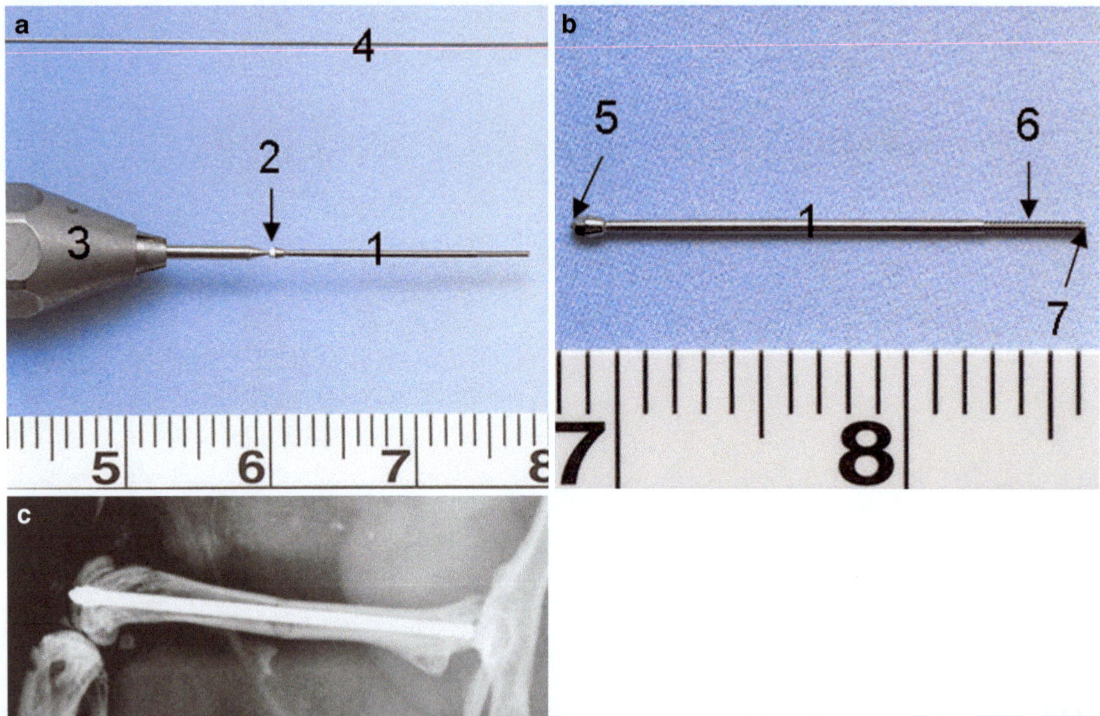

Fig. 14.6 (**a**, **b**) Intramedullary compression screw (*1*) containing a proximal cone-shaped head (*5*), a distal thread (*6*), and a longitudinal borehole at the distal end (*7*) to insert a guide wire (*4*).[24] The screw is inserted by using a screw-holder (*3*), which is connected to the screw by a torque-dependent breaking point (*2*). (**c**) X-ray of a fractured mouse femur after closed stabilization by the screw

by osteoporosis, the stability of the intramedullary screw osteosynthesis might be decreased in osteoporotic animals. Nevertheless, we could not observe significant implant failure in femurs of SAMP6 and ovariectomized (OVX) mice, which we stabilized by the intramedullary screw (T. Histing et al., unpublished data).

14.4.2 Open Diaphyseal Models

14.4.2.1 Open Intramedullary Locking Nail

Beside the locking nail described earlier, an additional locking nail has been developed for the fixation of femur fractures and segmental defects (up to 2 mm) (Fig. 14.7).[55] In contrast to the first locking nail, however, an open lateral approach is necessary for the osteotomy. The locking principle of this mouse nail is comparable to that of human nails. In accordance, interlocking bolts are used to achieve rotational and axial stability. A technically advanced targeting arm is required to insert the implant. Although an increased porosity and thinning of the cortex in osteoporotic bones might reduce the stability of the bolts, the integrity of the entire osteosynthesis is not critically affected by osteoporosis. In accordance to the situation in humans, this locking nail is also suitable for the fixation of osteoporotic bones in mice.

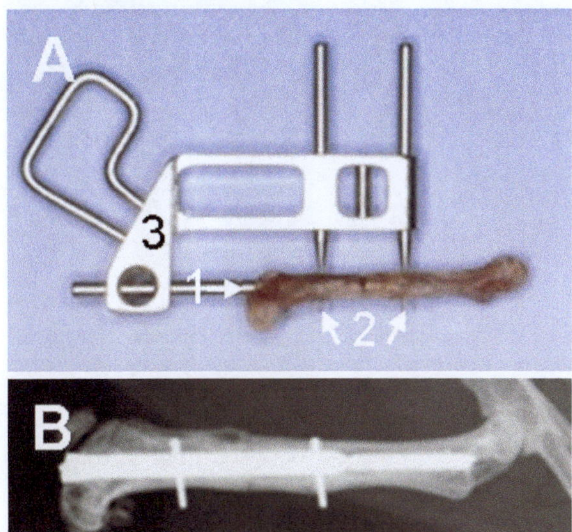

Fig. 14.7 (**a**) Open intramedullary locking nail[55]. The nail (*1*) is locked proximally and distally by two pins (*2*) using a specially designed targeting arm (*3*). (**b**) X-ray of an osteotomized mouse femur at 5 weeks after open stabilization by the locking nail

14.4.2.2 Pin-Clip Device

The pin-clip device includes the proximally and distally flattened intramedullary nail as described earlier and an extramedullary clip that leads to an additional axial stability of the osteosynthesis (Fig. 14.8). [35,54] The insertion of the clip requires a lateral surgical approach to the femur. Comparable to the open locking nail, the pin-clip technique can also be used for the stabilization of segmental bone defects (up to 1.8 mm). Thus, it is possible to analyze the healing process of critical size defects or even non-unions. Rotational testing showed a comparable torsional stiffness of osteotomized cadaver femurs that were fixed by the

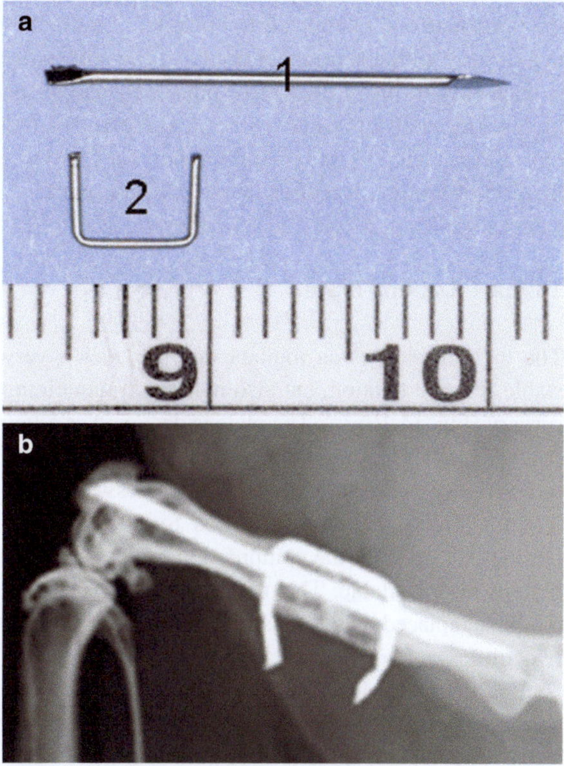

Fig. 14.8 (**a**) Pin-clip device.[35,47] The pin-clip device includes the proximally and distally flattened intramedullary nail (*1*) as described in Fig. 14.5 and an extramedullary clip (*2*) that leads to an additional axial stability of the osteosynthesis. (**b**) X-ray of an osteotomized mouse femur at 5 weeks after open stabilization by the pin clip[47]

intramedullary screw and the pin clip.[47] In contrast, the stiffness of femurs that was stabilized by the pin clip was found decreased when compared to what was stabilized by the open locking nail. From this viewpoint, the open locking nail might be considered more suitable for the fixation of osteoporotic bones than the pin clip. On the other hand, the osteosynthesis by the intramedullary screw, which provides a comparable stiffness to that achieved by the pin clip, was found sufficient for the stabilization of femur fractures in osteoporotic mice as well.

14.4.2.3 External Fixator

Biomechanical ex vivo testing of different osteosynthesis techniques indicated that the external fixator provides the highest rotational stability of all implants tested (Fig. 14.9).[36,47] Like the open locking nail and the pin clip, the external fixator also allows for stabilizing segmental bone defects of different gap sizes. Representing an external stabilization device, the fixator does not significantly injure the endosteum and the bone marrow. In contrast to humans, a traumatizing surgery with a significant injury of the soft tissue is necessary to insert the fixator pins. Because of the high stiffness of this osteosynthesis, the external fixator is considered to be an ideal implant for the stabilization of femoral fractures in osteoporotic mice.

14.4.2.4 Locking Plate

The locking plate is an implant that provides a very stable fracture fixation, but also requires traumatizing surgery (Fig. 14.10).[51-53] The plate is designed as a low contact locking compression plate, resulting in only minor injury to the periosteum. Nonetheless, the plate fixation affects the external callus formation at the implant site. Beside the compression plate, a flexible plate is also available. The medial part of this second model is replaced by two elastic splinting wires. These two different plate models allow the study of bone healing under stable or flexible conditions. The plate can also be used for the stabilization of different gap sizes. The locking principle of this implant, which causes the high stability of the osteosynthesis, qualifies the locking plate as an ideal fixation device for the stabilization of osteoporotic femurs in mice.

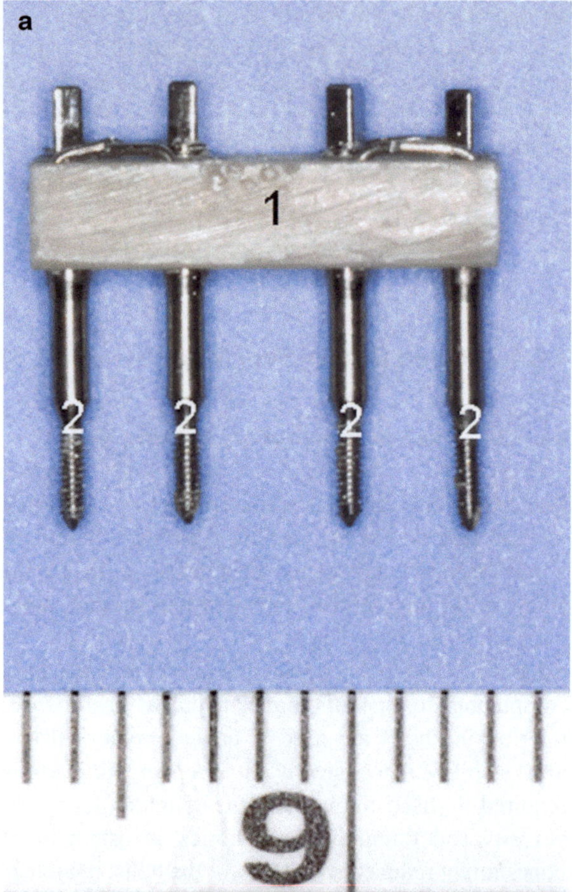

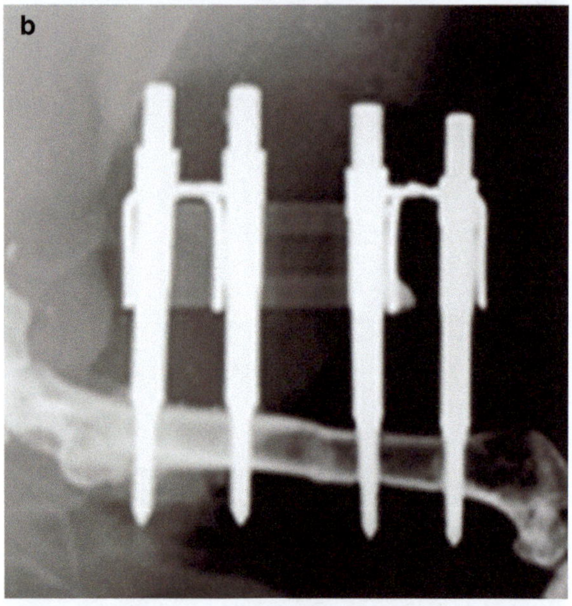

Fig. 14.9 (**a**) External fixator[47] consisting of a fixator block (*1*) and four micro-Schanz screws (*2*). (**b**) X-ray of an osteotomized mouse femur after open stabilization by the external fixator[47]

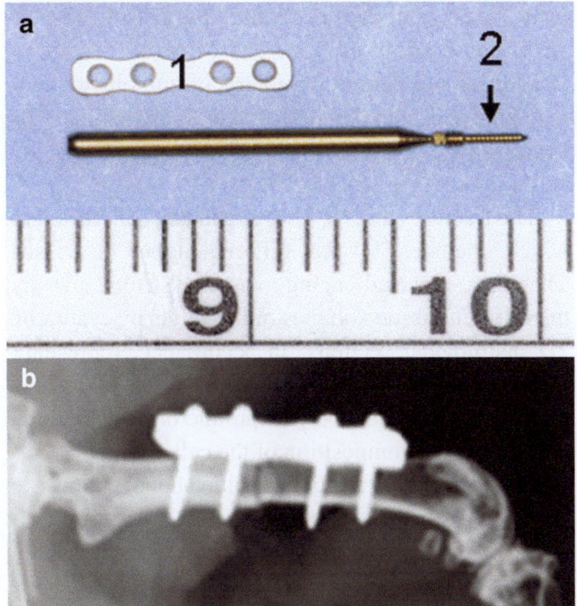

Fig. 14.10 (**a**) Locking plate.[47] The plate (*1*) is fixed to the bone by four micro-interlocking screws (*2*). (**b**) X-ray of an osteotomized mouse femur after open stabilization by the locking plate[47]

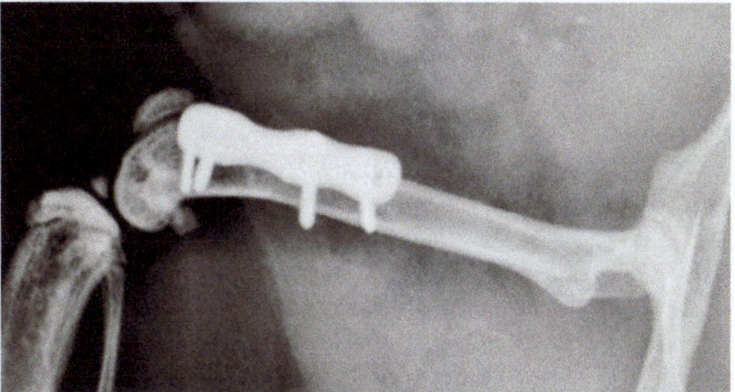

Fig. 14.11 X-ray of an osteotomy at the distal femur metaphysis that is stabilized by a locking plate

14.4.3 Metaphyseal Model

14.4.3.1 Locking Plate

In humans, most osteoporotic fractures occur at the metaphysis or the spine.[49] Apart from a metaphyseal defect model, in which a simple hole is drilled into the distal femur,[34] no metaphyseal fracture models have been reported to our knowledge in mice. Therefore, we aimed to develop a metaphyseal fracture model that includes a stable osteosynthesis and allows standardized studies on cancellous bone repair. According to the diaphyseal locking plate described earlier, we designed a metaphyseal locking plate in cooperation with the AO Development Institute, Davos, Switzerland (Fig. 14.11). Using a lateral approach, the distal part of the femur is osteotomized. Then, the plate is fixed to the bone by two screws proximal and two screws distal to the osteotomy. A pilot study showed no signs of implant loosening in both non-osteoporotic and osteoporotic animals. Histomorphometric analyses revealed a standardized healing pattern in all animals analyzed (T. Histing et al., unpublished data). These first results indicate that the herein introduced metaphyseal fracture model is useful to study cancellous bone healing in osteoporotic mice.

14.5 Methods for the Analysis of Bone Repair in Murine Femur Fracture

Several analysis methods have become available to assess bone repair in murine fracture models. These methods can be applied to non-osteoporotic as well as osteoporotic animals. While mice have to be killed to analyze bone healing by histological, biomechanical, cytological, and molecular methods, some *in vivo* imaging techniques have been introduced which do not require the sacrifice of the animals.

14.5.1 Imaging

Noninvasive imaging techniques include microcomputerized tomography (μCT), micro-positron emission tomography (μPET), and micro-magnetic resonance imaging (μMRI), as well as a variety of molecular imaging techniques, such as bioluminescence and near-infrared fluorescence analyses. Those can be used for noninvasive real-time studies on gene expression, protein degradation, cell migration, and cell death in living animals.[56-60]

The most common imaging techniques to analyze bone repair in mice are high-resolution radiography as well as two-dimensional (2D) and three-dimensional (3D) μCT.[24,59,60] These methods can be used in living animals as well; however, postmortem images of the resected bones are associated with a higher resolution

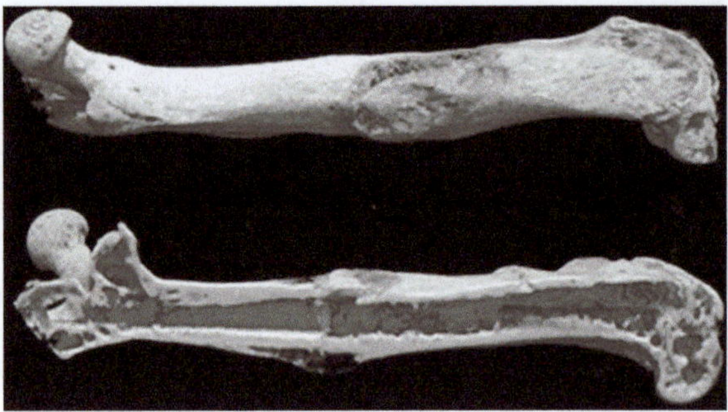

Fig. 14.12 *Ex vivo* 3D μCT of a mouse femur at 4 weeks of fracture healing

and no soft tissue artifacts.[59,60] Micro-x-rays can be used to quantify the size and density of the fracture callus, while additional parameters, such as tissue mineral density, total callus volume, and bone volume fraction of the callus, can be determined by μCT (Fig. 14.12).[61,63] In addition, the vasculature of the callus can be analyzed postmortem by 3D μCT angiography (using a chromate-based contrast agent).[64]

14.5.2 Histology

Histological analyses represent the gold standard to assess and quantify the size and tissue composition of the callus (histomorphometry) (Fig. 14.13).[65] Nomenclature, indices for assessment, and methodological approaches for histomorphometric analyses have been standardized and published by the American Society of Bone and Mineral Research.[66] In addition to histomorphometry, immunohistochemical analyses can be performed to investigate the expression of different proteins like cytokines and cell markers (Fig. 14.14).[62,67]

The fracture callus is a heterogeneous, 3D structure, which includes several different types of tissue. Therefore, it is challenging to assess the total size and the different tissue volumes of the callus by evaluating 2D histological sections. In accordance, representative, standardized longitudinal or transverse bone sections have to be defined to reproducibly calculate the size and tissue composition of the callus.[65]

Both decalcified and undecalcified bone sections can be used for histomorphometric analyses. A variety of different staining methods have been reported enabling the differentiation of the different tissue types (fibrous tissue, cartilage, osteoid, and mineralized bone).[65] For histological sections, the implant has to be removed except for the use of the "sawing and grinding technique," which allows histological analyses with the implant in situ.[53]

14.5.3 Biomechanics

Biomechanical testing is used to analyze the stiffness and ultimate strength of the fracture callus. These parameters can be determined by three-point (Fig. 14.15)

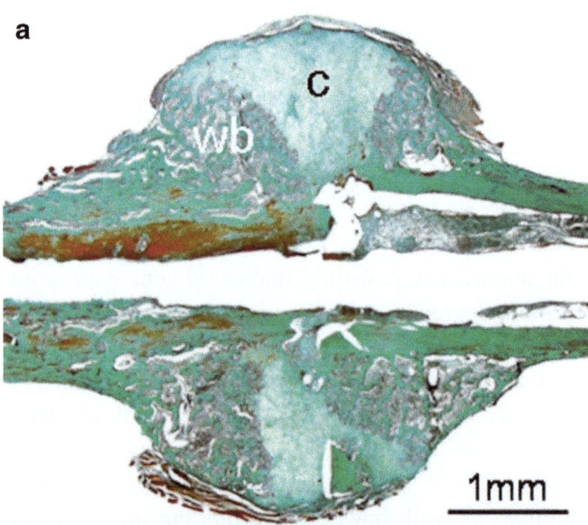

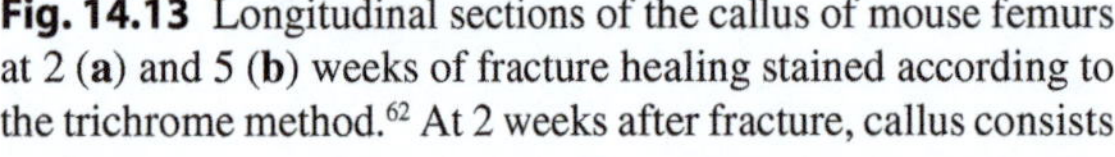

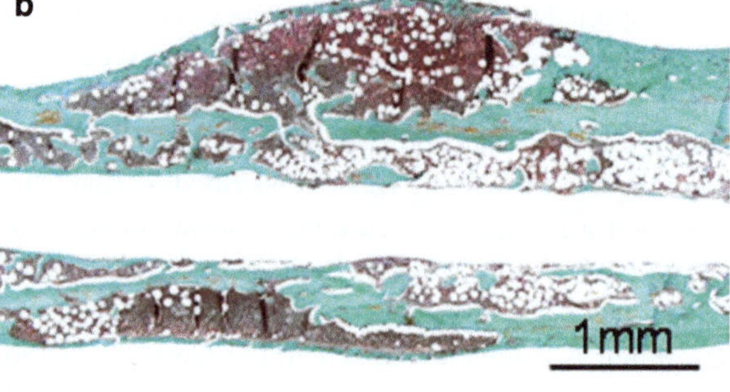

Fig. 14.13 Longitudinal sections of the callus of mouse femurs at 2 (**a**) and 5 (**b**) weeks of fracture healing stained according to the trichrome method.[62] At 2 weeks after fracture, callus consists predominately of cartilage (c) and woven bone (wb). At 5 weeks, cartilage has been completely replaced by bone

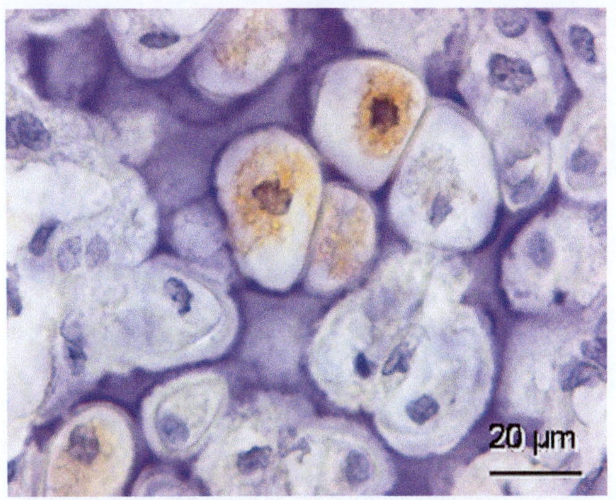

Fig. 14.14 Immunohistochemistry of vascular endothelial growth factor (VEGF) expression within the mouse callus (hypertrophic chondrocytes) at 2 weeks after fracture[67]

and four-point bending tests, torsion tests (Fig. 14.15), and distraction tests.[48,53,55,62]

Because of the small bone size, even minor differences in the testing setup critically affect the test results. Therefore, a standardized and accurate fixation of the bones in the testing device is mandatory. Of course, only highly sensitive testing devices are suitable for biomechanical testing of mice. The stiffness of the callus can be assessed from load displacement curves also by nondestructive testing methods.[68] In contrast, the ultimate load at failure of the bone can be determined only with destructive techniques.[62] The results of the biomechanical testing procedures can be expresses as absolute values.[68] To account for individual differences of the animals, however, data of the fractured bone are also often expressed as percentages of data of the contralateral, intact bone.[67]

14.5.4 Cytological and Molecular Analysis

A variety of different methods are available to investigate cellular and molecular aspects of bone repair. Biochemical methods for semiquantitative protein analyses, such as Western blotting and enzyme-linked immunosorbent assay (ELISA) techniques, can be used to support results of immunohistochemical analyses.[62,67] In situ hybridization as well as semiquantitative techniques, such as Northern blot analysis and reverse transcription polymerase chain reaction (RT-PCR), provide further information on the corresponding mRNA expression.[64,69,70] Cell counting methods like fluorescence activated cell sorting (FACS) analysis can be used to evaluate associations between bone repair and different bone marrow cells.[71]

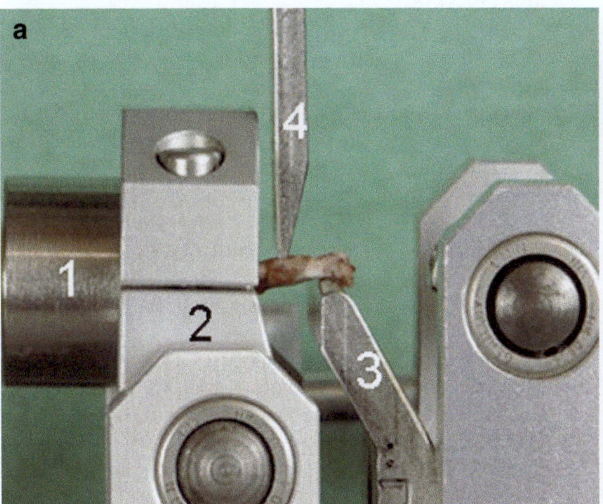

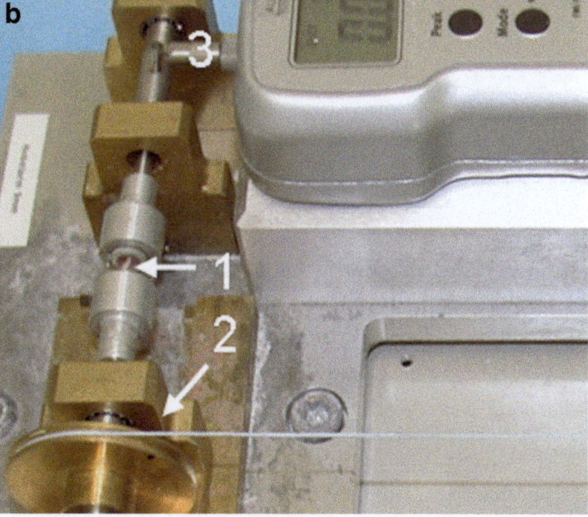

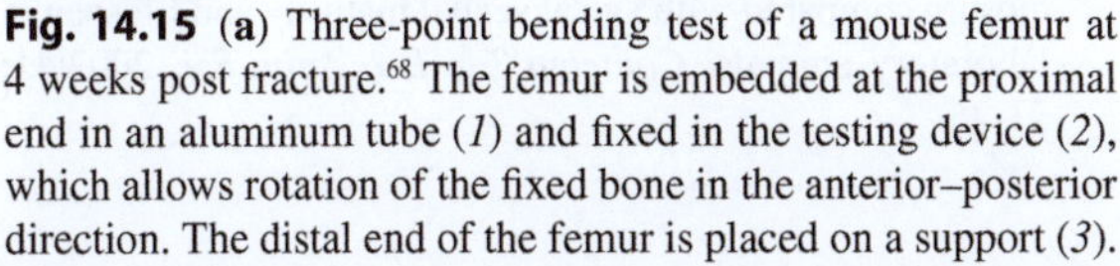

Fig. 14.15 (**a**) Three-point bending test of a mouse femur at 4 weeks post fracture.[68] The femur is embedded at the proximal end in an aluminum tube (*1*) and fixed in the testing device (*2*), which allows rotation of the fixed bone in the anterior–posterior direction. The distal end of the femur is placed on a support (*3*). A materials testing machine generates a dorsal deflection in the center of the femur (*4*). (**b**) Rotational testing setup:[47] The embedded femur (*1*) is rotated by a pulling tool (*2*). The torsion-dependent torque is quantified by a contact sensor (*3*)

Additional cell culture studies can be performed by harvesting cells of the fracture callus.[72]

14.6 Summary and Recommendations

Murine fracture models are an important tool to study the effect of osteoporosis on bone repair. Osteoporosis affects both the cortical bone and the cancellous bone. In accordance, diaphyseal fracture models should be used to analyze the impact of osteoporosis on cortical bone repair, while metaphyseal models allow the investigation of cancellous bone healing in osteoporotic animals. During the last years, a variety of different diaphyseal fracture models has become available for the mouse femur. In addition, a metaphyseal femur model has been recently introduced. As for large animal models, standardized study conditions are also required for mouse models. These include a stable fracture fixation, which can be achieved in osteoporotic bones by locking nails, locking plates, or external fixators. Due to the small size of mouse bones, surgery is demanding and requires sophisticated skills. A wide spectrum of different analytic methods is available to investigate the different aspects of bone repair in mice. The large number of gene-targeted animals and specific antibodies highlights the interest in mouse models for musculoskeletal research as well. Therefore, mouse models provide great opportunities to improve our knowledge on fracture healing in osteoporotic bones.

References

1. Wasnic RD. Epidemiology of osteoporosis in the United States of America. *Osteoporos Int*. 1997;7:S68-S72.
2. Boyle P, Leon ME, Autier P. Epidemiology of osteoporosis. *J Epidemiol Biostat*. 2001;6:185-192.
3. Cummings SR, Black DM, Rubin SM. Lifetime risks of hip, Colles', or vertebral fracture and coronary heart disease among white postmenopausal women. *Arch Intern Med*. 1989;149:2445-2448.
4. Barrios C, Brostrom LA, Stark A, Walheim G. Healing complications after internal fixation of trochanteric hip fractures: the prognostic value of osteoporosis. *J Orthop Trauma*. 1993;7:438-442.
5. Cornell CN. Internal fracture fixation in patients with osteoporosis. *J Am Acad Orthop Surg*. 2003;11:109-119.
6. Sterck JG, Klein-Nulend J, Lips P, Burger EH. Response of normal and osteoporotic human bone cells to mechanical stress *in vitro*. *Am J Physiol*. 1998;274:E1113-E1120.
7. Lill CA, Hesseln J, Schlegel U, Eckhardt C, Goldhahn J, Schneider E. Biomechanical evaluation of healing in a non-critical defect in a large animal model of osteoporosis. *J Orthop Res*. 2003;21:836-842.
8. Namkung-Matthai H, Appleyard R, Jansen J, et al. Osteoporosis influences the early period of fracture healing in a rat osteoporotic model. *Bone*. 2001;28:80-86.
9. Walsh WR, Sherman P, Howlett CR, Sonnabend DH, Ehrlich MG. Fracture healing in a rat osteopenia model. *Clin Orthop*. 1997;342:218-227.
10. Ashhurst DE, Hogg J, Perren SM. A method for making reproducible experimental fractures of the rabbit tibia. *Injury*. 1982;14:236-242.
11. Bonnarens F, Einhorn TA. Production of a standard closed fracture in laboratory animal bone. *J Orthop Res*. 1984;2:97-101.
12. Cheal EJ, Mansmann KA, DiGioia AM III, Hayes WC, Perren SM. Role of interfragmentary strain in fracture healing: ovine model of a healing osteotomy. *J Orthop Res*. 1991;9:131-142.
13. Davy DT, Connolly JF. The biomechanical behaviour of healing canine radii and ribs. *J Biomech*. 1982;15:235-247.
14. Hiltunen A, Vuorio E, Aro HT. A standardized experimental fracture in the mouse tibia. *J Orthop Res*. 1993;11:305-312.
15. Nunamaker DM, Richardson DW, Butterveck DM, Provost MT, Sigafoos RD. A new external skeletal fixation device that allows immediate full weightbearing: application in the horse. *Vet Surg*. 1986;15:1345-1355.
16. Toombs JP, Wallace LJ, Bjorling DE, Rowland GN. Evaluation of Key's hypothesis in the feline tibia: an experimental model for augmented bone healing studies. *Am J Vet Res*. 1985;46:513-518.
17. Nunamaker DM. Experimental models of fracture repair. *Clin Orthop Relat Res*. 1998;355:S56-S65.
18. Egermann M, Goldhahn J, Schneider E. Animal models for fracture treatment in osteoporosis. *Osteoporos Int*. 2005; 16:S129-S138.
19. Gennari L, Merlotti D, Nuti R. Perspectives in the treatment and prevention of osteoporosis. *Drugs Today*. 2009;45: 629-647.
20. Brockstedt H, Kassem M, Eriksen EF, Mosekilde L, Melsen F. Age- and sex-related changes in iliac cortical bone mass and remodeling. *Bone*. 1993;14:681-691.
21. Jacenko O, Olsen BR. Transgenic mouse models in studies of skeletal disorders. *J Rheumatol Suppl*. 1995;43:39-41.
22. Houdebine LM. Transgenic animal models in biomedical research. *Methods Mol Biol*. 2007;360:163-202.
23. Silver LM. *Mouse Genetics*. New York: Oxford University Press; 1995.
24. Holstein JH, Garcia P, Histing T, et al. Advances in the establishment of defined mouse models for the study of fracture healing and bone regeneration. *J Orthop Trauma*. 2009;23:S31-S38.
25. Lu C, Miclau T, Hu D, et al. Cellular basis for age-related changes in fracture repair. *J Orthop Res*. 2005;23:1300-1307.
26. Kilborn SH, Trudel G, Uhthoff H. Review of growth plate closure compared with age at sexual maturity and lifespan in laboratory animals. *Contemp Top Lab Anim Sci*. 2002;41: 21-26.

27. Manigrasso MB, O'Connor JP. Characterization of a closed femur fracture model in mice. *J Orthop Trauma*. 2004;18: 687-695.
28. Gazit D, Turgeman G, Kelley P, et al. Engineered pluripotent mesenchymal cells integrate and differentiate in regenerating bone: a novel cell-mediated gene therapy. *J Gene Med*. 1999;1:121-133.
29. Meinel L, Fajardo R, Hofmann S, et al. Silk implants for the healing of critical size bone defects. *Bone*. 2005;37:688-698.
30. Nakase T, Nomura S, Yoshikawa H, et al. Transient and localized expression of bone morphogenetic protein 4 messenger RNA during fracture healing. *J Bone Miner Res*. 1994;9:651-659.
31. Paccione MF, Warren SM, Spector JA, Greenwald JA, Bouletreau PJ, Longaker MT. A mouse model of mandibular osteotomy healing. *J Craniofac Surg*. 2001;12:444-450.
32. Stone CA. Unravelling the secrets of foetal wound healing: an insight into fracture repair in the mouse foetus and perspectives for clinical application. *Br J Plast Surg*. 2000; 53:337-341.
33. Zilberman Y, Kallai I, Gafni Y, et al. Fluorescence molecular tomography enables *in vivo* visualization and quantification of nonunion fracture repair induced by genetically engineered mesenchymal stem cells. *J Orthop Res*. 2008;26:522-530.
34. Uusitalo H, Rantakokko J, Ahonen M, et al. A metaphyseal defect model of the femur for studies of murine bone healing. *Bone*. 2001;28:423-429.
35. Garcia P, Holstein JH, Histing T, et al. A new technique for internal fixation of femoral fractures in mice: impact of stability on fracture healing. *J Biomech*. 2008;41:1689-1696.
36. Röntgen V, Blakytny R, Matthys R, et al. Fracture healing in mice under controlled rigid and flexible conditions using an adjustable external fixator. *J Orthop Res*. 2010;28:1456-1462.
37. Colnot C, Thompson Z, Miclau T, Werb Z, Helms JA. Altered fracture repair in the absence of MMP9. *Development*. 2003;130:4123-4133.
38. Augat P, Burger J, Schorlemmer S, Henke T, Peraus M, Claes L. Shear movement at the fracture site delays healing in a diaphyseal fracture model. *J Orthop Res*. 2003;21: 1011-1017.
39. Augat P, Simon U, Liedert A, Claes L. Mechanics and mechano-biology of fracture healing in normal and osteoporotic bone. *Osteoporos Int*. 2005;16:S36-S43.
40. Claes L, Eckert-Hübner K, Augat P. The effect of mechanical stability on local vascularization and tissue differentiation in callus healing. *J Orthop Res*. 2002;20:1099-1105.
41. Schell H, Epari DR, Kassi JP, Bragulla H, Bail HJ, Duda GN. The course of bone healing is influenced by the initial shear fixation stability. *J Orthop Res*. 2005;23:1022-1028.
42. Lienau J, Schell H, Epari DR, et al. CYR61 (CCN1) protein expression during fracture healing in an ovine tibial model and its relation to the mechanical fixation stability. *J Orthop Res*. 2006;24:254-262.
43. Lienau J, Schell H, Duda GN, Seebeck P, Muchow S, Bail HJ. Initial vascularization and tissue differentiation are influenced by fixation stability. *J Orthop Res*. 2005;23:639-645.
44. Nomura S, Takano-Yamamoto T. Molecular events caused by mechanical stress in bone. *Matrix Biol*. 2000;19:91-96.
45. Le AX, Miclau T, Hu D, Helms JA. Molecular aspects of healing in stabilized and non-stabilized fractures. *J Orthop Res*. 2001;19:78-84.
46. Auer JA, Goodship A, Arnoczky S, et al. Refining animal models in fracture research: seeking consensus in optimising both animal welfare and scientific validity for appropriate biomedical use. *BMC Musculoskelet Disord*. 2007;8:72.
47. Histing T, Holstein JH, Garcia P, et al. *Ex vivo* analysis of rotational stiffness of different osteosynthesis techniques in mouse femur fracture. *J Orthop Res*. 2009;27:1152-1156.
48. Holstein JH, Matthys R, Histing T, et al. Development of a stable closed femoral fracture model in mice. *J Surg Res*. 2009;153:71-75.
49. Strømsøe K. Fracture fixation problems osteoporosis. *Injury*. 2004;35:107-113.
50. Holstein JH, Menger MD, Culemann U, Meier C, Pohlemann T. Development of a locking femur nail for mice. *J Biomech*. 2007;40:215-219.
51. Matthys R, Perren SM. Internal fixator for use in the mouse. *Injury*. 2009;40:S103-S109.
52. Histing T, Garcia P, Matthys R, et al. An internal locking plate to study intramembranous bone healing in a mouse femur fracture model. *J Orthop Res*. 2010;28(3):397-402.
53. Gröngröft I, Heil P, Matthys R, et al. Fixation compliance in a mouse osteotomy model induces two different processes of bone healing but does not lead to delayed union. *J Biomech*. 2009;42:2089-2096.
54. Garcia P, Holstein JH, Maier S, et al. Development of a reliable non-union model in mice. *J Surg Res*. 2008;147: 84-91.
55. Garcia P, Herwerth S, Matthys R, Holstein JH, Histing T, Menger MD, Pohlemann T. The locking mouse nail - a new implant for standardized stable osteosynthesis in mice. *J Surg Res*. 2009 Dec 10.
56. Lee SW, Padmanabhan P, Ray P, et al. Stem cell-mediated accelerated bone healing observed with *in vivo* molecular and small animal imaging technologies in a model of skeletal injury. *J Orthop Res*. 2009;27:295-302.
57. Zachos TA, Bertone AL, Wassenaar PA, Weisbrode SE. Rodent models for the study of articular fracture healing. *J Invest Surg*. 2007;20:87-95.
58. Mayer-Kuckuk P, Boskey AL. Molecular imaging promotes progress in orthopedic research. *Bone*. 2006;39:965-977.
59. Cano J, Campo J, Vaquero JJ, Martínez JM, Bascones A. High resolution image in bone biology I. Review of the literature. *Med Oral Patol Oral Cir Bucal*. 2007;12:E454-E458.
60. Cano J, Campo J, Vaquero JJ, Martínez González JM, Bascones A. High resolution image in bone biology II. Review of the literature. *Med Oral Patol Oral Cir Bucal*. 2008;13:E31-E35.
61. Garcia P, Schwenzer S, Slotta JE, et al. Inhibition of angiotensin-converting enzyme stimulates fracture healing and periosteal callus formation - role of a local renin-angiotensin system. *Br J Pharmacol*. 2010;159:1672-1680.
62. Holstein JH, Menger MD, Scheuer C, et al. Erythropoietin (EPO): EPO-receptor signaling improves early endochondral ossification and mechanical strength in fracture healing. *Life Sci*. 2007;80:893-900.
63. Yang X, Ricciardi BF, Hernandez-Soria A, Shi Y, Pleshko Camacho N, Bostrom MP. allus mineralization and maturation are delayed during fracture healing in interleukin-6 knockout mice. *Bone*. 2007;41:928-936.
64. Duvall CL, Taylor WR, Weiss D, Wojtowicz AM, Guldberg RE. Impaired angiogenesis, early callus formation, and late stage

remodeling in fracture healing of osteopontin-deficient mice. *J Bone Miner Res*. 2007;22:286-297.
65. Gerstenfeld LC, Wronski TJ, Hollinger JO, Einhorn TA. Application of histomorphometric methods to the study of bone repair. *J Bone Miner Res*. 2005;20:1715-1722.
66. Parfitt AM, Drezner MK, Glorieux FH, et al. Bone histomorphometry: standardization of nomenclature, symbols, and units. Report of the ASBMR histomorphometry nomenclature committee. *J Bone Miner Res*. 1987;2:595-610.
67. Holstein JH, Klein M, Garcia P, et al. Rapamycin affects early fracture healing in mice. *Br J Pharmacol*. 2008;154:1055-1062.
68. Claes L, Schmalenbach J, Herrmann M, et al. Hyperhomocysteinemia is associated with impaired fracture healing in mice. *Calcif Tissue Int*. 2009;85:17-21.
69. Toyosawa S, Kanatani N, Shintani S, et al. Expression of dentin matrix protein 1 (DMP1) during fracture healing. *Bone*. 2004;35:553-561.
70. Uusitalo H, Hiltunen A, Söderström M, Aro HT, Vuorio E. Expression of cathepsins B, H, K, L, and S and matrix metalloproteinases 9 and 13 during chondrocyte hypertrophy and endochondral ossification in mouse fracture callus. *Calcif Tissue Int*. 2000;67:382-390.
71. Matsumoto T, Mifune Y, Kawamoto A, et al. Fracture induced mobilization and incorporation of bone marrow-derived endothelial progenitor cells for bone healing. *J Cell Physiol*. 2008;215:234-242.
72. Miller BS, Bronk JT, Nishiyama T, et al. Pregnancy associated plasma protein-A is necessary for expeditious fracture healing in mice. *J Endocrinol*. 2007;192:505-513.
73. Li B, Aspden RM. Composition and mechanical properties of cancellous bone from the femoral head of patients with osteoporosis or osteoarthritis. *J Bone Miner Res*. 1997;12:641-651.
74. Dickenson RP, Hutton WC, Stott JR. The mechanical properties of bone in osteoporosis. *J Bone Joint Surg Br*. 1981;63:233-238.
75. Jerome CP, Turner CH, Lees CJ. Decreased bone mass and strength in ovariectomized cynomolgus monkeys (*Macaca fascicularis*). *Calcif Tissue Int*. 1997;60:265-270.
76. Kasra M, Grynpas MD. Effect of long-term ovariectomy on bone mechanical properties in young female cynomolgus monkeys. *Bone*. 1994;15:557-561.
77. Lill CA, Gerlach UV, Eckhardt C, Goldhahn J, Schneider E. Bone changes due to glucocorticoid application in an ovariectomized animal model for fracture treatment in osteoporosis. *Osteoporos Int*. 2002;13:407-414.
78. Vanderschueren D, Van Herck E, Schot P, et al. The aged male rat as a model for human osteoporosis: evaluation by nondestructive measurements and biomechanical testing. *Calcif Tissue Int*. 1993;53:342-347.
79. Mosekilde L, Danielsen CC, Knudsen U. The effect of aging and ovariectomy on the vertebral bone mass and biomechanical properties of mature rats. *Bone*. 1993;14:1-6.
80. Peng Z, Tuukkanen J, Zhang H, Jamsa T, Vaananen HK. The mechanical strength of bone in different rat models of experimental osteoporosis. *Bone*. 1994;15:523-532.
81. Silva MJ, Brodt MD, Uthgenannt BA. Morphological and mechanical properties of caudal vertebrae in the SAMP6 mouse model of senile osteoporosis. *Bone*. 2004;35:425-431.
82. Silva MJ, Brodt MD, Ettner SL. Long bones from the senescence accelerated mouse SAMP6 have increased size but reduced whole-bone strength and resistance to fracture. *J Bone Miner Res*. 2002;17:1597-1603.
83. Niedhart C, Braun K, Graf Stenbock-Fermor N, et al. The value of peripheral quantitative computed tomography (pQCT) in the diagnosis of osteoporosis. *Z Orthop Ihre Grenzgeb*. 2003;141:135-142.
84. Simmons A, Simpson DE, O'Doherty MJ, Barrington S, Coakley AJ. The effects of standardization and reference values on patient classification for spine and femur dual-energy X-ray absorptiometry. *Osteoporos Int*. 1997;7:200-206.
85. Balena R, Toolan BC, Shea M, et al. The effects of 2-year treatment with the aminobisphosphonate alendronate on bone metabolism, bone histomorphometry, and bone strength in ovariectomized nonhuman primates. *J Clin Invest*. 1993;92:2577-2586.
86. Shen V, Dempster DW, Birchman R, et al. Lack of changes in histomorphometric, bone mass, and biochemical parameters in ovariohysterectomized dogs. *Bone*. 1992;13:311-316.
87. Bagi CM, Ammann P, Rizzoli R, Miller SC. Effect of estrogen deficiency on cancellous and cortical bone structure and strength of the femoral neck in rats. *Calcif Tissue Int*. 1997;61:336-344.
88. Chen H, Shoumura S, Emura S. Ultrastructural changes in bones of the senescence-accelerated mouse (SAMP6): a murine model for senile osteoporosis. *Histol Histopathol*. 2004;19:677-685.
89. Kimmel DB, Recker RR, Gallagher JC, Vaswani AS, Aloia JF. A comparison of iliac bone histomorphometric data in post-menopausal osteoporotic and normal subjects. *Bone Miner*. 1990;11:217-235.
90. Newman E, Turner AS, Wark JD. The potential of sheep for the study of osteopenia: current status and comparison with other animal models. *Bone*. 1995;16:277S-284S.
91. Ito M, Nishida A, Nakamura T, Uetani M, Hayashi K. Differences of three-dimensional trabecular microstructure in osteopenic rat models caused by ovariectomy and neurectomy. *Bone*. 2002;30:594-598.
92. Feik SA, Thomas CD, Clement JG. Age-related changes in cortical porosity of the midshaft of the human femur. *J Anat*. 1997;191:407-416.
93. Ritzel H, Amling M, Posl M, Hahn M, Delling G. The thickness of human vertebral cortical bone and its changes in aging and osteoporosis: a histomorphometric analysis of the complete spinal column from thirty-seven autopsy specimens. *J Bone Miner Res*. 1997;12:89-95.
94. Burr DB, Hirano T, Turner CH, Hotchkiss C, Brommage R, Hock JM. Intermittently administered human parathyroid hormone (1–34) treatment increases intracortical bone turnover and porosity without reducing bone strength in the humerus of ovariectomized cynomolgus monkeys. *J Bone Miner Res*. 2001;16:157-165.
95. Chavassieux P, Garnero P, Duboeuf F, et al. Effects of a new selective estrogen receptor modulator (MDL 103, 323) on cancellous and cortical bone in ovariectomized ewes: a biochemical, histomorphometric, and densitometric study. *J Bone Miner Res*. 2001;16:89-96.
96. Wilson AK, Bhattacharyya MH, Miller S, Mani A, Sacco-Gibson N. Ovariectomy-induced changes in aged beagles:

histomorphometry of rib cortical bone. *Calcif Tissue Int.* 1998;62:237-243.

97. Lauritzen DB, Balena R, Shea M, et al. Effects of combined prostaglandin and alendronate treatment on the histomorphometry and biomechanical properties of bone in ovariectomized rats. *J Bone Miner Res*. 1993;8:871-879.
98. Chen H, Zhou X, Emura S, Shoumura S. Site-specific bone loss in senescence-accelerated mouse (SAMP6): a murine model for senile osteoporosis. *Exp Gerontol*. 2009;44: 792-798.

Index

G. Duque and K. Watanabe (eds.), *Osteoporosis Research*,
DOI: 10.1007/978-0-85729-293-3,

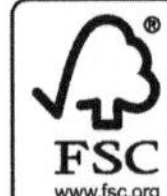

MIX
Papier aus verantwortungsvollen Quellen
Paper from responsible sources
FSC® C105338

If you have any concerns about our products,
you can contact us on
ProductSafety@springernature.com

In case Publisher is established outside the EU,
the EU authorized representative is:
Springer Nature Customer Service Center GmbH
Europaplatz 3, 69115 Heidelberg, Germany

Printed by Libri Plureos GmbH
in Hamburg, Germany